Recent Progress of Nanomedicine and Targeted Drug Delivery for Cancer Treatment

Recent Progress of Nanomedicine and Targeted Drug Delivery for Cancer Treatment

Editor

Huijie Zhang

MDPI • Basel • Beijing • Wuhan • Barcelona • Belgrade • Manchester • Tokyo • Cluj • Tianjin

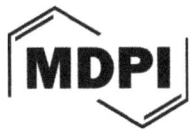

Editor
Huijie Zhang
School of Life Sciences and
Health Engineering
Jiangnan University
Wuxi
China

Editorial Office
MDPI
St. Alban-Anlage 66
4052 Basel, Switzerland

This is a reprint of articles from the Special Issue published online in the open access journal *Pharmaceuticals* (ISSN 1424-8247) (available at: www.mdpi.com/journal/pharmaceuticals/special_issues/Nanomedicine_Cancer).

For citation purposes, cite each article independently as indicated on the article page online and as indicated below:

LastName, A.A.; LastName, B.B.; LastName, C.C. Article Title. *Journal Name* **Year**, *Volume Number*, Page Range.

ISBN 978-3-0365-7041-9 (Hbk)
ISBN 978-3-0365-7040-2 (PDF)

© 2023 by the authors. Articles in this book are Open Access and distributed under the Creative Commons Attribution (CC BY) license, which allows users to download, copy and build upon published articles, as long as the author and publisher are properly credited, which ensures maximum dissemination and a wider impact of our publications.
The book as a whole is distributed by MDPI under the terms and conditions of the Creative Commons license CC BY-NC-ND.

Contents

Ms Farheen, Md Habban Akhter, Havagiray Chitme, Md Sayeed Akhter, Fauzia Tabassum and Mariusz Jaremko et al.
Harnessing Folate-Functionalized Nasal Delivery of Dox–Erlo-Loaded Biopolymeric Nanoparticles in Cancer Treatment: Development, Optimization, Characterization, and Biodistribution Analysis
Reprinted from: *Pharmaceuticals* **2023**, *16*, 207, doi:10.3390/ph16020207 1

Liangju Sheng, Xuanlei Zhu, Miao Sun, Zhe Lan, Yong Yang and Yuanrong Xin et al.
Tumor Microenvironment-Responsive Magnetic Nanofluid for Enhanced Tumor MRI and Tumor multi-treatments
Reprinted from: *Pharmaceuticals* **2023**, *16*, 166, doi:10.3390/ph16020166 31

Binghong He and Qiong Yang
Recent Development of LDL-Based Nanoparticles for Cancer Therapy
Reprinted from: *Pharmaceuticals* **2022**, *16*, 18, doi:10.3390/ph16010018 47

Jiabin Xu, Wenqiang Cao, Penglai Wang and Hong Liu
Tumor-Derived Membrane Vesicles: A Promising Tool for Personalized Immunotherapy
Reprinted from: *Pharmaceuticals* **2022**, *15*, 876, doi:10.3390/ph15070876 59

Sara Zaher, Mahmoud E. Soliman, Mahmoud Elsabahy and Rania M. Hathout
Sesamol Loaded Albumin Nanoparticles: A Boosted Protective Property in Animal Models of Oxidative Stress
Reprinted from: *Pharmaceuticals* **2022**, *15*, 733, doi:10.3390/ph15060733 87

Ibrahim A. Mousa, Taha M. Hammady, Shadeed Gad, Sawsan A. Zaitone, Mohamed El-Sherbiny and Ossama M. Sayed
Formulation and Characterization of Metformin-Loaded Ethosomes for Topical Application to Experimentally Induced Skin Cancer in Mice
Reprinted from: *Pharmaceuticals* **2022**, *15*, 657, doi:10.3390/ph15060657 109

Mengjie Rui, Min Cai, Yu Zhou, Wen Zhang, Lianglai Gao and Ke Mi et al.
Identification of Potential RBPJ-Specific Inhibitors for Blocking Notch Signaling in Breast Cancer Using a Drug Repurposing Strategy
Reprinted from: *Pharmaceuticals* **2022**, *15*, 556, doi:10.3390/ph15050556 135

Hibah M. Aldawsari, Sima Singh, Nabil A. Alhakamy, Rana B. Bakhaidar, Abdulrahman A. Halwani and Nagaraja Sreeharsha et al.
Adenosine Conjugated Docetaxel Nanoparticles—Proof of Concept Studies for Non-Small Cell Lung Cancer
Reprinted from: *Pharmaceuticals* **2022**, *15*, 544, doi:10.3390/ph15050544 155

Yang Qu, Zhiqi Wang, Miao Sun, Tian Zhao, Xuanlei Zhu and Xiaoli Deng et al.
A Theranostic Nanocomplex Combining with Magnetic Hyperthermia for Enhanced Accumulation and Efficacy of pH-Triggering Polymeric Cisplatin(IV) Prodrugs
Reprinted from: *Pharmaceuticals* **2022**, *15*, 480, doi:10.3390/ph15040480 171

Yajing Ren, Chenlin Miao, Liang Tang, Yuxiang Liu, Pinyue Ni and Yan Gong et al.
Homotypic Cancer Cell Membranes Camouflaged Nanoparticles for Targeting Drug Delivery and Enhanced Chemo-Photothermal Therapy of Glioma
Reprinted from: *Pharmaceuticals* **2022**, *15*, 157, doi:10.3390/ph15020157 189

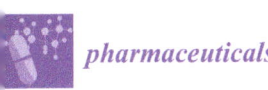

Article

Harnessing Folate-Functionalized Nasal Delivery of Dox–Erlo-Loaded Biopolymeric Nanoparticles in Cancer Treatment: Development, Optimization, Characterization, and Biodistribution Analysis

Ms Farheen [1], Md Habban Akhter [1,*], Havagiray Chitme [1], Md Sayeed Akhter [2], Fauzia Tabassum [3], Mariusz Jaremko [4] and Abdul-Hamid Emwas [5]

1. School of Pharmaceutical and Population Health Informatics (SoPPHI), DIT University, Dehradun 248009, India
2. Department of Clinical Pharmacy, College of Pharmacy, King Khalid University, Abha 62529, Saudi Arabia
3. Department of Pharmacology, College of Dentistry and Pharmacy, Buraydah Private College, Buraydah 51418, Saudi Arabia
4. Smart-Health Initiative (SHI) and Red Sea Research Center (RSRC), Division of Biological and Environmental Sciences and Engineering (BESE), King Abdullah University of Science and Technology (KAUST), Thuwal 23955, Saudi Arabia
5. Core Labs, King Abdullah University of Science and Technology (KAUST), Thuwal 23955, Saudi Arabia
* Correspondence: habban.akhter@dituniversity.edu.in

Abstract: The aim of the present study is to develop Doxorubicin–Erlotinib nanoparticles (Dox–Erlo NPs) and folate-armored Dox–Erlo-NP conjugates for targeting glioma cancer. Glioma is one of the most common progressive cancerous growths originating from brain glial cells. However, the blood–brain barrier (BBB) is only semi-permeable and is highly selective as to which compounds are let through; designing compounds that overcome this constraint is therefore a major challenge in the development of pharmaceutical agents. We demonstrate that the NP conjugates studied in this paper may ameliorate the BBB penetration and enrich the drug concentration in the target bypassing the BBB. NPs were prepared using a biopolymer with a double-emulsion solvent evaporation technique and functionalized with folic acid for site-specific targeting. Dox–Erlo NPs and Dox–Erlo-NP conjugates were extensively characterized in vitro for various parameters. Dox–Erlo NPs and Dox–Erlo-NP conjugates incurred a z-average of 95.35 ± 10.25 nm and 110.12 ± 9.2 nm, respectively. The zeta potentials of the Dox–Erlo NPs and Dox–Erlo-NP conjugates were observed at −18.1 mV and −25.1 mV, respectively. A TEM image has shown that the NPs were well-dispersed, uniform, de-aggregated, and consistent. A hemolytic assay confirmed hemocompatibility with the developed formulation and that it can be safely administered. Dox–Erlo-NP conjugates significantly reduced the number of viable cells to 24.66 ± 2.08% and 32.33 ± 2.51% in U87 and C6 cells, respectively, and IC50 values of 3.064 µM and 3.350 µM in U87 and C6 cells were reported after 24 h, respectively. A biodistribution study revealed that a significant concentration of Dox and Erlo were estimated in the brain relative to drug suspension. Dox–Erlo-NP conjugates were also stable for three months. The findings suggest that the developed Dox–Erlo-NP conjugates may be a promising agent for administration in glioma therapy.

Keywords: brain targeting; nanoparticles; folate receptor; glioma cancer; doxorubicin; erlotinib; blood–brain barrier

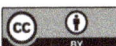

1. Introduction

Glioma results from the growth of malignant tissue in the brain or spinal cord and is extremely difficult to treat. Any drug targeting glioma must overcome the blood–brain barrier and effectively target any of a variety of cells proliferating at different rates while also providing a satisfactory safety profile. Gliomas destroy surrounding tissue and are associated with a devastating loss of functionality and a poor prognosis, with the mean survival rate from the time of diagnosis being <2 years [1]. The tumors show a limited response to conventional chemotherapy, and the development of therapies to specifically target the malignant cerebral or spinal tissue is extremely challenging due to the nature of the blood bran barrier (BBB) and the wide variety of malignant cells, different locations of tumors, and high rates of cell proliferation. Current therapeutic approaches are based on neurosurgical procedures, advanced radiotherapy, and a variety of emerging chemotherapies. Among novel drug therapies, nano-particle compounds are the most promising as these formulations penetrate the blood–brain barrier (BBB) and the blood–brain tumor barrier (BBTB) more effectively than conventional drugs. They allow for more selective tumor targeting as well as a reduction in the size and frequency of dosage, thus improving the options for the development of tailored formulations and less invasive therapies for this patient population. When successful, targeted drug therapies that are tailored to the specific malignancies of individual patients will provide hope to this patient population as a whole, promising to meaningfully extend their individual lifetimes following a glioma diagnosis [1].

Despite advances in nanotechnology and the development of multimodal therapies, disease prognosis remains a main challenge for therapeutic, drug-based interventions. Gliomas in the brain represent 57% of all gliomas, while 48% are malignancies associated with the central nervous system [2]. A range of tumors may develop within each category, each requiring tailored intervention. The current standard of therapy for gliomas includes chemotherapy and radiotherapy with temozolomide, a combination of radiation and chemotherapy followed by surgical resection [3]. The surgery is carried out to excise the tumor; however, successful excision is no guarantee against re-growth or metastasis. The invasive nature of surgical procedures is also associated with risk to surrounding tissue, and the development of efficient, effective, and safe drug-based therapies tailored to target individual tumors is therefore highly desirable and may lead to a real improvement in survival rates and quality of life for this patient population [4].

Conventional chemotherapy is inefficient in treating gliomas because of the two barriers in the brain: the blood–brain barrier (BBB), and the blood–brain tumor barrier (BBTB). These barriers limit the transportation of dissolved, active therapeutic agents to the brain while also inhibiting drug excretion, i.e., the removal of metabolites and drug residues via the blood stream, thus limiting the effects on the tumor while also increasing the risk of damage to other, healthy tissue. Chemotherapeutic agents are toxic formulations known to cause multiple adverse responses due to their lack of tissue specificity, the high doses required to successfully target malignant tissue, and the required frequency of dosage. In addition, the limited excretion of metabolites and drug residues from the treated tissues leads to drug deposition and the accumulation of damaged tissues in the normal and neighboring cells/tissues, adding to the toxic burden and exacerbating the harmful effects of already toxic drugs [5,6].

In accordance with estimates for 2021, 83,570 people in the U.S.A. alone were expected to be diagnosed with a brain tumor. Of this number, 24,530 were expected to be malignant tumors and 59,040 were expected to be non-malignant tumors, with brain tumors being established as the likely cause of death in 18,600 of these cases [7]. More alarmingly, the most recent evidence suggests that there was a massive growth in the global occurrence of glioblastoma between 1995 and 2015, with more than double the rate of 2.4 to 5.0 per 100,000 individuals in the U.K. Glioblastoma occurrence is predicted to also increase dramatically in the U.S.A. over the next 30 years [8].

Erlotinib [N-(3-ethynylphenyl)-6,7-bis(2-methoxyethoxy)-4-quinazolinamine] is a quinazoline compound with antineoplastic activity that functions as an epidermal growth factor receptor (EGFR) antagonist and protease inhibitor. The main action mechanism of this drug is the inhibition of the phosphorylation of tyrosine kinase associated with tumor growth. However, this compound has a limited ability to overcome the constraints of the BBB and BBTB; it may therefore not be a suitable alternative for glioma patients [9].

Doxorubicin (Dox) is one of the most commonly recommended agents for the treatment of benign and malignant tumors, including solid and liquid tumors. Its action mechanism involves the inhibition of the topoisomerase II inhibitor, leading to a transient arrest of the cell cycle in the G2 to M phases. However, as is the case with quinazoline, this drug has limited BBB and BBTB penetrability [10].

In recent decades, nano-scale technology has emerged as a useful tool in a range of sciences and industrial applications, including pharmacology and the production of pharmaceuticals [11]. The size of nanoparticles (NPs) generally varies in the range of 1–100 nm, thus meeting one criterion for successful drug penetration of the BBB and the BBTB. As drug carriers, nanoparticles protect therapeutic agents from degradation in the biological fluid, provide bio-stability, prevent early release, and enable the transport of drug compounds to the intended tissues/cells [12]. The surface area and mass ratio of NPs are higher than macro-scale particles, resulting in the unique features of very small size and high drug-loading/encapsulation capacities, making nanoparticles important candidates as carriers of both diagnostic and therapeutic agents [13,14]. NP technologies applied to biomedical sciences enable the tailoring of drugs to specific tissues in a controlled manner, thus opening up the development of drug tailoring for individual patients and novel diagnostic tools [15]. So far, NPs have demonstrated advantages in the targeting of glioma tumors by enabling BBB and BBTB penetration for site-specific delivery, enabling precise drug-to-tissue tailoring, minimizing off-target effects, and reducing drug dose and frequency, and reducing the duration of drug administration, which also helps to improve patient compliance [16,17].

The BBB was first identified by Ehrlich in 1885 through a dye test. It comprises endothelial cells such as astrocytes, pericytes, and neuronal cells. Endothelial cells primarily restrict the passive transport of substances from blood to the brain. The permeability of brain blood vessels can be increased only when the BBB is ruined; however, some blood vessels nurturing a tumor form the BBTB. The BBTB causes less hindrance to the transport of substances in a brain tumor. The blood vessels bear over-expressed receptors, which could facilitate the ligand-gated active targeting of substances in the tumor microenvironment. To overcome the BBB and achieve a successful therapeutic delivery in the brain, ligand-targeted NPs have an overwhelming response in the diagnosis and treatment of glioma [18]. Luque-Michel et al. injected mice with polymeric NPs loaded with both superparamagnetic iron oxide NPs and Dox and, using an MRI, observed the high accumulation of nanocarriers in a glioma tumor region, leading to the successful suppression of tumor growth [19].

It is well established that the folate receptors (FR) are over-expressed in a range of solid tumor cells, viz., non-small cell lung cancers, colorectal, pancreatic, ovarian, breast, kidney, gastric, and prostate cancers, including glial tumors of the brain and central nervous system [20]. Folate receptors are glycoprotein-based receptors with a molecular weight in the range of 38–45 kDa, and folic conjugate has been proven to have higher rates of uptake than conventional therapies through folate-receptor-mediated endocytosis in tumor cells [21]. A high level of expression of folate receptors has been observed in solid tumors of the body. These sites may therefore represent an ideal target domain for nanocarriers [22]. In the development of drugs, folic acids (FA) are biotechnological ligands as they retain a high affinity for folate receptors and enable the targeted delivery of drugs to a tumor. Like antibodies, FAs are superior targeting ligands due to their relatively smaller size and lack of immunogenicity. They are readily available and have relatively simple conjugation properties. Folic acids have been used for a while as targeting ligands for nanoparticle uptake in cancer cell lines and are extensively explored as a targeting ligand for cell lines and tumors that over-express folate [23].

A biopolymer is a macromolecule composed of repeating structural units of monomers with covalent bonds that form a chain-like structure. Recently, biopolymers have gained wider attention with a view to develop pharmaceutical nanocomposites meeting the essential requirements of having antimicrobial properties: having stability and flexibility and being biocompatible, biodegradable, and bioresorbable [24]. Biopolymers have the major advantage of being easily broken down in the biological system by naturally occurring microorganisms and enzymes. Additionally, as their by-products are organic and without detrimental impact on the biological system, they are highly promising carriers for therapeutic drugs. As a result, a significant body of work has emerged on polysaccharide-based biopolymers for biomedical applications, replacing synthetic nanomaterials to hopefully improve efficacy and safety profiles and reduce the harmful side effects of anti-cancer drugs.

In the present study, biopolymers obtained from a natural source—the bark of *Cinnamomum zeylanicum*—were used to achieve drug encapsulation and the delivery of the active compound to the targeted site, facilitating its entry into the brain tumor [25]. This is the first time we have prepared a combined formulation of Erlo and Dox in functional biopolymer. We expect this formulation to have the dual advantage of diminishing resistance development in cancer cells and eliciting ameliorating, anti-cancer effects via the inhibition of epidermal growth factor receptor (EGFR) and damage to DNA. The functionalized nanoparticles were delivered via a naturally obtained *Cinnamomum zeylanicum* biopolymer, while the formulation was evaluated in vitro for physicochemical characteristics such as particle size, surface charge, % drug release. The biocompatibility of NPs was assessed using a hemolysis assay. We also examined the formula's biodistribution and cell viability against glioma cell lines and performed stability studies in vitro.

2. Results

2.1. Formulation Optimization

The experimental design applied a novel tool to achieve statistical optimization and enable the minimization of method-induced variability while yielding a high-quality product with uniform and homogeneous particle size distribution, as well as methodical stability for other parameters under study. As in many other experimental designs, the Box–Behnken design was used to optimize and investigate the principal effects, interactions, and quadratic effects of the independent variables on responses, viz., particle size, PDI, and %drug release. This design is effective for exploring quadratic response surfaces and constructing second-order polynomial models [26]. The Dox–Erlo NPs were optimized using the Box–Behnken design and a preliminary formulation was developed based on the trial-and-error method to identify the desirable components and select the appropriate concentration for the independent variables. According to this examination, a surfactant concentration lower than 1.00% w/v yielded larger NP sizes owing to a minimum size reduction attributed to poor emulsification, resulting in low drug encapsulation and impaired drug release. Furthermore, NPs in the >3.00% w/v size range demonstrated a diminished overlay and an extremely poor drug profile. To obtain the required particle sizes for the formulation, sonication below 3.00 min of sonication time is required. Size reductions of the nanoparticles were observed to be low. Above 12.00 min small particles were in line to accumulate, leading to instability issues, possibly due to an excess reduction of particle size. Thus, the selection of low and high levels of excipient concentrations was based solely on primary investigations. In this context, the surfactant levels were low (−1), medium (0), and high, (+1); at 0.50, 1.50, and 2.50% (w/v), respectively. Polymer concentrations were 1.00, 2.00, and 3.00% (w/v); and the sonication time levels were low, (−1), medium (0), and high (+1); corresponding to 3.00, 7.50, and 12.00 min, respectively, as is depicted in Table 1. The obtained independent variable data in the Box–Behnken design and their corresponding responses according to experimental runs are shown in Table 2.

Table 1. Box–Behnken design variables for formulation of Dox–Erlo NPs.

Independent Variables	Level Used		
	Low (−1)	Medium (0)	High (+1)
Polymer concentration (A), % w/v	1.00	2.00	3.00
PVA (B), % w/v	0.50	1.50	2.50
Sonication Time (C), min	3.00	7.50	12.00
Dependent variables			
Particle size (R1)		Minimize	
PDI (R3)		Minimize	
Drug release (R2)		Maximize	

Table 2. Observed responses in Box–Behnken design for Dox–Erlo NP preparations with their predicted and actual values.

Run Order	(A)	(B)	(C)	Actual Value of R1	Predicted Value of R1	Actual Value of R2	Predicted Value of R2	Actual Value of R3	Predicted Value of R3
1	3.00	1.50	12.00	121.00	128.00	89.00	89.50	0.1230	0.1208
2	2.00	0.50	3.00	230.00	230.13	78.00	77.00	0.2230	0.2253
3	2.00	1.50	7.50	180.00	190.00	71.00	75.00	0.1430	0.1332
4	3.00	0.50	7.50	240.00	236.12	71.00	72.00	0.2210	0.2235
5	1.00	1.50	3.00	159.00	152.00	65.00	64.50	0.2310	0.2332
6	1.00	1.50	12.00	100.00	96.25	63.00	63.00	0.2070	0.2117
7	2.00	2.50	3.00	227.00	230.13	57.00	58.50	0.2130	0.2132
8	2.00	1.50	7.50	201.00	190.00	74.00	75.00	0.1300	0.1332
9	2.00	1.50	7.50	189.00	190.00	79.00	75.00	0.1290	0.1332
10	3.00	1.50	3.00	170.00	173.75	83.00	83.00	0.1950	0.1903
11	2.00	1.50	7.50	200.00	190.00	76.00	75.00	0.1230	0.1332
12	2.00	2.50	12.00	130.00	129.88	73.00	74.00	0.1120	0.1097
13	1.00	0.50	7.50	136.00	142.87	59.00	60.50	0.2980	0.2935
14	1.00	2.50	7.50	156.00	159.88	45.00	44.00	0.2230	0.2205
15	3.00	2.50	7.50	127.00	120.12	79.00	77.50	0.1520	0.1565
16	2.00	0.50	12.00	232.00	228.88	68.00	66.50	0.2380	0.2377
17	2.00	1.50	7.50	180.00	190.00	75.00	75.00	0.1410	0.1332

(A) Polymer concentration, % w/v; (B) surfactant concentration, % w/v; and (C) sonication time, min. R1—Particle size; R2—drug release %; and R3—PDI.

The linear correlation plots (A, C, E) and their residual plots (B, D, F) between actual vs. predicted values of particle size, PDI, and % drug release, are indicated in Figure 1. Fitting data to the various models—viz., cubic, 2FI, linear, and quadratic—in the Box–Behnken design indicated the quadratic model for each response. The best-fitted model for each response was selected using ANOVA by regression analysis the calculation of F values. The response surface morphology of the BBD expresses the individual, combined, and quadratic impacts on the dependent variables, viz., particle size (nm), PDI, and % drug release (Figure 2). The outcome of the regression analysis for particle size (R1), % drug release (R2), and the PDI (R3) of formulation are provided in Table 3. The analysis of variance of the calculated models for responses are shown in Table 4.

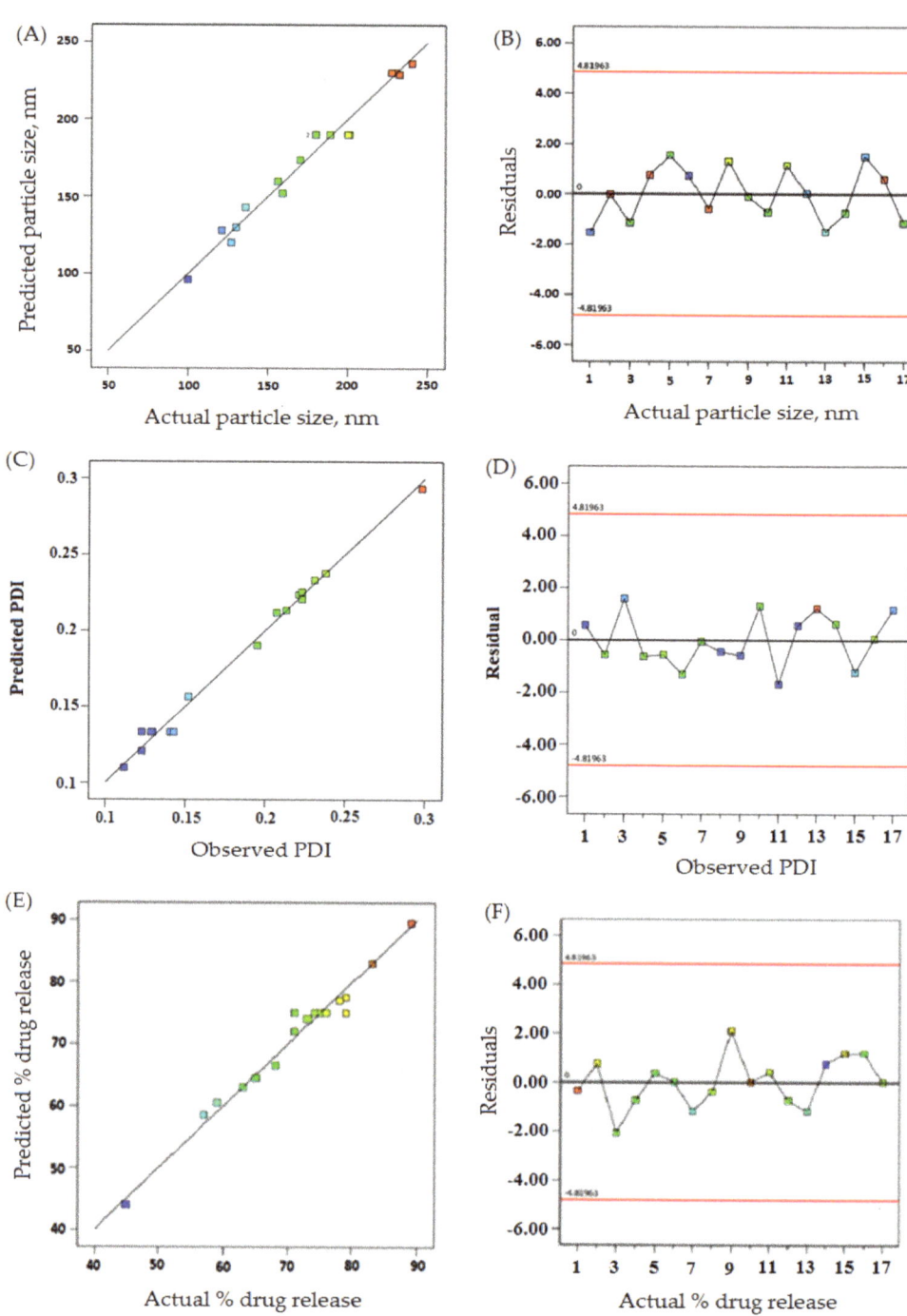

Figure 1. The actual vs. predicted values represented as linear correlation plots (**A,C,E**), and associated residual plots (**B,D,F**) providing responses according to particle size, PDI, and %drug release.

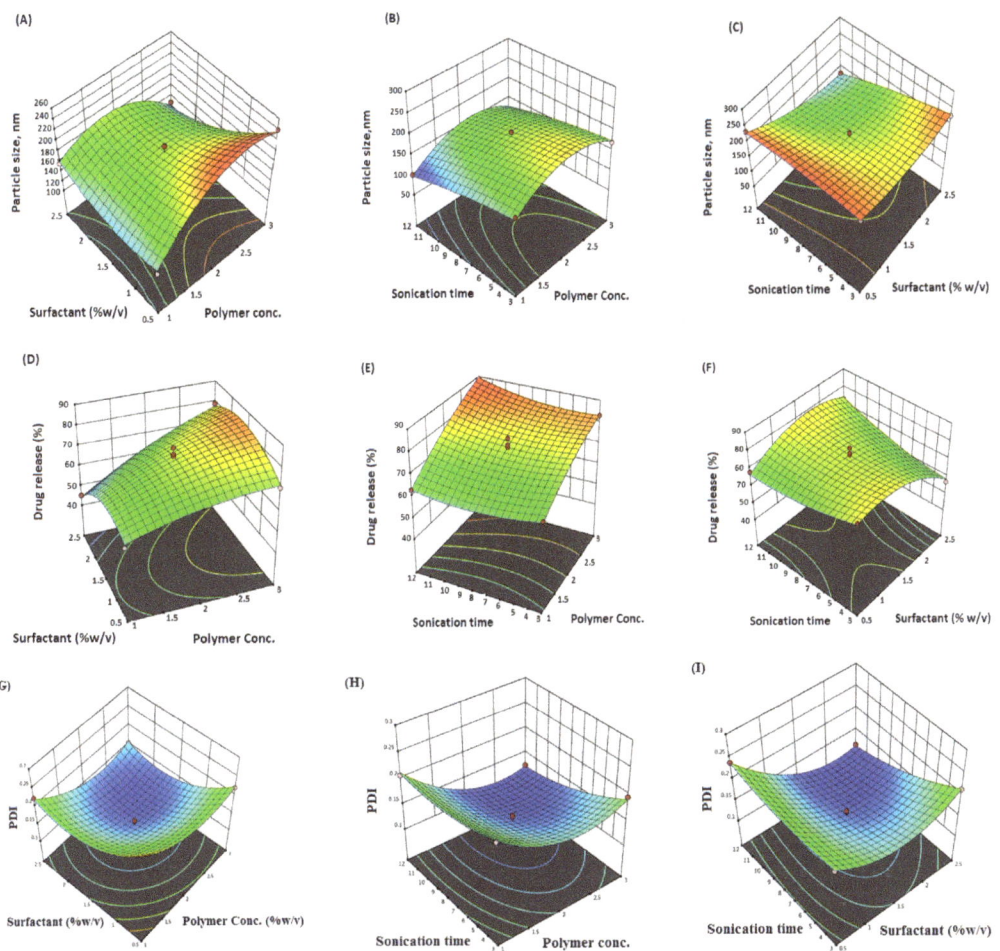

Figure 2. Three-dimensional (3D) surface response plot (**A–F**) indicating comparative effects of polymer, surfactant, and sonication time on responses, particle size (**A–C**), % drug release (**D–F**), and PDI (**G–I**).

Table 3. Summary results of regression analysis for response fitting of quadratic models for R1, R2, and R3.

Quadratic Model	R-Squared	Adjusted R-Squared	Predicted R-Squared	SD	% CV
Response (R1)	0.9768	0.9469	0.8327	9.94	5.68
Response (R2)	0.9740	0.9405	0.8524	2.60	3.68
Response (R3)	0.9914	0.9802	0.9502	0.0076	4.18

Regression equation of the fitted quadratic model

Particle size (R1) = $+190.00 + 13.37 \times A - 24.75 \times B - 25.38 \times C - 33.25 \times A \times B + 2.50 \times A \times C - 24.75 \times B \times C - 46.25 \times A^2 + 21.00 \times B^2 - 6.25 \times C^2$

% Drug release (R2) = $+75.00 + 11.25 \times A - 2.75 \times B + 1.25 \times C + 5.50 \times A \times B + 2.00 \times A \times C + 6.50 \times B \times C - 2.75 \times A^2 - 8.75 \times B^2 + 2.75 \times C^2$

PDI (R3) = $+0.1332 - 0.0335 \times A - 0.0350 \times B - 0.0228 \times C + 0.0015 \times A \times B - 0.0120 \times A \times C - 0.0290 \times B \times C + 0.0414 \times A^2 + 0.489 \times B^2 + 0.0144 \times C^2$

Table 4. Analysis of variance (sum of square, degree of freedom, mean square, F-value, and *p*-value) for response, particle size, drug release, and PDI.

Result of the Analysis of Variance	Particle Size (nm)	Drug Release (%)	PDI
	1. Regression analysis		
Sum of squares	29,090.22	1776.26	0.6131
Degree of freedom (df)	9	9	17
Mean squares	3232.25	197.36	0.0361
F-value	32.68	29.09	113.60
p-Value	<0.0001	<0.0001	<0.0001
	2. Lack-of-fit tests		
Sum of squares	270.25	13.50	0.0001
df	3	3	3
Mean squares	90.08	4.50	0.0000
F-value	0.8539	0.5294	0.5471
p-Value	0.5330	0.6858	0.6762
Correlation of variation (% CV)	5.68	3.68	4.18
	3. Residual		
Sum of squares	692.25	47.50	0.0004
df	7	7	7
Mean squares	98.89	6.79	0.0001
SD	9.94	2.60	0.0076

2.2. Response 1: Effect on Particle Size

The effects on particle size of various excipients used in the formulation are explained by the quadratic equation (Table 2). In the above equation of particle size (Table 2), the terms A, B, C, AB, AC, BC, A^2, B^2, and C^2 are significant. The model's F-value, 32.68, suggested a significant model. The statistical *p*-values < 0.05 indicate significant model terms, while *p* > 0.05 indicates insignificant model terms. The lack-of-fit F-value of 0.85 expressed remained insignificant for this quadratic model.

The size of particles in the formulations were reported from 100 to 240 nm in formulations number 6 to 3 (Table 2). The surfactant concentration revealed positive and negative effects on particle size. For example, formulations number 2 and 4 exhibited particle sizes of 230 nm and 240 nm, respectively, at a 0.5% concentration of surfactant. On the other hand, a particle size of 227 nm at a 2.5% concentration of surfactant was found for formulation number 7. Formulation number 6 and formulation number 1 demonstrated a particle size of 100 nm and 121 nm, respectively, at a 1.5% surfactant concentration (Table 2).

The concentration of the polymer provided a positive effect on particle size. Raising the polymer concentration to 3% w/v led to an increased size of particle. For example, formulations number 6 and 13, having a polymer concentration of 1% w/v, had particle sizes of 100 nm and 136 nm, respectively. On the other hand, formulations number 11 and 7 demonstrated particle sizes of 200 nm and 227 nm, respectively, with a 2% w/v polymer concentration. Again, increasing the polymer concentration (3% w/v) led to larger particle size: 240 nm.

On the other hand, sonication time demonstrated a negative impact on particle size. The formulations number 6 and 1 achieved particle sizes of 121 nm and 100 nm, respectively, with 12 min of sonication. With the same sonication time, formulation 16 exhibited a 232 nm particle size, probably due to a combined effect. Formulations 2 and 10 achieved a particle size of 230 nm and 170 nm, respectively, by sonication for 3 min.

2.3. Response 2: Effect on % Drug Release

The impact on % drug release of various excipients used in the formulation is explained by quadratic equation (Table 3).

In the above equation, the terms A, B, C, AB, AC, BC, A^2, and B^2 are significant. The Model F-value, 29.09, indicated a significant model for the % drug release. The lack-of-fit F-value of 0.53 entails insignificant for the model to fit. The polymer concentration positively impacted the % drug release. Formulation number 14 demonstrated that a 45% drug release had a 1% w/v polymer concentration. The increase of polymer concentration to 2% w/v led to an increased drug release: 71% and 75%, as seen in formulations number 3 and 17, respectively. Furthermore, after an increase in the polymer concentration of the formulation to 3% w/v, an increase in drug release was observed, such as cases of 89% and 83% in formulations number 1 and 10, respectively (Table 2).

2.4. Response 3: Effect on the PDI

The effect on the PDI of various excipients used in the formulation is explained by the quadratic equation (Table 3).

Surfactant concentration provided both positive and negative effects on the PDI. The observed PDI values were achieved: 0.123 and 0.231 at 1.5% and 2.5% of w/v surfactant concentration, corresponding to formulations number 1 and 5, respectively. Similarly, the polymer concentration provided both a positive and a negative effect on the PDI. When increasing the concentration of the polymer from 1 to 3% w/v, the PDI was initially increased and later decreased. For example, the polymer concentration of 3% w/v, as seen in formulations 4 and 5, indicated PDI values of 0.221 and 0.231, respectively. On the other hand, sonication time had a less negative impact on the PDI of formulations (Table 2).

In view of the above obtained outcomes, the optimized formulation was generated using a point-prediction technique with a Box–Behnken design. The optimized formula for preparation included a polymer concentration (2.94% w/v), surfactant concentration (2.20% w/v), and sonication time (11.39 min). The experimental design predicted a particle size of 92.76 nm, a % drug release of 89.31%, and a PDI of 0.102. The experimental or observed values of particle size, % drug release, and PDI were 95.35 ± 10.25 nm, 70.42 ± 7.25%, and 0.109, respectively.

2.5. Characterization of Dox–ErloNPs

2.5.1. Particle Size and Zeta Potential

The particle size and zeta potential of Dox–Erlo NPs and Dox–Erlo-NP conjugates are shown in Figure 3A,B. Dox–Erlo NPs demonstrated a particle size of 95.35 ± 10.23 nm. On the other hand, Dox–Erlo-NP conjugates appeared at a particle size of 110.12 ± 9.2 nm. The zeta potential of Dox–Erlo NPs and the Dox–Erlo-NP conjugates were −18.1 mV and −25.1 mV, respectively, as is shown in Figure 3C,D. The size range of the Dox–Erlo NPs and the Dox–Erlo-NP conjugates was between 50 and 150 nm (Figure 4A,B). The entrapment efficiency % of Erlo and Dox was 80 ± 2.3% and 78 ± 4.8%, respectively, and the polydispersity index (PDI) of the Dox–Erlo NP formulation was reported be 0.1027. The predicted NP size of the optimized formulation was 92.7661 nm, vs. an experimental particle size of 95.35 ± 10.25, reporting a percentage error of 2.79%. On the other hand, the % drug release of the optimized NPs was 89.91%, vs. the experimental value of 79.203 ± 0.24%, demonstrating a percentage error of 11.90%. The PDI of the predicted formulation was 0.102, compared to a PDI of 0.10, for the experimental value, demonstrating a percentage error of 6.8% (shown in Table 5).

Table 5. The optimized composition using experimental design for the development of Dox–Erlo NPs with experimental and predicted responses.

Variable Composition	Responses	Predicted Value	Experimental Value	% Error
A (2.94 % w/v)	R1	92.76 nm	95.35 ± 10.25 nm	2.79
B (2.20 % w/v)	R2	89.91%	79.203 ± 0.24%	11.90
C (11.39 min)	R3	0.102	0.109	6.8

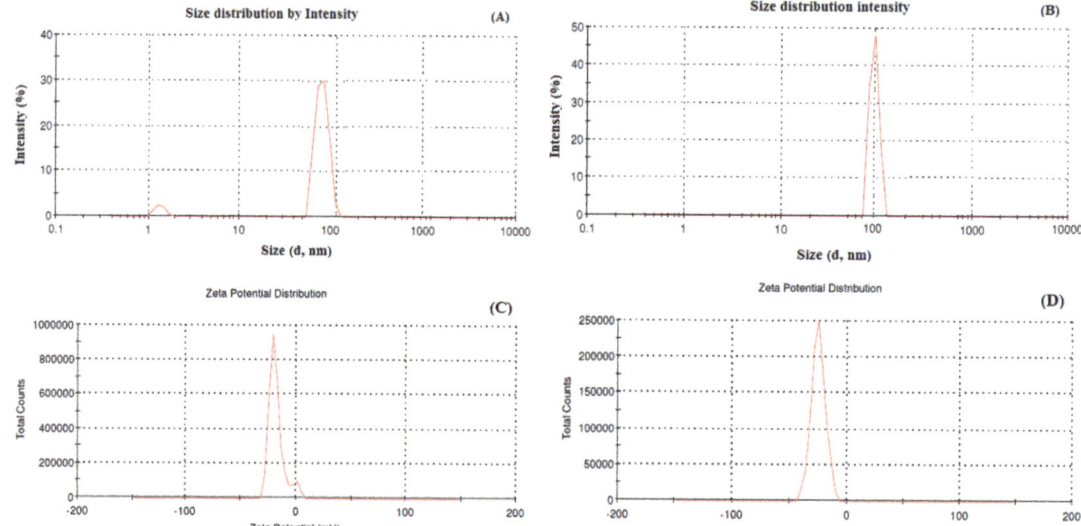

Figure 3. Particle size and size distribution analysis of Dox–Erlo NPs (**A**), particle size and size distribution analysis of Dox–Erlo-NP conjugates (**B**), zeta potential of Dox–Erlo NPs (**C**) and Dox–Erlo-NP conjugates (**D**).

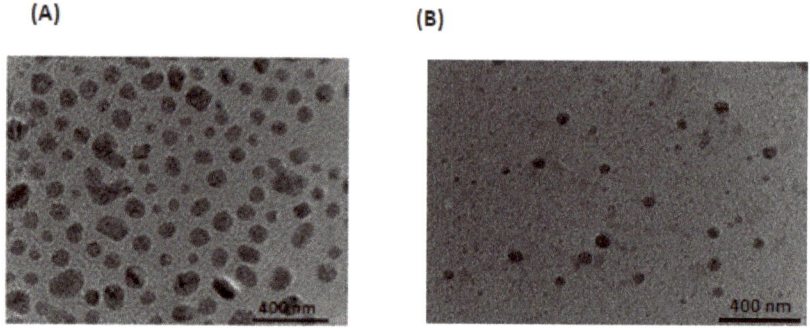

Figure 4. Transmission electron microscopic image of Dox–Erlo NPs (**A**), Dox–Erlo NPs conjugate (**B**).

2.5.2. DSC of Dox–Erlo NPs

DSC is used for the physicochemical characterization of the nature of substance. The DSC peaks of Erlo, cinnamon biopolymer, polyvinyl alcohol, Dox–Erlo NPs, and Dox–Erlo-NP conjugates are shown in Figure 5. The pure Erlo has a characteristic peak at 234.544 °C. Polyvinyl alcohol has shown a peak at 316.97 °C. Further, the endothermic peak, obtained at 168.136 °C, corresponds to the mannitol that was detected in the Dox–Erlo-NP conjugate in Figure 5.

2.5.3. FT-IR Spectral Analysis

FT-IR spectroscopy characterized the chemical stability of NPs encapsulated in the core of the biopolymer. The FT-IR spectra of Erlo, biopolymer, polyvinyl alcohol, Dox–Erlo NPs, and Dox–Erlo-NP conjugates are indicated in Figure 6. The structure of Erlo shows a 2-methoxy ethoxy group (C-O stretching) and amino-group (N-H stretching) of quinazoline ring. The biopolymer demonstrated a peak around 2743.12 cm^{-1}, and 2918.33 cm^{-1} belongs to the carboxylic acid group. The Erlo drug demonstrated absorption bands at

3267.14 cm^{-1}, corresponding to N-H stretching, and at 1081.18 cm^{-1}, attributed to C-O stretching (Figure 6).

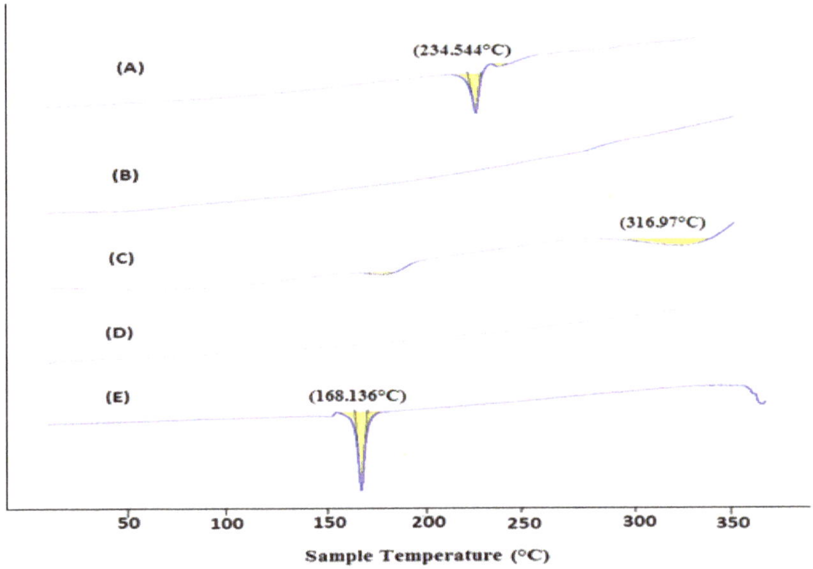

Figure 5. DSC thermogram of Erlo (A), cinnamon biopolymer (B), polyvinyl alcohol (C), Dox–Erlo NPs (D), and Dox–Erlo-NP conjugates (E).

2.5.4. Proton Nuclear Magnetic Resonance (^{1}H NMR)

The formation of an amide bond between the primary amine group (-NH2) of folic acid and the carboxylic acid group from the Dox–Erlo NPs through a conjugation reaction is shown in Figure 7A. The ^{1}H NMR spectroscopy of the amide linkage formation in Dox–Erlo-NP conjugates is shown in Figure 7A,B. An appearance of the signals at 8.3921 ppm indicated the formation of an amide bond through a reaction between the activated ester group of the polymeric nanoparticles and the primary amine group of folic acid (Figure 7B).

2.5.5. X-ray Diffraction Analysis

The confirmation of the physicochemical drug behavior encapsulation in the NPs was further illustrated with help of X-ray analysis. The X-ray diffraction patterns of Erlo, cinnamon biopolymer, Dox–Erlo NPs, and Dox–Erlo-NP conjugates are shown in Figure 8. The high-intensity characteristic peaks in the Erlo were observed at 2θ angles of 18.74°, 20.38°, 21.07°, 25.26°, 36.04°, and 40.33°, indicating their crystalline nature (Figure 8A). The low-intensity peaks in the biopolymer were observed at 2θ angles of 18.84°, 22.72°, 23.48°, and 25.41°. Moreover, the peaks prevailed in the biopolymer, as is shown in Figure 8B, suggesting a less-crystalline nature. However, the peaks of crystalline nature were produced at a very low intensity or disappeared in the diffraction patterns of Dox–Erlo NPs and the Dox–Erlo conjugates, indicating that Erlo and Dox were in amorphous or molecular states in the NPs.

2.5.6. In Vitro Drug Release

In vitro release studies were performed for Erlo and Dox from Dox–Erlo NPs and Dox–Erlo-NP conjugates at a pH of 7.4 (simulating a physiological pH) and a pH of 5.4 (mimicking the pH of acidic, intracellular, endosomal cancer cells), respectively. The maximum amounts of Dox released from the Dox–Erlo NPs and Dox–Erlo-NP conjugates at a pH of 7.4 were 59.54 ± 0.10% and 58.34 ± 0.073%, respectively. On the other hand, at a pH of 5.4, the maximum amounts of Dox release from the Dox–Erlo NPs and Dox–Erlo-NP conjugates were 76.29 ± 0.19% and 74.24 ± 0.24%, respectively. The amounts of Erlo released from Dox–Erlo NPs and Dox–Erlo-NP conjugates at a pH of 7.4 were 70.42 ± 0.05% and 68.47 ± 0.29%, respectively. Similarly, at a pH of 5.4, the amounts of Erlo released at the end of 47 h were 82.11 ± 0.30% and 78.43 ± 0.39%, respectively, as is shown in Figure 9A,B.

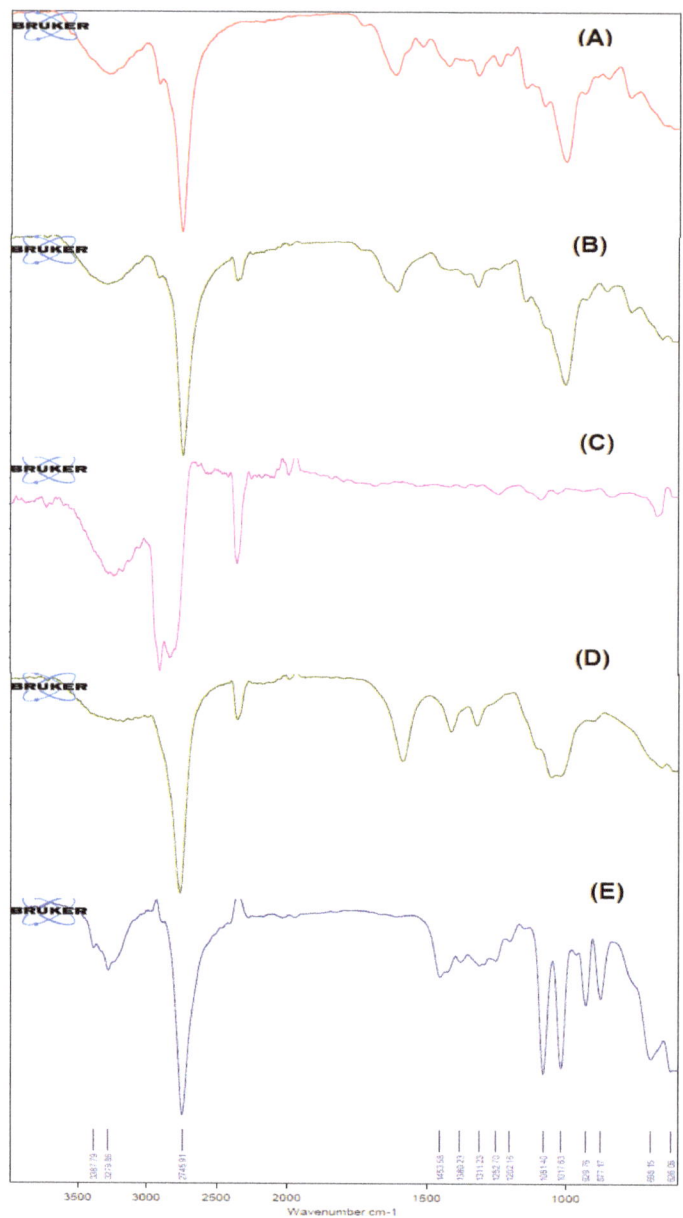

Figure 6. The FT–IR Spectra of Erlo (**A**), cinnamon polymer (**B**), polyvinyl alcohol (**C**), Dox–Erlo NPs (**D**), and Dox–Erlo NP conjugates (**E**).

(A)

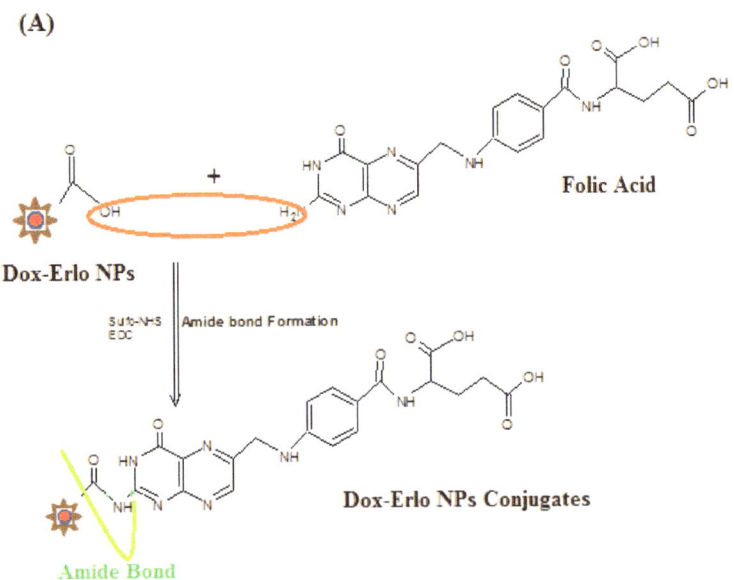

(B)

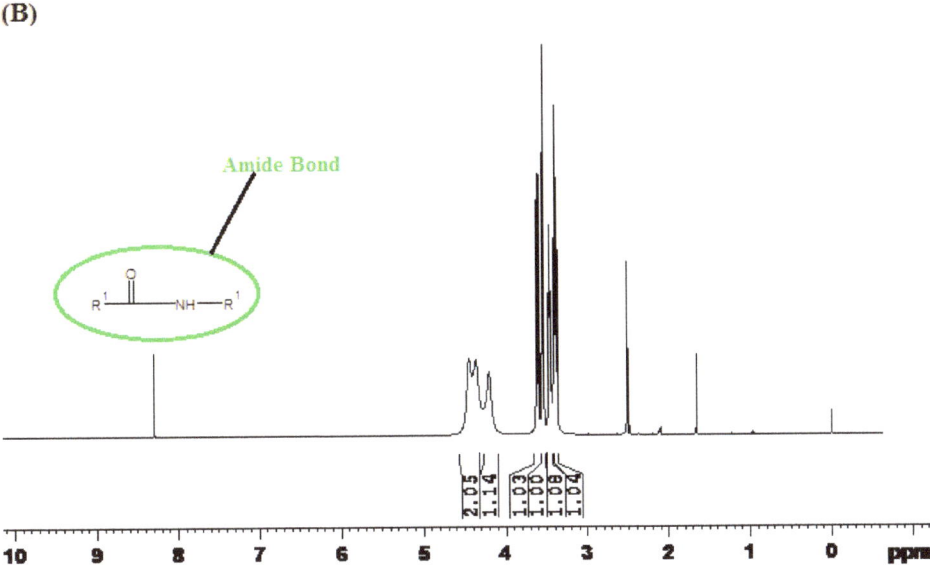

Figure 7. Schematic diagram of amide bond formation of Dox–Erlo NPs (A) and the ^{1}H NMR spectrum of Dox–Erlo-NP conjugates (B).

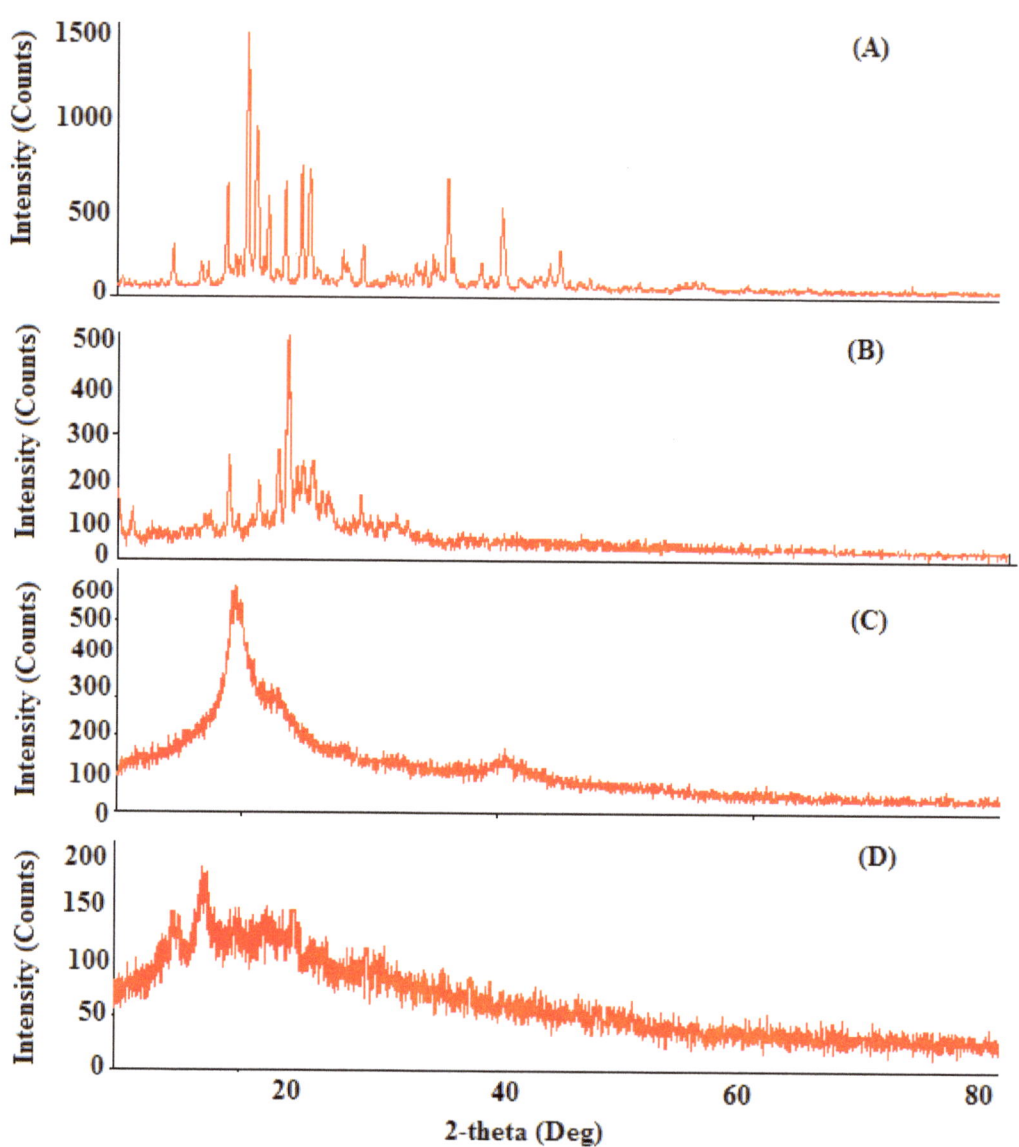

Figure 8. The XRD diffraction analyses of Erlo (**A**), cinnamon biopolymer (**B**), Dox–Erlo NPs (**C**), and Dox–Erlo-NP conjugates (**D**).

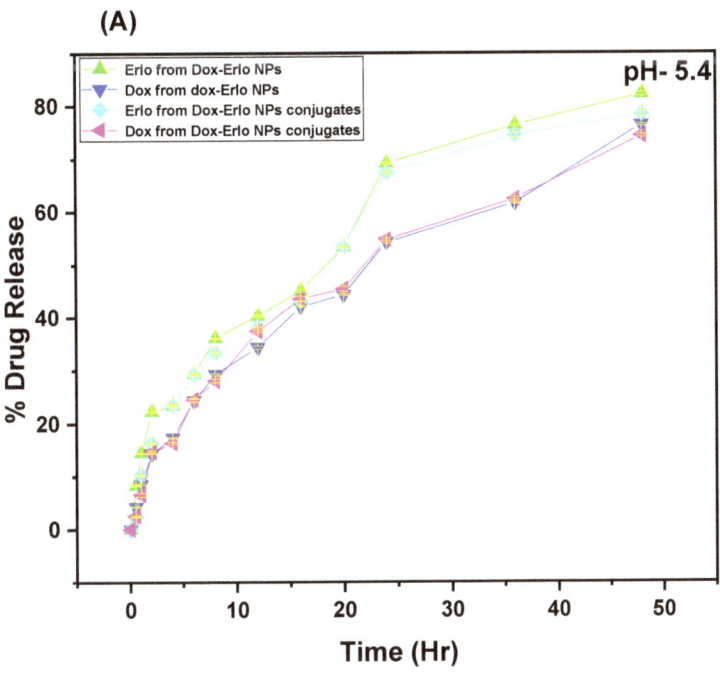

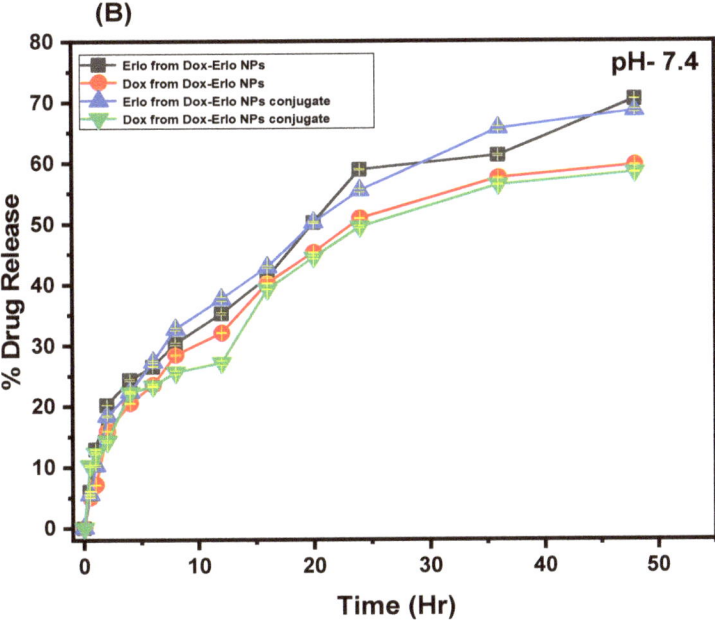

Figure 9. In vitro drug releases of Erlo and Dox from the plain drug, Dox–Erlo NPs, and Dox–Erlo-NP conjugates at a pH of 5.4 (**A**) and a pH of 7.4 (**B**).

2.5.7. Kinetic Release Model

The releases of Erlo and Dox from Dox–Erlo NPs and their conjugates were fitted to the different release kinetic model. The exponent (n) expressed aFickian or non-Fickian pattern of drug release. The exponent value for the zero-order release/Case II transport, $n = 1$; non-Fickian diffusion, $0.5 < n < 1$; or relaxational release, $n > 1$ is considered. The model of good fit was judged based on the regression coefficient value (R^2). The regression coefficient (R^2) values for such models were determined, for example: zero order ($R^2 = 0.9002$), first order ($R^2 = 0.9744$), Higuchi ($R^2 = 0.9096$), Korsmeyer–Peppas ($R^2 = 0.9793$), and Hixson–Crowell ($R^2 = 0.9593$) were estimated. It was observed that Korsmeyer–Peppas showed a good fit to the model of ($R^2 = 0.9793$) for the Erlo release from Dox–Erlo-NP conjugates at apH of5.4. The n-value was 0.4805 and the k-value was 3.0543. The release of Dox from Dox–Erlo-NP conjugates at a pH of 5.4 fitted in a different kinetic model, and the regression coefficients for various kinetic models were provided: zero order ($R^2 = 0.8541$), First order ($R^2 = 0.9231$), Higuchi matrix ($R^2 = 0.9233$), Korsmeyer–Peppas ($R^2 = 0.9751$), and Hixson–Crowell ($R^2 = 0.9025$) [Table 6]. The Korsmeyer–Peppas was the best-fitted model, with a regression value of ($R^2 = 0.9751$), an n-value of 0.5951, and a k-value of 2.4551. The release mechanism indicated an anomalous, non-Fickian diffusion of Dox, both via diffusion and biopolymeric matrix erosion; on the other hand, Erlo was released via biopolymeric matrix erosion.

Table 6. Kinetic drug release of Erlo and Dox release from Dox–Erlo-NP conjugates at pH 5.4.

Erlo Release from Dox–Erlo-NP Conjugates at pH 5.4		
Zero order	0.9002	1.65021
First order	0.9744	−0.0355
Higuchi matrix	0.9096	9.7543
Korsmeyer–Peppas	0.9793	3.0543
Hixson–Crowell	0.9593	0.0090
Dox release from Dox–Erlo-NP conjugates at pH 5.4		
Model Fitting	R^2	k
Zero order	0.8541	1.2361
First order	0.9231	−0.0195
Higuchi Matrix	0.9233	8.3559
Korsmeyer–Peppas	0.9751	2.5251
Hixson–Crowell	0.9025	0.0056

In the determination of the Erlo release from the Dox–Erlo-NP conjugates at a pH of 7.4, the regression coefficient values for the zero order ($R^2 = 0.8704$), first order ($R^2 = 0.9537$), Higuchi matrix ($R^2 = 0.9190$), Korsmeyer–Peppas ($R^2 = 0.9782$), and Hixson–Crowell ($R^2 = 0.9306$) were determined. Among these models, Korsmeyer–Peppas demonstrated the highest regression value ($R^2 = 0.9782$), with a release exponent n-value of 0.5294 and a k-value of 2.733 selected. Further, the regression coefficients for Dox release from Dox–Erlo-NP conjugates at a pH of 7.4 were determined using the same models: zero order ($R^2 = 0.8718$), first order ($R^2 = 0.9294$), Higuchi ($R^2 = 0.9062$), Korsmeyer–Peppas ($R^2 = 0.9709$), and Hixson–Crowell ($R^2 = 0.9125$). Due to the emergence of a highest regression coefficient value for the Korsmeyer–Peppas model, it was selected as the model of good fit. It indicated an n-value of 0.41 and a k-value of 2.9451 [Table 7]. The mechanism of drug release expressed that Dox was released via Fickian diffusion following both diffusion and biopolymeric matrix erosion. On the other hand, the Erlo release mechanism followed an anomalous or non-Fickian diffusion through biopolymeric matrix erosion [27].

Table 7. Kinetic drug release of Erlo and Dox release from Dox–Erlo-NP conjugates at pH 7.4.

Erlo Release from Dox–Erlo-NP Conjugates at pH 7.4		
Model Fitting	R^2	k
Zero order	0.8704	1.3919
First order	0.9537	−0.0244
Higuchi Matrix	0.9190	8.8754
Korsmeyer–Peppas	0.9782	2.7330
Hixson–Crowell	0.9306	0.0067
Dox release from Dox–Erlo NPs conjugates at pH 7.4		
Model Fitting	R^2	k
Zero order	0.8718	1.1629
First order	0.9294	−0.0183
Higuchi Matrix	0.9062	8.3554
Korsmeyer–Peppas	0.9709	2.9451
Hixson–Crowell	0.9125	0.0052

2.5.8. Hemolysis Study

Hemolysis experiments were carried out to ensure the biocompatibility of the in-house-built NPs and NP conjugates in the bloodstream and to obtain information about the charge–particle interaction with biomolecules in terms of thrombosis and hemolysis in vivo. These interactions enable damage to erythrocytes and thereby acquit hemoglobin from erythrocytes. It was observed that increasing the NP doses led to an increased release of hemoglobin from the erythrocytes. The hemolytic analysis revealed that RBC damages were less than 6–8% in any of the concentrations (1.5 mg, 3 mg, and 6 mg) used in the experiment relating to placebo NPs, Dox–Erlo NPs, and Dox–Erlo-NP conjugates.

2.5.9. Cytotoxicity Assay

The results of the MTT assay analysis of plain drugs, Dox–Erlo-NPs, and Dox–Erlo-NP conjugates on glioma cell lines (U87 and C6) at varying concentrations (0.20 µM, 0.40 µM, 0.80 µM, 1.6 µM, 3.2 µM, and 6.4 µM) are shown in Figure 10A,B. The Dox–Erlo-NP conjugates significantly depleted the count of viable cells to 24.66 ± 2.08% when compared to Dox–ErloNPs (66 ± 2.6%) and plain drugs (85.33 ± 5.5%) in glioma U87 cells. Oppositely, Dox–Erlo-NP conjugates reduced the viable cell count to 32.33 ± 2.51% when compared to Dox–ErloNPs (65 ± 1%) and plain drugs (87 ± 3.46%) in glioma C6 cells. Furthermore, cell death was expressed in terms of the IC50 related to the dose of drug, which killed 50% of cancer cells in a specified time period, i.e., the inhibitory concentration (IC50). The IC50 values of plain Dox–Erlo, Dox–ErloNPs, and Dox–Erlo-NP conjugates were 26.589 µM, 9.830 µM, and 3.064 µM, respectively, after 24 h in the U87 cell line. The IC50 values of plain Dox–Erlo, Dox–ErloNPs, and Dox–Erlo-NP conjugates were determined to be 32.60 µM, 8.625 µM, and 3.350 µM, respectively, after 24 h in the C6 glioma cell line, shown in Figure 10A,B.

2.5.10. Biodistribution Study

The tissue homogenates from various organs such as the liver, kidney, brain, and blood of rats were extracted and analyzed via HPLC for the presence of Dox and Erlo. It was found that a significant amount of Dox and Erlo were estimated in the brain as compared to drug suspension ($p < 0.05$). The biodistribution studies of the formulation in various organs are expressed in Figure 11.

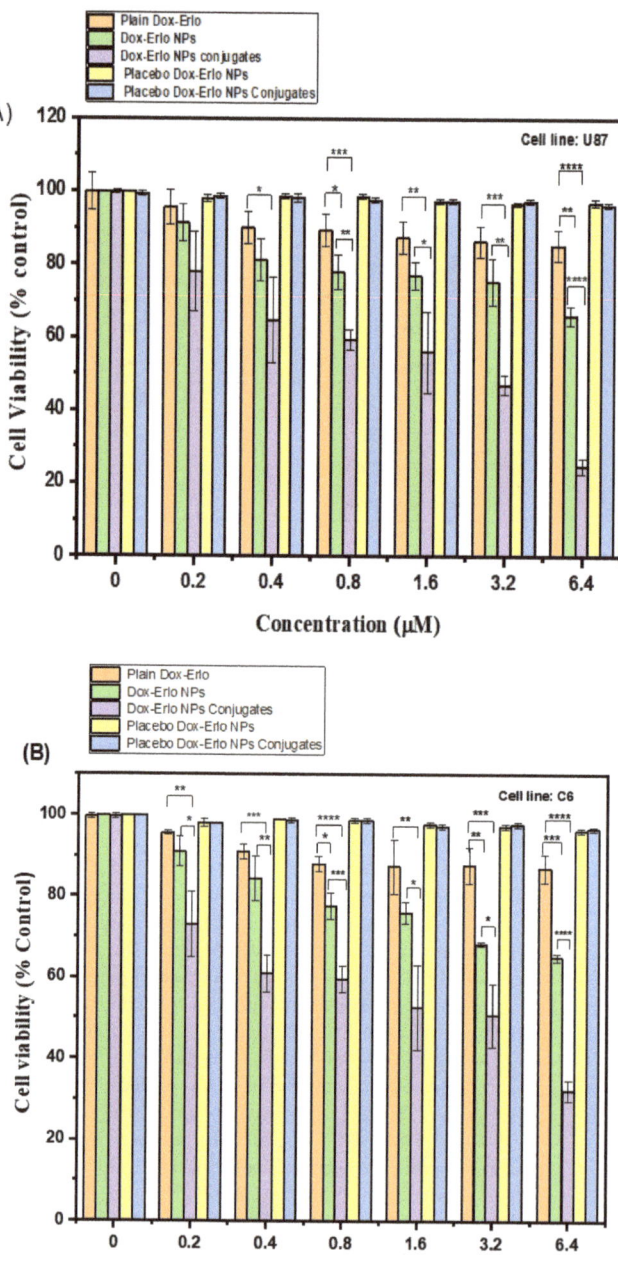

Figure 10. The percentage cell viability following 24 h of treatment with various doses of plain Dox-Erlo, Dox–ErloNPs, Dox-Erlo-NP conjugates, placebo Dox–Erlo NPs, and placebo Dox–Erlo-NP conjugates on U87 (**A**) and C6 (**B**) glioma cell lines. The experiments were performed in triplicate with mean ± S.D (n = 3). Significance value * ($p < 0.05$), ** ($p < 0.01$), *** ($p < 0.001$), **** ($p < 0.0001$) relative to pure Dox-Erlo.

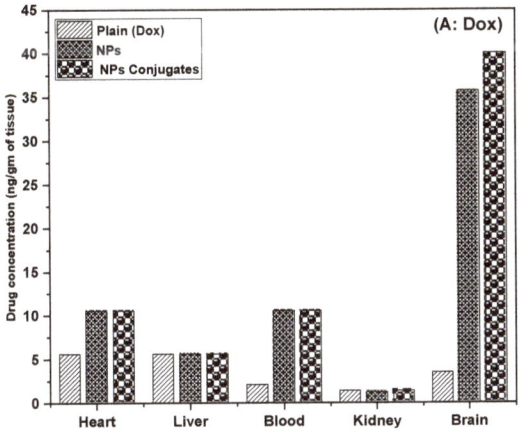
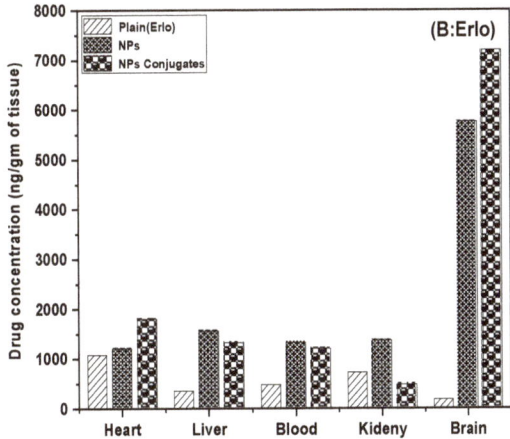
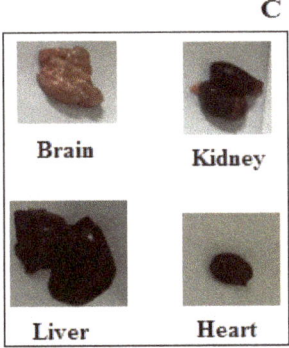

Figure 11. Graph representing the biodistribution of Dox (**A**) and Erlo (**B**) from plain, Dox–Erlo NPs, and Dox–Erlo-NP conjugates. Isolated organs of animals after 24 h of dose (**C**).

2.5.11. Stability Study

The stability study was performed as per guideline issues under a stability study [28]. The Dox–Erlo-NP conjugates' stability experiments under a specific set of conditions are expressed in Table 8. The particle size observed was 109.45 ± 12.48 nm at 25 ± 2 °C, 65 ± 5% RH at the end of 90 days. However, at an elevated temperature of 40 ± 2 °C, 75 ± 5% RH, a particle size of 115.33 ± 12.38 nm was observed. Similarly, the surface charge on the Dox–Erlo-NP conjugates at temperatures of 25 ± 2 °C, 65 ± 5% RH and 40 ± 2°C, 75 ± 5% RH were recorded as −21.1 ± 4.01 and −20.4± 3.20 mV, respectively. The entrapment efficiencies after a stability period of 90 days were calculated at 76 ± 5.3% and 73 ± 3.3%, respectively.

Table 8. Stability indicating data of Dox–Erlo-NP conjugates with regard to particle size, zeta potential, and % entrapment efficiency.

Sampling Period (in Days)	Particle Size (nm)		Zeta Potential (mV)		% Entrapment Efficiency	
	(25 ± 2 °C, 65 ± 5% RH)	(40 ± 2 °C, 75 ± 5% RH)	(25 ± 2 °C, 65 ± 5% RH)	(40 ± 2 °C, 75 ± 5% RH)	(25 ± 2 °C, 65 ± 5% RH)	(40 ± 2 °C, 75 ± 5% RH)
0	95.35 ± 10.23	95.35 ± 10.33	−18.1 ± 2.40	−18.1 ± 2.40	80 ± 2.3%	80 ± 4.6%
30	99.39 ± 11.03	100.46 ± 9.2	−18.3 ± 3.40	−19.3 ± 2.31	79.3 ± 3.4%	79 ± 3.2%
60	104.22 ± 13.44	106.25 ± 14.25	−19.2 ± 3.24	−20.2 ± 2.05	78 ± 3.8%	77 ± 4.4%
90	109.45 ± 12.48	115.33 ± 12.38	−21.1 ± 4.01	−20.4± 3.20	76 ± 5.3%	73 ± 3.3%

3. Discussion

The treatment of a glioma is impeded via the invasiveness or the inadequacy of drugs penetrating the BBB [29]. The current study was designed to develop, characterize, and evaluate Dox–Erlo NPs and folate-armored Dox–Erlo-NP conjugates for targeting glioma cancer via a nose-to-brain route. The study aimed to improve the targeted specificity and promote the penetration of NPs to glioma cells to achieve the desired therapeutic concentration.

This biopolymeric, nanocarrier-based drug delivery is a novel approach for drug targeting to a specific region as it offers biodegradability and biocompatibility and is non-toxic to the vital organs of the body, as was disclosed in the hemocompatibility study. The folate-armored, polymeric nanocarrier has shown better biodistribution in the brain due to its higher permeability and penetration of the BBB. The developed biopolymer nanoconjugates were effective in glioma therapy as they enabled a controlled drug release over a prolonged time and a tunable size, by which they could approach the target domain, minimize off-target effects, and increase bio-stability. The TEM studies of the nanoconjugate were well-dispersed, uniform, de-aggregated, and consistent in size. The low PDI value showed that the developed preparations were consistent, homogeneous, and had a narrow size distribution. The zeta potential value indicated a negative surface charge on the nanoparticle formulation; the nanoparticles showed no agglomeration due to a same-charge surface repellence of each other, creating a resistive force that led to the enhanced stability of the nanosize system [30].

It has been proven that the over-expressed folate receptor on the tumor cells' surface could be a specific target site for delivering cytotoxic agents [31]. In our study, the conjugation of folic acid to Erlo–Dox preparations was found to be at a higher concentration in the brain when compared to a non-conjugated preparation. This substantiates the higher efficacy of folate-conjugated nanoparticles when compared to plain NPs. The conjugated NPs' formulation exhibited a remarkable cell death and higher concentration in the brain when compared to the unconjugated NPs, consistent with the previous literature. The conjugation of folate with NPs was confirmed by ^{1}H NMR analysis. The results clearly indicated that conjugated NPs can be a promising, tumor-targeting carrier candidate. No endothermic peak in DSC was detected for the drug in Dox–Erlo NPs and conjugated NPs, suggesting that drug has been incorporated in the NPs. The DSC chromatogram of mannitol was detected in the Dox–Erlo-NP conjugates [32].

The functional peaks of the drug in FT-IR becoming flattened in the Dox–Erlo NPs and Dox–Erlo-NP conjugates indicated that the drug was encapsulated in the biopolymeric core [33]. ^{1}H NMR evidently revealed the conjugation of the primary amine group of folic acid with the carboxylic acid group of the polymeric NPs. In ^{1}H NMR, the appearance of the signals at 8.3921 ppm indicated the formation of an amide bond by a reaction between the activated ester group of the polymeric nanoparticles and the primary amine group of the folic acid. Dox–Gefit-NP conjugates were synthesized, as indicated by the formation of amide bond. The appearance of this peak confirmed the conjugation of folic acid [34].

The prepared nanoparticles were nano-sized, having a desirable diameter of 95.35 ± 10.25 nm and 110.12 ± 9.2 nm for the NPs and conjugates, respectively, and exhibited a sustained release of the drug under physiological conditions [35,36].The zeta potential value indicated a negative surface charge on the nanoparticle formulation and no non-agglomerated NPs, probably due to the same-charge surface repellence of each other, with the resultant resistive force leading to an enhanced stability of the nanosize system [37]. Furthermore, the mean PDI of the NPs in our study was 0.109, showing that the developed preparations were consistent, homogeneous, had a narrow particle-size distribution, were monodispersed, and were satisfactory [38,39].

Free Dox and Erlo can cause brain toxicity, cardiotoxicity, and kidney or liver damage. In this study, converting them to NPs and encapsulating them within a biopolymer helped to prevent the toxic side effects of systemic Dox and Erlo administration. The encapsulation of the drug was confirmed by DSC, with FTIR analysis as standard practice. It is being proven that biopolymers demonstrate non-toxicity and short immunogenicity, are bio-absorbable, and have subsequently good biocompatibility. Hence, their use can minimize the potential hazards of cytotoxicity. In the present study, a *Cinnamomum zeylanicum* biopolymer was extracted and used as a nanoparticle-carrier material to achieve a higher concentration of the drug at the targeted tumor site with reduced toxicity. The cytotoxicity study result showed no toxicity of the biopolymer, signifying that the biopolymer is safe and biocompatible [40].

The results of the % drug release assessment demonstrated that Erlo released faster than Dox from NPs. During the initial phase of drug release, an abrupt release was demonstrated, followed a controlled release for a long time. This may be due to Erlo becoming entrapped in the exterior layer, while Dox was encapsulated in the interior core of the NPs [41]. Further, it was observed that release of Erlo and Dox was found to be higher at an acidic, intracellular, endosomal pH of 5.4 when compared to a pH of 7.4. It is worthwhile to disclose herein that the microenvironment of a tumor is slightly more acidic than the physiological fluid [42]. The higher drug release at an endosomal pH of 5.4 in the slightly acidic microenvironment of the tumor may be attributed to the fact that the protonation of the biopolymer and drugs resulted in a higher dissolution of Dox and Erlo from the internal polymeric complex of the NPs in the acidic environment. The pH-dependent drug release is highly desirable for cancer-tissue targeting and also minimizes non-selective drug release in systemic circulation. It also provides sufficient drug concentration upon cellular internalization, which is mediated via endosomal escape and lysosomal fusion [43–45]. After fitting the drug-release data in kinetic models, the exponent value *n* of Erlo from Dox–Erlo NPs at a pH of 5.4 and a pH of 7.4 and Dox from Dox–Erlo NPs at a pH of 5.4 showed that the release mechanism was diffusion (non-Fickian). However, Dox at a pH of 7.4 demonstrated a Fickian drug release mechanism. The findings indicate that Erlo and Dox release from Dox–Erlo-NP conjugates was ascertained via diffusion from polymeric core. The hemolysis assay disclosed that the maximum concentration of formulation was 6 mg; when tested for hemocompatibility, this did not cause significant hemolysis. The hemolysis study was resembled preceding work in the literature [46,47]. The developed formulations were conceived to be as least toxic or non-toxic and are regarded as safe and hemocompatible for in vivo administration. As per the experimental observation, the stability of the Dox–Erlo-NP conjugates were maintained, as indicated by an insignificant alteration in particle size, zeta potential, and entrapment efficiency after an analysis of the sample at fixed intervals of time during a storage period of 90 days ($p > 0.05$). This further indicates that in-house-built Dox–Erlo NPs were robust and consistently in line with the ICH stability-testing guidelines [48,49].

The efficacy of the formulation was studied by assessing the IC50 values and the percent of depletion of cancer cells [50]. The cell-killing potency of the formulations was dose and time-dependent. The MTT assay interpreted that the Dox–Erlo-NP conjugates successfully decreased the % cell viability according to the concentration of the drug in NPs and the drug delivery into the cells [51]. The existing literature demonstrates that using a synergistic combination of EGFR inhibitor viz., Erlotinib provides the cells susceptible to apoptosis with exposure to the DNA-destructive agent doxorubicin [52].

The analytical estimation showed that drug concentration was achieved in the vital organs (the heart, liver, and kidney) with small quantities of Dox and Erlo when compared to the targeted brain, which may be attributed to the partitioning behavior of the nanosized Dox–Erlo NPs and the Dox–Erlo-NP conjugates via endothelial fenestration. Overall, the concentrations of Dox and Erlo achieved in the target organ, i.e., in the brain, were significantly higher than in other organs of the body ($p < 0.05$), indicating the specific delivery of the formulated conjugate in the targeted region of glioma cancer [53].

4. Material and Methods

4.1. Materials

Erlotinib (Mol wt = 393.436, purity of $\geq$95%) was a gift sample from Natco Pharma Ltd. UPSIDC (Dehradun, India). Doxorubicin also a gift sample from Neon Laboratories Pvt. Ltd. (Ghaziabad, India).The cinnamon biopolymer was purchased from Shree Ram Overseas (New Delhi, India). The polyvinyl alcohol (PVA) was received from Sisco Research Laboratory Pvt. Ltd. (Mumbai, India). The cross-linking agents EDC [1-(3 Dimethylaminopropyl)-3-Ethyl Carbodiimide Hydrochloride] and Sulpho-NHS [N-Hydroxysuccinimide] were received from Sisco Research Laboratories Pvt. Ltd. (Mumbai, India). The solvent, Dimethyl Sulfoxide (DMSO), was obtained from Merck Pvt. Ltd. (Mumbai, India), and acetone was obtained from SD Fine Chem Pvt. Ltd. (Mumbai, India), HPLC-grade water and other reagents were used as received.

4.2. Cytotoxicity Study

Materials

The specified materials for the study of cytotoxicity, such as culture media, penicillin streptomycin, MTT (4, five-dimethylthiazol-2yl)-2, five-diphenyl tetrazolium bromide), fetal bovine serum (FBS), and Dulbecco's Modified Eagle Medium (DMEM) were bought from Himedia (Mumbai, India). The phosphate-buffered saline (PBS) was purchased from (Himedia, India). The cell lines C6 and U87 were received from NCCS, Pune, India. Cells were stored at 37 °C and 5% CO_2 in a humidified CO_2 incubator to maintain continuous growth.

4.3. Formulation Optimization Using Statistical Design

The optimization of formulation was carried out through Design-Expert Software (Design-Expert version 12, State-Ease® Inc., Minneapolis, MN, USA) using Box–Behnken design (BBD).The expert design used a three-level, three-factor BBD which produced seventeen experimental runs for optimizing the formulation. The investigative impact of independent variables, viz., (A) polymer concentration; (B) surfactant concentration; and (C) sonication time on thefactors (R1) particle size (nm); (R2) PDI, and (R3) drug release (%) were studied. The levels of independent variables under study were used as low (−1), intermediate (0), and high (+1), and their impact on the responses R1, R2, and

R3 are shown in Table 1. This design comprehensively explained the major, combined, and quadratic effect of factors A, B, and C on various selected responses in the study of the formulation. The optimization of formulation based on Design-Expert version 12, State-Ease® Inc. (Minneapolis, MN, USA) was reported in various preceding works [54].

4.4. Preparation of Dox–Erlo-Loaded NPs

Dox–Erlo-loaded biopolymeric NPs were developed by implementing a modified, double-emulsion solvent-evaporation technique [55]. The technique involved the preparation of an Erlo solution in an organic phase (1 mg/mL), a Dox solution in an aqueous phase (5 µg/mL), a biopolymer in an aqueous phase (29.4 mg/mL), and the preparation of an aqueous PVA solution. Primarily, the solutions of Erlo (1 mg/mL) and Dox (5 µg/mL) were transferred slowly using an injectable needle in the aqueous biopolymer solution (2.94% w/v) and emulsified slowly using a probe sonicator (Hielscher ultrasonicator, Berlin, Germany) (02 min, 30 KHz power, 50 W, 01 cycle) to obtain a polymeric core of the drug as a primary emulsion (o/w). Second, this primary emulsion was transferred into the aqueous PVA solution (2.20 % w/v) slowly, using an injection needle at a rate of 0.5 mL/min. This was then emulsified for 11 min with the probe sonicator (30 KHz power, 80 W, 01 cycle) to obtain a secondary emulsion comprising a nanoparticle suspension. Thereafter, the preparation was stirred magnetically at 1000× g rpm for 4 h at ambient temperature to allow for the evaporation of the organic phase. Further, NPs were held open overnight to obtain hard and dry particles. The nanoparticles were then ultracentrifuged at 15,000× g rpm (OptimaTM LE-80K Ultracentrifuge) for 30 min and washed (n = 3) to free the NPs of un-entrapped drug and free biopolymer matter. The Dox–Erlo-loaded nanoparticle was then re-dispersed in water and lyophilized to dryness for future characterization. The NP preparation steps are illustrated in Figure 12.

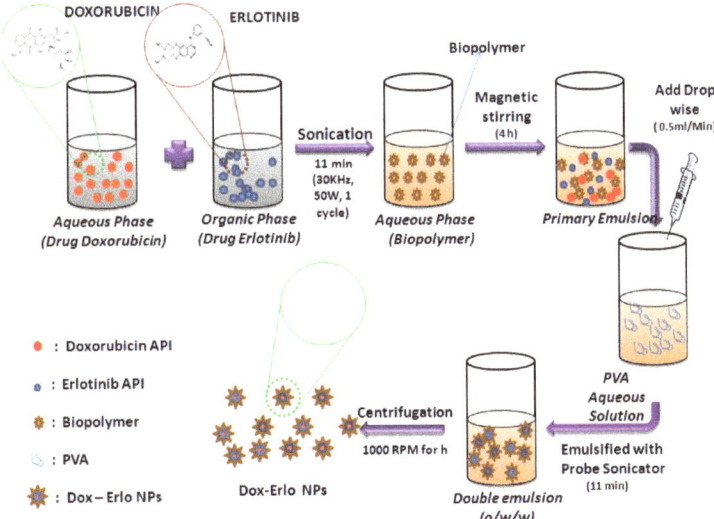

Figure 12. Schematic representation of the preparation of Dox–Erlo NPs by double-emulsion evaporation method.

4.5. Surface Modification of Dox–Erlo Biopolymeric NPs

The nanoparticles were re-dispersed to 10 mg/mL in double-distilled water and incubated with 0.1% of 1-(3 Dimethylaminopropyl)-3-Ethyl Carbodiimide Hydrochloride (EDC. HCl) and N-hydroxysuccinimide (sulpho-NHS, 0.05% w/v), for 5 h in a biological shaker to activate the carboxylic group. In the course of the first step of the coupling reaction, an unstable intermediate was formed on reaction with the EDC cross-linker, which further reacted with sulpho-NHS and formed a stable ester. After incubation, the amine-reactive stable ester (sulpho-NHS NPs) was washed three times with distilled water. In the consequent step, the stable ester (sulpho-NHS NPs) was re-dispersed with folic acid (0.1% w/v) and incubated overnight to hasten the coupling reaction at ambient temperature in an end-to-end biological shaker. The folate-conjugated Dox–Erlo NPs were subjected to centrifugation for half an hour at 15,000× g rpm; thereafter, the supernatant was withdrawn and washed to remove traces of un-conjugated EDC and sulpho-NHS. The conjugated Dox–Erlo NPs were dried via lyophilization for further use. The surface-modification steps of the NPs are shown in Figure 13.

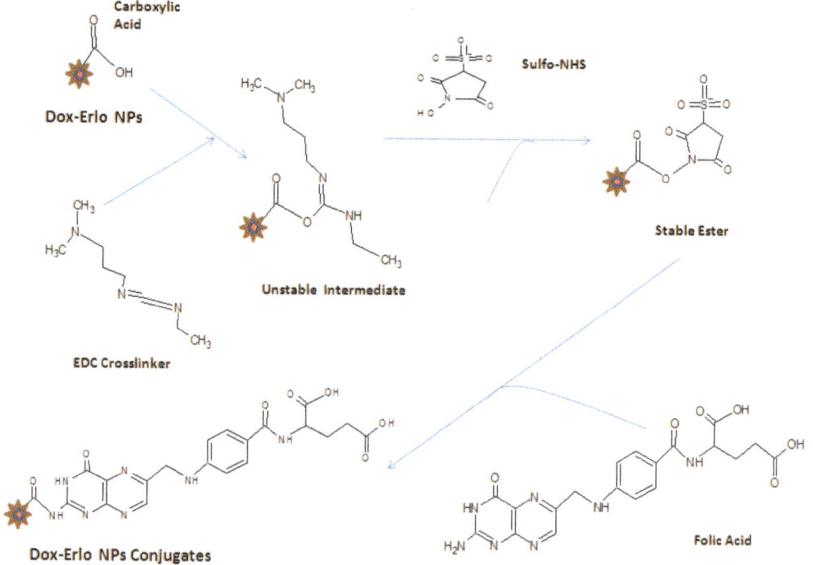

Figure 13. Surface modification of Dox–Erlo NPs.

4.6. Characterization of Dox–ErloNanoparticles

4.6.1. Particle Analysis and Z-Average

The distribution of particles and the Z-average of Dox–Erlo NPs were analyzed by utilizing a Zetasizer 1000 HS (Malvern Instruments, Worcestershire, UK). As per the standard procedure, the Dox–Erlo NPs were re-distributed in HPLC-grade water (0.5 mg/mL) and sonicated for one minute for one cycle at 60 Hz. The sizing analyses were computed and recorded three times ($n = 3$).

4.6.2. Drug Entrapment and Loading in NPs

Erlo and Dox entrapment in the Dox–Erlo NPs was evaluated by the centrifugation of the formulation at an elevated speed of 15,000× g rpm at 4 °C for 30 min (C24, REMI Refrigerated Centrifuge, Mumbai, India). The amount of un-incorporated drug was estimated by reading the absorbance of the supernatant at 342 nm and 480 nm using a UV-visible spectrophotomer.

The % entrapment efficiency and the loading of drug were estimated using following equation:

$$\% \ Entrapment \ efficiency = \frac{Total \ amount \ of \ drug - amount \ of \ drug \ in \ the \ supernatant}{Total \ amount \ of \ drug} \times 100 \quad (1)$$

4.6.3. High-Resolution Transmission Electron Microscopy (HR-TEM)

The morphological characterization of the nanoparticles was studied using a JEOL, JEM 2100 Plus, (Japan) operated at 80 to 200 kV at an ultra-high resolution (UHR). The re-dispersed nanoparticles (0.5 mg/mL) were sonicated for 1 min by dispersion in water. Further, one drop of nanoparticles was stretched over a permeable film grid and dried for ten minutes. Microscopic images were observed and captured at 80 to 200 kV.

4.6.4. Fourier Transform Infrared Spectroscopy (FT-IR)

The FT-IR spectra of Erlo, biopolymer, PVA, Dox–Erlo NPs, and Dox–Erlo-NP conjugates were characterized by FT-IR (Tensor 37, Bruker, MA, USA). Sample of weights of 5 mg were directly placed into the light-beam path and spectra were recorded in a scanning range of 4000–400 cm^{-1}.

4.6.5. Differential Scanning Calorimetry (DSC)

The DSC technique was used to compute the melting point and physical state of the drugs Dox, Erlo, biopolymer, PVA, Dox–Erlo NPs, and Dox–Erlo-NP conjugates by using DSC (Pyris 4 DSC, Perkin Elmer, Waltham, MA, USA). This technique estimated the difference in temperature between a test sample and a reference as a function of the time and temperature when the samples underwent temperature scanning in a range of 50–350 °C in a controlled atmosphere.

4.6.6. X-ray Diffraction (XRD)

XRD analyses of Dox, Erlo, biopolymer, PVA, Dox–Erlo NPs, and Dox–Erlo-NP conjugates were characterized by a PAN analytical X'pert PRO, (Netherland) working at 40 kV, 30 mA, and 2-theta angle ranges (0° to 80°) using monochromatic CuKa-radiation (k = 1.5406 Å).

4.6.7. Proton-Nucleic Magnetic Resonance (^{1}H-NMR)

The ^{1}H-NMR spectra of Dox–Erlo NPs and Dox–Erlo-NP conjugates were acquired on a Bruker Avance—II (Terre Haute, IN, USA) at 400 MHz. The chemical shifting was reported in ppm for the structure elucidation of Dox–Erlo-NP conjugates, which were compared with the Dox–Erlo NPs to confirm the conjugation by using a DMSO solvent and investigating the surface chemistry of the nano-conjugate [56].

4.6.8. In Vitro Release Studies

In vitro Dox and Erlo release of the developed formulations of Dox–Erlo NPs and Dox–Erlo-NP conjugates were assessed by diluting the nanoparticles in PBS at a physiological pH of 7.4 and at an acidic, intracellular, endosomal pH of 5.4. The encapsulated drug NPs were kept enclosed in a dialysis bag (Mol. wt cut-off = 60–8 kDa) with the ends tightened. The dialysis bag was then immersed in 50 mL of PBS at a pH of 7.4 and maintained at 37 ± 0.5 °C with a gentle shaking at 50 rpm. A sample (1 mL) was adjourned at programmed intervals and replaced with an equal volume of fresh PBS at a pH of 7.4 and a pH of 5.4. Samples were examined using UV-visible light with wavelengths of 342 nm and 480 nm.

4.6.9. Hemolysis Study

The hemolysis study was carried out by collecting blood from adult rats in EDTA-coated tubes, followed by centrifugation at 2000 rpm for 10 min to separate the cells and plasma. Further, the sediment cells were washed ($n = 3$) with PBS at a pH of 7.4. Various concentrations of NPs (placebo NPs, Dox–Erlo NPs, and Dox–Erlo-NP conjugates), including 1.5 mg, 3 mg, and 6 mg, were incubated with RBCs of number 1.5×10^7 at 37 °C for 1 h. The samples were subsequently subjected to centrifugation for ten minutes at 2000 rpm. The supernatant was analyzed at 540 nm using UV-visible spectroscopy. An RBC hemolysis of 100% with Triton X-100 was considered to be a positive control and an RBC hemolysis of 0% after treatment with PBS was considered to be a negative control [57]. If the hemolysis was less than 10%, it was regarded as non-toxic. The following formula was used to calculate the hemolysis %:

$$\% \text{ Hemolysis} = [(\text{Abs(treatment)} - \text{Abs(PBS)}) / \text{Abs(Triton} \times -100)] \times 100 \qquad (2)$$

4.6.10. Cytotoxicity Study

The test for the efficacy of the nanosystem composition in terms of therapeutic accumulation and internalization was investigated in cell lines C6 (ATCC, CCL107) and U87 (ATCC, HTB14) of glioma tumors in vitro. The cell-viability study of Dox–Erlo NP and Dox–Erlo-NP conjugate nanosystem was carried out using an MTT assay. The culture cells were treated with DMSO, and the formazan reagent formed (solubilized) was estimated using a spectrophotometer. MTT acts only on biologically active cells, and the activity of cells indicates the cells' viability [58]. In this method, cell lines were added to a 96-well plate (106 cells/well) containing DMEM media and then incubated overnight at 37 °C in a humidified atmosphere in which the air was enriched with (5% v/v) CO_2 tofacilitate the attachment of cells to the bottom of each well. Upon the well attachment of cultured cells, cells were treated with concentrations (between 0.20 and 6.4 µM) of Dox–Erlo-NPs and Dox–Erlo-NP conjugates and incubated for 24 h.

After the completion of the treatment, the media were removed carefully and incubation was repeated with 10 mL of MTT for 3 h. After the completion of the incubation, the optical density was measured at 570 nm in a microplate reader. Each experiment was performed in triplicate ($n = 3$). Untreated cells were related to the control group (100% cell viability), and the IC50 of the cells was determined. IC50 is the drug concentration that slows cell growth by 50% when compared to a control. It is calculated using a regression analysis of cell-viability studies.

Cell viability (%) was expressed as the mean viability (%) ± standard deviation (SD) ($n = 3$) using the following formula:

The cell viability (%) was represented as mean ± SD ($n = 3$) using following formula;

$$\text{Percent cell viability} = \text{OD treated} / \text{OD controlled} \times 100 \qquad (3)$$

4.6.11. Biodistribution Studies

Animals were procured from an animal house prior to the experiment and maintained in polymeric cage as per animal ethical guidelines. The animals were housed at room temperature and exposed to 12 h of light/dark. They were kept on food and water ad libitum. Institutional Animal Ethics Committee (IAEC) guidelines were followed in conducting animal experiments as per the guidelines by DIT University, Dehradun, Uttarakhand, India (Ref no. DITU/IAEC/21-22/07-05). To investigate biodistribution, the administration of a single dose of a formulation such as pure Erlo, pure Dox, Dox–Erlo NPs, or Dox–Erlo-NPs conjugates having 1 mg Erlo and 5 µg of Dox was performed via the nose-to-brain delivery of 20 µL once per day for 14 days in four groups of male Wistar rats ($n = 3$). Different organs, viz., the liver, heart, kidney, blood, and brain were removed from each group ($n = 3$) 24 h after the last dose. The removed tissues were blotted with tissue paper, weighed, and homogenized in 1 mL of ice-cold sodium chloride solution per 1 g of tissue. Thereafter, aliquots were separated and kept at −20 °C until analysis. The Dox and Erlo contents were estimated by using HPLC, using the procedure shown in the section on HPLC methodology.

4.6.12. Stability Study

This study was carried out as per ICH guidelines on three months of Dox–Erlo-NP conjugates. A stability study of the in-house-built formulation was performed to ensure the physiochemical alteration in the quality of Dox–Erlo-NP conjugates. The samples were kept in a stability chamber at an ambient temperature, 25 ± 2 °C, 65 ± 5% RH; and at a higher temperature, 40 ± 2 °C, 75 ± 5% RH, for 90 days. The evaluations were conducted at intervals of 0, 30, 60, and 90 days.

4.6.13. Statistical Analysis

Quantitative data are presented as the mean ± standard deviation (SD). Statistical comparisons between different treatments were analyzed with a one-way ANOVA using Graph Pad Prism. A value of $p < 0.05$ was considered statistically significant.

5. Conclusions

Dox–Erlo NPs were successfully developed for the first time, prepared using a *Cinnamomum zeylanicum* biopolymer. The optimization procedure was accomplished using a three-factor and three-level Box–Behnken experimental design. The optimized composition had a biopolymer content of 2.94% w/v, a surfactant content of a 2.2% w/v, and a sonication time of 11.39 min. In this optimum composition, formulation was characterized by a particle size of 95.35 nm, a PDI of 0.102, and % drug release of 89.91%. The analytical findings confirmed that both drugs were loaded in the biopolymeric core of the NPs. The biodistribution study revealed that folate-functionalized NP conjugates showed improved Dox and Erlo transport across biological barriers and potentially enriched the drug concentration in the brain. The higher cell death in an MTT assay recorded for the NP conjugates over the drug suspension against C6 and U87 cell lines resulted in an enhanced anti-tumor efficacy. The hemolysis study demonstrated that Dox–Erlo-NP conjugates were suitable for in vivo administration. Based on the findings of the studies, it is further suggested that Dox–Erlo-NP conjugates could be an option for effective drug delivery to glioma cancer.

6. Patents

This work has been patented as Indian Patent Application No. 202111038933. Publication Date, 10 September 2021.

Author Contributions: Conceptualization, M.H.A. and M.F.; methodology, M.H.A. and M.F.; software, M.H.A. and M.F.; validation, M.H.A. and M.F.; formal analysis, M.H.A., M.F. and H.C.; investigation, M.H.A. and H.C.; resources, M.J., A.-H.E. and M.S.A.; data curation, M.F., M.H.A. and H.C.; writing—original draft preparation, M.F.; writing—review and editing, M.H.A., H.C., M.J. and A.-H.E.; visualization, M.S.A., M.J., F.T. and A.-H.E.; supervision, M.H.A. and H.C.; project administration, M.H.A. and H.C.; funding acquisition, M.S.A., M.J., F.T. and A.-H.E. All authors have read and agreed to the published version of the manuscript.

Funding: This work was supported by the Dean of Scientific Research, King Khalid University, Saudi Arabia [grant numbers: RGP.1/242/43].

Institutional Review Board Statement: The animal study protocol was approved by the Institutional Animal Ethics Committee (IAEC) guidelines of Faculty of Pharmacy, DIT University (Ref no. DITU/IAEC/21-22/07-05, approved on 1 July 2021) for studies involving animals.

Informed Consent Statement: Not applicable.

Data Availability Statement: Not applicable.

Acknowledgments: This work was supported by the Faculty of Pharmacy, DIT University, Dehradun. The authors extend their appreciation to the Deanship of Scientific Research at King Khalid University for funding this work through the Small Groups Project under grant number (RGP.1/242/43). M.J. and Abdel thanks to King Abdullah University of Science and Technology, Saudi Arabia for financial support.

Conflicts of Interest: The authors declare no conflict of interest.

References

1. Akhter, M.H.; Rizwanullah, M.; Ahmad, J.; Amin, S.; Ahmad, M.Z.; Minhaj, M.A.; Mujtaba, M.A.; Ali, J. Molecular Targets and Nanoparticulate Systems Designed for the Improved Therapeutic Intervention in Glioblastoma Multiforme. *Drug Res.* **2021**, *71*, 122–137. [CrossRef] [PubMed]
2. Aaron, C.; Ashley, D.M.; López, G.Y.; Malinzak, M.; Friedman, H.S.; Khasraw, M. Management of glioblastoma: State of the art and future directions. *CA Cancer J. Clin.* **2020**, *70*, 299–312.
3. Clarke, J.; Butowski, N.; Chang, S. Recent Advances in Therapy for Glioblastoma. *Arch. Neurol.* **2010**, *67*, 279–283. [CrossRef] [PubMed]
4. Hassan, Y.A.; Alfaifi, M.Y.; Shati, A.A.; Elbehairi, S.E.I.; Elshaarawy, R.F.M.; Kamal, I. Co-delivery of anticancer drugs via poly(ionic crosslinked chitosan-palladium) nanocapsules: Targeting more effective and sustainable cancer therapy. *J. Drug Del. Sci. Technol.* **2022**, *69*, 103151. [CrossRef]
5. Jani, P.; Suman, S.; Subramanian, S.; Korde, A.; Gohel, D.; Singh, R.; Sawant, K. Development of mitochondrial targeted theranostic nanocarriers for treatment of gliomas. *J. Drug Del. Sci. Technol.* **2021**, *64*, 102648. [CrossRef]
6. Akhter, M.H.; Madhav, N.S.; Ahmad, J. Epidermal growth factor receptor based active targeting: A paradigm shift towards advance tumor therapy. *Artif. Cells Nanomed. Biotechnol.* **2018**, *46*, 1188–1198. [CrossRef]
7. Miller, K.D.; Ostrom, Q.T.; Kruchko, C.; Patil, N.; Tihan, T.; Cioffi, G.; Fuchs, H.E.; Waite, K.A.; Jemal, A.; Siegel, R.L.; et al. Brain and other central nervous system tumor statistics. *CA Cancer J. Clin.* **2021**, *71*, 381–406. [CrossRef]
8. Finch, A.; Solomou, G.; Wykes, V.; Pohl, U.; Bardella, C.; Watts, C. Advances in Research of Adult Gliomas. *Int. J. Mol. Sci.* **2021**, *22*, 924. [CrossRef]
9. Seshacharyulu, P.; Ponnusamy, M.P.; Haridas, D.; Jain, M.; Ganti, A.K.; Batra, S.K. Targeting the EGFR signaling pathway in cancer therapy. *Expert Opin. Ther. Targets* **2012**, *16*, 15–31. [CrossRef]
10. Norouzi, M.; Yathindranath, V.; Thliveris, J.A.; Kopec, B.M.; Siahaan, T.J.; Miller, D.W. Doxorubicin-loaded iron oxide nanoparticles for glioblastoma therapy: A combinational approach for enhanced delivery of nanoparticles. *Sci. Rep.* **2020**, *10*, 11292. [CrossRef]
11. Wong, I.Y.; Bhatia, S.N.; Toner, M. Nanotechnology: Emerging tools for biology and medicine. *Genes. Dev.* **2013**, *27*, 2397–2408. [CrossRef] [PubMed]
12. Akhter, M.H.; Khalilullah, H.; Gupta, M.; Alfaleh, M.A.; Alhakamy, N.A.; Riadi, Y.; Shadab, M. Impact of Protein Corona on the Biological Identity of Nanomedicine: Understanding the Fate of Nanomaterials in the Biological Milieu. *Biomedicines* **2021**, *9*, 1496. [CrossRef] [PubMed]
13. Jong, W.H.D.; Borm, P.J.A. Drug delivery and nanoparticles:applications and hazards. *Int. J. Nanomed.* **2008**, *3*, 133–149. [CrossRef]
14. Ahmad, J.; Ameeduzzafar, M.Z.; Ahmad, J.; Akhter, M.H. Surface-Engineered Cancer Nanomedicine: Rational Design and Recent Progress. *Curr. Pharm. Des.* **2020**, *26*, 1181–1190. [CrossRef]
15. Akhter, M.H.; Rizwanullah, M.; Ahmad, J.; Ahsan, M.J.; Mujtaba, M.A.; Amin, S. Nanocarriers in advanced drug targeting: Setting novel paradigm in cancer therapeutics. *Artif. Cells Nanomed. Biotechnol.* **2018**, *46*, 873–884. [CrossRef] [PubMed]
16. Akhter, M.H.; Beg, S.; Tarique, M.; Malik, A. Receptor-based targeting of engineered nanocarrier against solid tumors: Recent progress and challenges ahead. *Biochim. Et Biophys. Acta-Gen. Subj.* **2021**, *1865*, 129777. [CrossRef]
17. Patra, J.K.; Das, G.; Fraceto, L.; Campos, E.V.R. Nano based drug delivery systems: Recent developments and future prospects. *J. Nanobiotechnol.* **2018**, *16*, 71. [CrossRef] [PubMed]
18. Li, J.; Zhao, J.; Tan, T.; Liu, M.; Zeng, Z.; Zeng, Y.; Zhang, L.; Fu, C.; Chen, D.; Xie, T. Nanoparticle Drug Delivery System for Glioma and Its Efficacy Improvement Strategies: A Comprehensive Review. *Int. J. Nanomed.* **2020**, *5*, 2563–2582. [CrossRef] [PubMed]
19. Luque-Michel, E.; Lemaire, L.; Blanco-Prieto, M.J. SPION and doxorubicin-loaded polymeric nanocarriers for glioblastoma theranostics. *Drug Deliv. Transl. Res.* **2021**, *11*, 515–523. [CrossRef]
20. Alibolandi, M.; Farzad, S.A.; Mohammadi, M.; Abnous, K.; Taghdisi, S.M.; Kalalinia, F.; Ramezani, M. Tetrac-decorated chitosan-coated PLGA nanoparticles as a new platform for targeted delivery of SN38. *Artif. Cells Nanomed. Biotechnol.* **2018**, *46*, 1003–1014. [CrossRef]
21. Cheung, A.; Bax, H.J.; Josephs, D.H.; Ilieva, K.M.; Pellizzari, G.; Opzoomer, J.; Bloomfield, J.; Fittall, M.; Grigoriadis, A.; Figini, M.; et al. Targeting folate receptor alpha for cancer treatment. *Oncotarget* **2016**, *7*, 52553–52574. [CrossRef] [PubMed]
22. Karim, S.; Akhter, M.H.; Burzangi, A.S.; Alkreathy, H.; Alharthy, B.; Kotta, S.; Shadab, M.; Rashid, M.A.; Afzal, O.; Altamimi, A.S.A.; et al. Phytosterol-Loaded Surface-Tailored Bioactive-Polymer Nanoparticles for Cancer Treatment: Optimization, In Vitro Cell Viability, Antioxidant Activity, and Stability Studies. *Gels* **2022**, *8*, 219. [CrossRef] [PubMed]
23. Zwicke, G.L.; Mansoori, G.A.; Jeffery, C.J. Utilizing the folate receptor for active targeting of cancer nanotherapeutics. *Nano Rev.* **2012**, *3*, 10. [CrossRef] [PubMed]
24. Jacob, J.; Haponiuk, J.T.; Thomas, S.; Gopi, S. Biopolymer based nanomaterials in drug delivery systems: A review. *Mater. Today Chem.* **2018**, *9*, 43–55. [CrossRef]
25. Sadasivuni, K.K.; Saha, P.; Adhikari, J.; Deshmukh, K.; Ahamed, M.B.; Cabibihan, J.J. Recent advances in mechanical properties of biopolymer composites: A review. *Polym. Compos.* **2020**, *41*, 32–59. [CrossRef]
26. Venugopala, V.; Kumara, K.J.; Muralidharanc, S.; Parasuramanb, S.; Raja, P.V.; Kumara, K.V. Optimization and in-vivo evaluation of isradipine nanoparticles using Box-Behnken design surface response methodology. *OpenNano* **2016**, *1*, 1–15. [CrossRef]

27. Dash, S.; Murthy, P.N.; Nath, L.; Chowdhury, P. Kinetic modelling on drug release from cnotrolled drug delivery system. *Acta Pol. Pharm.* **2010**, *67*, 217–223.
28. Akhter, M.H.; Ahmad, A.; Ali, J.; Mohan, G. Formulation and Development of CoQ10-Loaded s-SNEDDS for Enhancement of Oral Bioavailability. *J. Pharm. Innov.* **2014**, *9*, 121–131. [CrossRef]
29. Zhang, C.; Song, J.; Lou, L.; Qi, X.; Zhao, L.; Fan, B.; Sun, G.; Lv, Z.; Fan, Z.; Jiao, B.; et al. Doxorubicin-loaded nanoparticle coated with endothelial cells-derived exosomes for immunogenic chemotherapy of glioblastoma. *Bioeng. Transl. Med.* **2020**, *3*, e10203. [CrossRef]
30. Amasya, G.; Ozturk, C.; Aksu, B.; Tarimci, N. QbD based formulation optimization of semi-solid lipid nanoparticles as nano-cosmeceuticals. *J. Drug Deliv. Sci. Technol.* **2021**, *66*, 102737. [CrossRef]
31. Bellotti, E.; Cascone, M.G.; Barbani, N.; Rossin, D.; Rastaldo, R.; Giachino, C.; Cristallini, C. Targeting Cancer Cells Overexpressing Folate Receptors with New Terpolymer-Based Nanocapsules: Toward a Novel Targeted DNA Delivery System for Cancer Therapy. *Biomedicines* **2021**, *9*, 1275. [CrossRef] [PubMed]
32. Lakkadwala, S.; Singh, J. Co-delivery of doxorubicin and erlotinib through liposomal nanoparticles for glioblastoma tumor regression using an in vitro brain tumor model. *Colloids Surf. B Biointerfaces* **2019**, *173*, 27–35. [CrossRef] [PubMed]
33. Eid, A.; Uddin, N.; Girgis, S. Formulation and optimization of Biodegradable Insulin Loaded Nanoparticles. *Int. J. Pharm. Sci. Health Care* **2019**, *3*, 12–35. [CrossRef]
34. Cheng, L.; Ma, H.; Shao, M.; Fan, Q.; Lv, H.; Peng, J.; Hao, T.; Li, D.; Zhao, C.; Zong, X. Synthesis of folate-chitosan nanoparticles loaded with ligustrazine to target folate receptor positive cancer cells. *Mol. Med. Rep.* **2017**, *16*, 1101–1108. [CrossRef]
35. Parijat, P.; Kamal, D.; Harish, D. Erlotinib loaded chitosan nanoparticles: Formulation, physicochemical characterization and cytotoxic potential. *Int. J. Biolog. Macromol.* **2019**, *139*, 1304–1316.
36. Zhou, X.; Tao, H.; Shi, K.H. Development of a nanoliposomal formulation of erlotinib for lung cancer and in vitro/in vivo antitumoral evaluation. *Drug Des. Devel. Ther.* **2017**, *18*, 1–8. [CrossRef]
37. Sharma, G.; Modgil, A.; Layek, B.; Arora, K.; Sun, C.; Law, B.; Singh, J. Cell penetrating peptide tethered bi-ligand liposomes for delivery to brain in vitro: Biodistribution and transfection. *J. Control. Release* **2013**, *167*, 1–10. [CrossRef]
38. Hosseini, S.M.; Abbasalipourkabir, R.; Jalilian, F.A.; Asl, S.S.; Farmany, A.; Roshanaei, G.; Arabestani, M.R. Doxycycline-encapsulated solid lipid nanoparticles as promising tool against Brucella melitensis enclosed in macrophage: A pharmacodynamics study on J774A.1 cell line. *Antimicrob. Resist Infect. Control* **2019**, *3*, 8–62. [CrossRef]
39. Li, X.; Wang, J.; Li, S.; Liu, Z. Development and Evaluation of Multifunctional Poly (Lactic-co-glycolic acid) Nanoparticles Embedded in Carboxymethyl-Glucan Porous Microcapsules as a Novel Drug Delivery System for Gefitinib. *Pharmaceutics* **2019**, *11*, 469. [CrossRef]
40. MacDiarmid, J.A.; Langova, V.; Bailey, D.; Pattison, S.T.; Pattison, S.L.; Christensen, N.; Armstrong, L.R.; Brahmbhatt, V.N.; Smolarczyk, K.; Harrison, M.T.; et al. Targeted Doxorubicin Delivery to Brain Tumors via Minicells: Proof of Principle Using Dogs with Spontaneously Occurring Tumors as a Model. *PLoS ONE* **2016**, *11*, e0151832. [CrossRef]
41. He, Y.; Su, Z.; Zhang, C. Co-delivery of erlotinib and doxorubicin by pH-sensitive charge conversion nanocarrier for synergistic therapy. *J. Control. Release* **2016**, *229*, 80–92. [CrossRef] [PubMed]
42. Kato, Y.; Ozawa, S.; Miyamoto, C.; Maehata, Y.; Suzuki, A.; Maeda, T.; Baba, Y. Acidic extracellular microenvironment and cancer. *Cancer Cell Int.* **2013**, *13*, 89. [CrossRef] [PubMed]
43. Begines, B.; Ortiz, T.; Pérez-Aranda, M.; Martínez, G.; Merinero, M.; Argüelles-Arias, F.; Alcudia, A. Polymeric Nanoparticles for Drug Delivery: Recent Developments and Future Prospects. *Nanomaterials* **2020**, *10*, 1403. [CrossRef]
44. Zhou, L.; Cheng, R.; Tao, H.; Ma, S.; Guo, W.; Meng, F.; Liu, H.; Liu, Z.; Zhong, Z. Endosomal pH-activatable poly(ethylene oxide)-graft-doxorubicin prodrugs: Synthesis, drug release, and biodistribution in tumor-bearing mice. *Biomacromol* **2011**, *12*, 1460–1467. [CrossRef] [PubMed]
45. Chen, Y.C.; Chianga, C.F.; Chenc, L.F.; Liangad, P.C.; Hsiehb, W.Y.; Linae, W.L. Polymersomes conjugated with des-octanoyl ghrelin and folate as a BBB-penetrating cancer cell-targeting delivery system. *Biomaterials* **2014**, *35*, 4066–4081. [CrossRef]
46. Tzeyung, A.S.; Shadab, M.; Bhattamisra, S.K.; Madheswaran, T.; Alhakamy, N.A.; Aldawsari, H.M.; Radhakrishnan, A.K. Fabrication, optimization, and Evaluation of Rotigotine-Loaded Chitosan Nanoparticles for Nose-To-Brain Delivery. *Pharmaceutics* **2019**, *11*, 26. [CrossRef]
47. Pan, D.; Vargas-Morales, O.; Zern, B.; Anselmo, A.C.; Gupta, V.; Zakrewsky, M.; Mitragotri, S.; Muzykantov, V. The Effect of Polymeric Nanoparticles on Biocompatibility of Carrier Red Blood Cells. *PLoS ONE* **2016**, *11*, e0152074. [CrossRef]
48. ICH Q1A (R2). Stability Testing Guidelines: Stability Testing of New Drug Substances and Products. ICH Step 5. CPMP/ICH/2736/99. Available online: https://www.ema.europa.eu/en/documents/scientific-guideline/ich-q-1-r2-stability-testing-new-drug-substances-products-step-5_en.pdf (accessed on 13 July 2022).
49. Zhao, Z.; Liu, W.; Jiang, Y.; Wan, Y.; Du, R.; Li, H. Solidification of heavy metals in lead smelting slag and development of cementitious materials. *J. Clean. Prod.* **2022**, *359*, 132134. [CrossRef]
50. Xu, H.; Rahimpour, S.; Nesvick, C.L.; Zhang, X.; Ma, J.; Zhang, M.; Zhang, G.; Wang, L.; Yang, C.; Hong, C.S.; et al. Activation of hypoxia signaling induces phenotypic transformation of glioma cells: Implications for bevacizumab antiangiogenic therapy. *Oncotarget* **2015**, *6*, 3592. [CrossRef]
51. Kumar, S.; Besra, S.E. The Growth Suppressing Activity Of Spathodea Campanulata Bark On C6 & U87mg Involve Induction Of Apoptosis And Cell Cycle Arrest. *World J. Pharm. Res.* **2020**, *9*, 2517.

52. Huang, C.; Luo, Y.; Zhao, J.; Yang, F.; Zhao, H.; Fan, W.; Ge, P. Shikonin Kills Glioma Cells through Necroptosis Mediated by RIP-1. *PLoS ONE* **2013**, *8*, e66326. [CrossRef] [PubMed]
53. Lakkadwala, S.; Rodrigues, B.S.; Sun, C.; Singh, J. Biodistribution of TAT or QLPVM coupled to receptor targeted liposomes for delivery of anticancer therapeutics to brain in vitro and in vivo. *Nanomed.* **2020**, *23*, 102112. [CrossRef] [PubMed]
54. Shadab, M.; Alhakamy, N.A.; Aldawsari, H.M.; Husain, M.; Khan, N.; Alfaleh, M.A.; Asfour, H.Z.; Riadi, Y.; Bilgrami, A.L.; Akhter, M.H. Plumbagin-Loaded Glycerosome Gel as Topical Delivery System for Skin Cancer Therapy. *Polymers* **2021**, *13*, 923.
55. Akhter, M.H.; Kumar, S.; Nomani, S. Sonication tailored enhance cytotoxicity of naringenin nanoparticle in pancreatic cancer: Design, optimization, and in vitro studies. *Drug Dev. Ind. Pharm.* **2020**, *46*, 659–672. [CrossRef]
56. Emwas, A.H.; Roy, R.; McKay, R.T.; Tenori, L.; Saccenti, E.; Gowda, G.A.N.; Raftery, D.; Alahmari, F.; Jaremko, L.; Jaremko, M.; et al. NMR Spectroscopy for Metabolomics Research. *Metabolites* **2019**, *9*, 123. [CrossRef]
57. Lakkadwala, S.; Rodrigues, B.D.S.; Sun, C.; Singh, J. Dual functionalized liposomes for efficient co-delivery of anti-cancer chemotherapeutics for the treatment of glioblastoma. *J. Cont. Rel.* **2019**, *307*, 247–260. [CrossRef]
58. Zhou, Z.; Kennell, C.; Jafari, M.; Lee, J.Y.; Ruiz-Torres, S.J.; Waltz, S.E.; Lee, J.H. Sequential delivery of erlotinib and doxorubicin for enhanced triple negative Breast cancer treatment using polymeric nanoparticle. *Int. J. Pharm.* **2017**, *530*, 300–307. [CrossRef]

Disclaimer/Publisher's Note: The statements, opinions and data contained in all publications are solely those of the individual author(s) and contributor(s) and not of MDPI and/or the editor(s). MDPI and/or the editor(s) disclaim responsibility for any injury to people or property resulting from any ideas, methods, instructions or products referred to in the content.

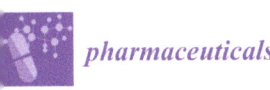

Article

Tumor Microenvironment-Responsive Magnetic Nanofluid for Enhanced Tumor MRI and Tumor multi-treatments

Liangju Sheng [1,†], Xuanlei Zhu [2,†], Miao Sun [2], Zhe Lan [1], Yong Yang [3], Yuanrong Xin [2,*] and Yuefeng Li [1,*]

1. College of Medicine, Jiangsu University, Zhenjiang 212013, China
2. College of Pharmacy, Jiangsu University, Zhenjiang 212013, China
3. College of Mechanical Engineering, Suzhou University of Science and Technology, Suzhou 215009, China
* Correspondence: liyuefeng@ujs.edu.cn (Y.L.); xinyuanrong@ujs.edu.cn (Y.X.)
† These authors contributed equally to this work.

Abstract: We prepared a tumor microenvironment-responsive magnetic nanofluid (MNF) for improving tumor targeting, imaging and treatment simultaneously. For this purpose, we synthesized sulfonamide-based amphiphilic copolymers with a suitable pK_a at 7.0; then, we utilized them to prepare the tumor microenvironment-responsive MNF by self-assembly of the sulfonamide-based amphiphilic copolymers and hydrophobic monodispersed Fe_3O_4 nanoparticles at approximately 8 nm. After a series of characterizations, the MNF showed excellent application potential due to the fact of its high stability under physiological conditions and its hypersensitivity toward tumor stroma by forming aggregations within neutral or weak acidic environments. Due to the fact of its tumor microenvironment-responsiveness, the MNF showed great potential for accumulation in tumors, which could enhance MNF-mediated magnetic resonance imaging (MRI), magnetic hyperthermia (MH) and Fenton reaction (FR) in tumor. Moreover, in vitro cell experiment did not only show high biocompatibility of tumor microenvironment-responsive MNF in physiological environment, but also exhibit high efficacy on inhibiting cell proliferation by MH-dependent chemodynamic therapy (CDT), because CDT was triggered and promoted efficiently by MH with increasing strength of alternating magnetic field. Although the current research is limited to in vitro study, these positive results still suggest the great potential of the MNF on effective targeting, diagnosis, and therapy of tumor.

Keywords: tumor microenvironment-responsive; magnetic nanofluid; improved magnetic resonance imaging; neutral-responsive Fenton reaction; enhanced chemodynamic therapy

Citation: Sheng, L.; Zhu, X.; Sun, M.; Lan, Z.; Yang, Y.; Xin, Y.; Li, Y. Tumor Microenvironment-Responsive Magnetic Nanofluid for Enhanced Tumor MRI and Tumor multi-treatments. *Pharmaceuticals* **2023**, *16*, 166. https://doi.org/10.3390/ph16020166

Academic Editor: Huijie Zhang

Received: 1 December 2022
Revised: 12 January 2023
Accepted: 18 January 2023
Published: 23 January 2023

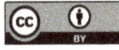

Copyright: © 2023 by the authors. Licensee MDPI, Basel, Switzerland. This article is an open access article distributed under the terms and conditions of the Creative Commons Attribution (CC BY) license (https://creativecommons.org/licenses/by/4.0/).

1. Introduction

In tumor diagnosis and treatment, superparamagnetic iron oxide (SPIO) nanoparticles play a unique and important role, because they possesses versatile applications for clinical diagnosis and tumor adjunctive therapy [1,2]. For tumor diagnosis, SPIO nanoparticles have been used widely as a contrast agent (CA) in magnetic resonance imaging (MRI), as it could improve the contrast in anatomical imaging to highlight the situation and structure of a tumor by shortening the spin−spin relaxation time (T_2) of the proton [3]. For tumor therapy, magnetic hyperthermia (MH) is a noninvasive hyperthermia that inhibits tumor growth by the Brownian relaxation and Néel relaxation of SPIO nanoparticles under an alternating magnetic field (AMF) [4]. Furthermore, many studies also found that SPIO nanoparticles could induce apoptosis of tumor cells directly by producing ferrous ions, which can generate toxic reactive oxygen species (ROS) by the Fenton reaction (FR) [5]. Although SPIO nanoparticles present much potential, their effectiveness in tumor diagnosis and therapy still depends on their accumulation in the tumor, which is similar to that of a chemotherapeutic drug. Learning from the progress of stimuli-responsive polymeric nanocarriers for tumor targeting [6,7], the targeted accumulation of SPIO nanoparticles in a tumor could also be improved by constructing stimuli-responsive magnetic nanofluid (MNF) through the self-assembly of SPIO nanoparticles and stimuli-responsive polymers.

Because tumor angiogenesis and aerobic glycolysis have been recognized as features of most malignant solid tumors, regardless of their tissue origin or genetic background [8], pH-sensitive nanocarriers have attracted tremendous interest in tumor diagnosis and subsequent treatment over the past decades [9,10]. In order to construct pH-sensitive nanocarriers, many types of pH-sensitive polymers have been designed and synthesized, as they possess ionizable basic or acidic residues [11], resulting in varied physicochemical properties (solubility or chain conformation) with a change in the surrounding pH [12]. However, slight pH differences between a tumor stroma (pH = 7.1–6.7) [13] and the physiological condition (pH = 7.35–7.45) is impossible to be recognized by most pH-sensitive deliveries, which usually consist of pH-sensitive polymers and occur during phase transition in endocytic organelles with a lower pH value (pH $\leq$ 6.0), such as endosomes and lysosomes [9,10]. There are only a few pH-sensitive polymers with dissociation constants (pK_a) around neutral pH, such as cationic polymers with repeating ionizable tertiary amines [14,15] or anionic polymers with suitable sulfonamide groups [16,17]. Until now, the most successful pH-sensitive polymers used in targeting tumor microenvironment were cationic polymers with ionizable tertiary amine blocks, showing a hydrophobic–hydrophilic phase transition in weakly acidic microenvironments [18,19], which disassemble rapidly in tumor microenvironment, leading to their application in targeted tumor chemotherapy [20] and enhanced tumor fluorescence imaging [19]. Unfortunately, ionized cationic polymer exhibit a potential risk of hemolysis in vivo, as its positive charge could easily damage membranes of red blood cells [21]. Therefore, a sulfonamide-based anionic polymer with suitable pK_a within a tumor microenvironment pH value (7.1–6.7) should be an optimized option to prepare MNF with tumor microenvironment responsiveness.

According to the property of an anionic polymer, its hydrophilic–hydrophobic phase transition can be triggered under a certain pH value, which is usually lower than the pK_a of anionic polymer [11]. As a result, a pH-responsive MNF with a suitable pK_a (7.1–6.7) should lose its colloidal stability in tumor stroma, resulting in the efficient accumulation and retention of SPIO in tumor tissue. Furthermore, tumor tissue had existing amounts of endogenous hydrogen ion (H^+) and hydrogen peroxide (H_2O_2). Due to the phase transition of anionic polymers in tumor stroma, encapsulated SPIO nanoparticles obtained the opportunity to interact with surrounding H^+, resulting in the release of ferrous ion (Fe^{2+}). Next, the endogenous H_2O_2 in the tumor tissue could be decomposed under the catalysis of Fe^{2+}, implying the possibility of FR in the tumor microenvironment. When the phase transition of anionic polymer blocks occurred completely, stranded SPIO nanoparticles could form many aggregations with a large size spontaneously. According to previous studies, a closed packing structure of the multiple SPIO nanoparticles exhibited its attractive effects on improving the negative signal contrast of pathological tissue [22] and enhanced the efficiency of MH [23] simultaneously. Therefore, sulfonamide-based MNF with a pH responsiveness not only possesses a specific advantage in tumor targeting but also shows other potentials for improving the sensitivity of tumor MRIs and enhancing the antitumor efficacy by a combination of MH- and FR-mediated chemodynamic therapy (CDT).

In this study, we designed and fabricated a tumor microenvironment-responsive MNF, which maintained stability in blood vessels and formed aggregations in tumor microenvironment to enhance tumor MH, ROS generation and MRIs simultaneously, as shown in Figure 1.

In order to prepare the tumor microenvironment-responsive MNF, we synthesized a sulfonamide-based amphiphilic copolymer, polycaprolactone-b-poly(sulfadimethoxine acrylamide) (PCL-b-pSMA) by reversible addition–fragmentation chain transfer (RAFT) polymerization, according to relevant studies [24,25], which showed pK_a of approximately 7.0. Then, the MNF was fabricated by the simple self-assembly of the PCL-b-pSMA and hydrophobic Fe_3O_4 nanoparticles. Due to the fact of the pH sensitivity of PCL-b-pSMA at a neutral pH value, the MNF in the aqueous phase displayed a similar pH responsiveness at a neutral pH value ($\approx$7.0). According to the pH sensitivity of the MNF on neutral medium, we further investigated its application potentials for MH, FR and MRI for tumor theranostics. The relevant results show that the MNF under neutral conditions exhibited a better performance in enhancing the specific absorption rate (SAR), increasing the generation of hydroxyl radical (•OH) and improving the T_2 relaxivity (r_2), simultaneously, compared to its counterpart in a physiological environment. Based on these advantages, we further studied the effects of the tumor microenvironment-responsive MNF on MH-induced cell death and ROS generation under different strengths of AMF ($H_{applied}$). As the intercellular ROS level and cell mortality rate under MH showed a high degree of correlation, this study suggests that the MNF can stimulate CDT by MH and inhibit cell proliferation efficiently by integrating MH and CDT effectively. Therefore, the tumor microenvironment-responsive MNF possesses a versatile potential for tumor targeting, diagnosis and treatment.

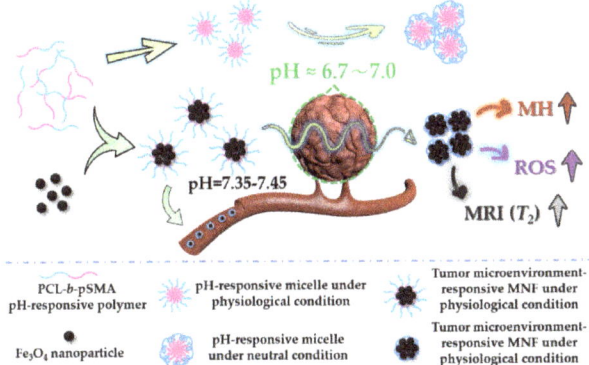

Figure 1. Schematic illustration of the tumor microenvironment-responsive MNF, which was prepared by self-assembly of Fe_3O_4 nanoparticles and pH-responsive polymer. According to the phase transition of the pH-responsive micelles under a neutral condition, the tumor microenvironment-responsive MNF could maintain an individual state and form aggregations in tumor microenvironment to improve tumor MH, ROS generation and MRI simultaneously.

2. Results and Discussion

2.1. Synthesis and Characterization of the pH-Responsive Amphiphilic Copolymer

As an anionic polymer usually possesses hydrophilicity in neutral and physiological conditions, we selected the polycaprolactone (PCL) segment as the hydrophobic block of the amphiphilic copolymer because of its high biocompatibility. The synthetic route, as shown in Figure S1 (Supplementary Materials), contained ring opening polymerization (ROP), an esterification reaction and RAFT polymerization simultaneously. By the ROP, the PCL was synthesized successfully, which was confirmed by the H proton nuclear magnetic resonance (^{1}H NMR) spectrum, as shown in Figure S2. S-1-dodecyl-S'-(a,a'-dimethyl-a''-acetic acid)trithiocarbonate (DDMAT) was used as the chain transfer agent (CTA) for the RAFT polymerization. The following product was PCL-DDMAT by the esterification reaction between PCL and DDMAT, which was also confirmed by its structure using the ^{1}H NMR spectrum, as shown in Figure S3.

The final reaction was the RAFT polymerization for the preparation of the pH-responsive amphiphilic copolymer. In this study, we selected sulfadimethoxine acrylamide (SMA) as the pH-sensitive monomer, because the poly(methacryloyl sulfadimethoxine) showed a pK_a at approximately 7.0 in a relevant study [24]. Utilizing DMSO-d_6 as a solvent, we characterized the structures of the PCL-b-pSMA and SMA, as shown in Figure 2. According to previous studies [24,26,27], all of the characteristic peaks of the SMA were identified and marked in Figure 2A (bottom spectrum). Based on the ^{1}H NMR results of the SMA (Figure 2A, bottom spectrum) and PCL-DDMAT (Figure S3), we further identified all of the characteristic peaks of the PCL-b-pSMA, also shown in Figure 2A (top spectrum). Apparently, because of the polymerization of SMA, the characteristic peaks of the acrylamide in the SMA disappeared; meanwhile, all of the characteristic peaks of the SM broadened. In addition to the characteristic peaks of SM, the characteristic peaks of PCL can also observed in Figure 2A (top spectrum), which confirms the successful polymerization of SMA as a product of the PCL-DDMAT.

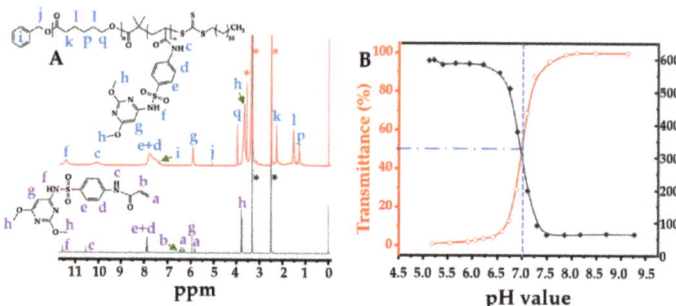

Figure 2. Structure and pH responsive of the PCL-b-pSMA: (**A**) ^{1}H NMR spectrum of PCL-b-pSMA, marking all characteristic peaks; (**B**) pH-dependent transmittance curve and diameter variation of PCL-b-pSMA, showing a pK_a at 7.0.

After researching the structure of the PCL-b-pSMA, we characterized the pK_a of the PCL-b-pSMA, as shown in Figure 2B. According to relevant studies [28,29], the cloud point method was utilized to determine the pK_a of the PCL-b-pSMA, as shown in Figure 2B (red line), by quantifying the turbidity of the PCL-b-pSMA under different pH buffers at 500 nm. We prepared the micelles of the PCL-b-pSMA in an alkaline solution first; then, we observed its light transmittance using a UV-Vis spectrophotometer under a decreasing pH from 9.13 to 5.18. Apparently, the transmittance of the PCL-b-pSMA micelles with a high concentration ($\approx$3 mg mL^{-1}) was influenced by the environmental pH value. In the alkaline environment, the PCL-b-pSMA micelles showed almost 100% transmittance. When the pH value decreased to 7.5, its transmittance decreased slightly. However, the turbidity increased sharply with the decrease of the pH from 7.27 to 6.88, and the corresponding light transmittance decreased from 87.7% to 29.3%. When the pH value decreased further ($\leq$6.59), the PCL-b-pSMA formed obvious sediment, and the corresponding light transmittance was near 0%. As PCL is a typical hydrophobic polymer, the high transmittance of the PCL-b-pSMA depends on the hydrophilicity of the pSMA in an alkaline solution. When the solution pH value downregulated from a weak alkaline to faintly acid, the increasing turbidity of the PCL-b-pSMA micelles indicated the rapid phase transition of the pSMA from hydrophilicity to hydrophobicity.

The phase transition of the pSMA not only decreased the transmittance of the PCL-b-pSMA micelles at the macro level but also reduced their stability at the micro level, which could be observed by dynamic light scattering (DLS), which was assessed under a low concentration of the PCL-b-pSMA micelles (0.3 mg mL^{-1}). As shown in Figure 2B (gray line), the DLS result exhibited the effect of the pH value on the PCL-b-pSMA micelle's hydrated diameter. According to the result, the hydrated diameter of the PCL-b-pSMA micelles in an alkaline solution decreased slightly from 64.7 (pH $\approx$ 9.21) to 62.9 nm (pH $\approx$ 7.43) with the decreasing pH value. When the surrounding pH value decreased to 7.05, the diameter of the PCL-b-pSMA micelles increased sharply to 198.9 nm. With the pH decreasing further (pH $\approx$ 6.85), the particle size of the PCL-b-pSMA micelles increased to 379.4 nm, indicating the agglomeration of the PCL-b-pSMA micelles. Finally, the diameter of these agglomerated micelles reached almost 600 nm in an acidic environment, which corresponded to the very low transmittance of its counterpart, with 10 times the concentration. According to the results shown in Figure 2B, we estimated the pK_a value of the PCL-b-pSMA at 7.0, because the PCL-b-pSMA micelles presented 50% transmittance at that pH value.

Furthermore, we observed the PCL-b-pSMA micelles under a physiological and neutral pH value directly by transmission electron microscopy (TEM), as shown in Figure 3A,B. By the negative staining of phosphotungstic acid, many bright spheres could easily be observed, which represented the inner core of the PCL-*b*-pSMA micelles. Apparently, the PCL-*b*-pSMA micelles in the buffer with a physiological pH value displayed high colloidal stability, because their inner cores (bright spheres) could be separated from each other by a hydrophilic shell composed of pSMA. On the contrary, in the neutral buffer (pH ≈ 7.05), the PCL-*b*-pSMA micelles did not display a larger inner core, but also collected together spontaneously, as shown in Figure 3B, indicating that the colloidal stability of the PCL-*b*-pSMA micelles was broken.

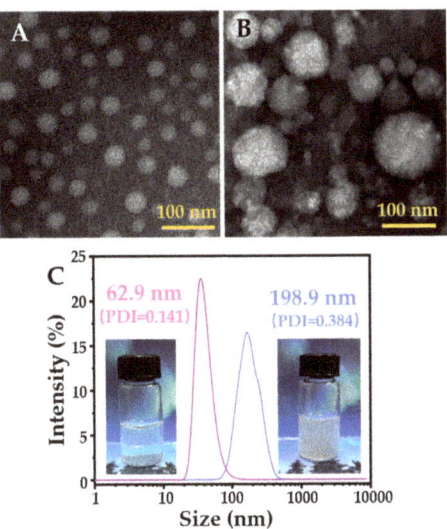

Figure 3. Morphologies (TEM) and particle size distributions (DLS) of PCL-*b*-pSMA micelles in the aqueous phase (0.3 mg mL^{-1}) with different pH values: (**A**) TEM result of PCL-*b*-pSMA micelles in the buffer with a physiological pH value (pH = 7.43); (**B**) TEM result of PCL-*b*-pSMA micelles in neutral buffer (pH = 7.05); (**C**) DLS results of the samples in (**A**,**B**).

Based on the TEM results, we investigated these TEM samples again by digital photos and DLS again; all are shown in Figure 3C. It was clear that the PCL-*b*-pSMA micelles in neutral solution looked similar to a milk solution; meanwhile, its counterpart in the physiological buffer with the same concentration showed excellent transmittance. Corresponding to these photos, the PCL-*b*-pSMA micelles in the physiological buffer in the neutral solution presented a smaller diameter (62.9 nm) and a narrower particle size distribution (PDI = 0.141) than their counterparts in the neutral solution, which explains the high transmittance of the former and the low transmittance of the latter.

Due to the fact of the results of the transmittance, DLS, TEM and digital photos, we prepared an anionic pH-responsive amphiphilic copolymer with a pK_a of approximately 7.0, which should be suitable for the preparation of a tumor microenvironment-responsive MNF.

2.2. Characterization of the Tumor Microenvironment-Responsive MNF

In order to prepare the tumor microenvironment-responsive MNF, we firstly synthesized hydrophobic Fe$_3$O$_4$ nanoparticles at approximately 8 nm. After, the MNF was prepared by the simple self-assembly between the amphiphilic PCL-*b*-pSMA and hydrophobic Fe$_3$O$_4$ nanoparticles. It was clear that the Fe$_3$O$_4$ nanoparticles in hexane (0.1 mg mL^{-1}) presented monodispersity with a uniform particle size, as shown in Figure 4A, due to the fact of their high hydrophobicity. In order to improve the water dispersibility of the hydrophobic Fe$_3$O$_4$ nanoparticles, the polymeric micelles provided a powerful platform to load the hydrophobic molecules into their hydrophobic cores. Therefore, we prepared the MNF by the self-assembly of the hydrophobic Fe$_3$O$_4$ nanoparticles and the amphiphilic

PCL-b-pSMA, with a corresponding weight ratio of 3/7. The obtained pH-responsive MNF could be dispersed in an alkaline buffer (pH ≈ 9.0) directly. We further observed the morphology of the MNF at a certain concentration (0.5 mg mL^{-1}), which is shown in Figure 4B. Apparently, in the aqueous phase, the hydrophobic Fe_3O_4 nanoparticles formed round packed clusters unlike the monodispersed nanoparticles in hexane (Figure 4A), which confirmed the successful fabrication of micellar MNF by encapsulation of the PCL-b-pSMA.

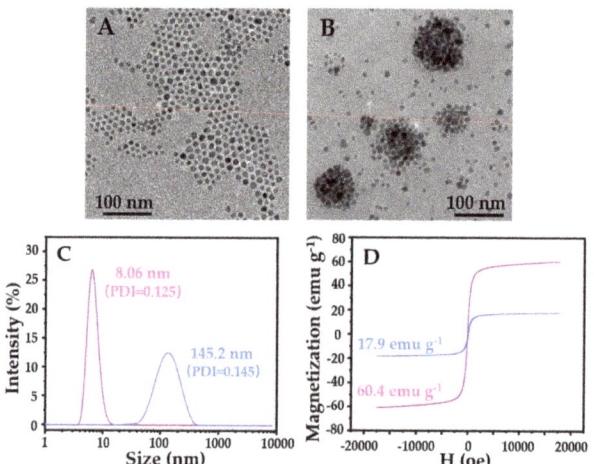

Figure 4. Characterization of the Fe_3O_4 nanoparticles and MNF, including the morphologies (TEM), particle size distributions (DLS) and magnetic properties (magnetic hysteresis loops): (A) TEM result of the hydrophobic Fe_3O_4 nanoparticles in hexane (0.1 mg mL^{-1}); (B) TEM result of the MNFs in alkaline buffer (pH ≈ 9.0, 0.5 mg mL^{-1}); (C) DLS results of the samples in (A,B); (D) magnetic properties of the desiccative Fe_3O_4 nanoparticles (60.4 emu g^{-1}) and MNF (17.9 emu g^{-1}).

In addition to TEM, we also used DLS to characterize the diameters of the Fe_3O_4 nanoparticles and MNF, as shown in Figure 4C. Apparently, the DLS result confirmed the Fe_3O_4 nanoparticles with a uniform particle size of approximately 8 nm, again, because of their low particle size distribution (PDI = 0.125). In addition, the DLS result also confirmed that the MNF possessed a larger particle size (145.2 nm) and a wider particle size distribution (PDI = 0.145) than those of the Fe_3O_4 nanoparticles, which corresponded to the TEM results in Figure 4A,B. Furthermore, the magnetic hysteresis curves of the Fe_3O_4 nanoparticles and MNF were characterized, as shown in Figure 4D. The Fe_3O_4 nanoparticles presented obvious superparamagnetism, corresponding to their diameters at approximately 8 nm. Consequently, the MNF also showed superparamagnetism without significant remanent magnetization. Meanwhile, the Fe_3O_4 nanoparticles exhibited a high saturation magnetism (M_s = 60.4 emu g^{-1}); on the contrary, the MNF showed a relatively low high saturation magnetism (M_s = 17.9 emu g^{-1}). To understand the phenomenon, we measured the Fe_3O_4 content in the MNF by thermogravimetric analysis (TGA). As shown in Figure S4, the content of the Fe_3O_4 nanoparticles was 29.3 wt%, which was close to its feed ration. Therefore, it was reasonable that the saturation magnetism of the MNF was 30% of that of the Fe_3O_4 nanoparticles. According to these results, the MNF was prepared successfully by loading the hydrophobic Fe_3O_4 nanoparticles into the inner core of the polymeric micelles.

In order to verify the pH responsiveness of the MNF, we also studied the macroscopic states and microscopic morphologies of the MNF in different buffers with the same concentration (0.5 mg mL^{-1}), as shown in Figure 5.

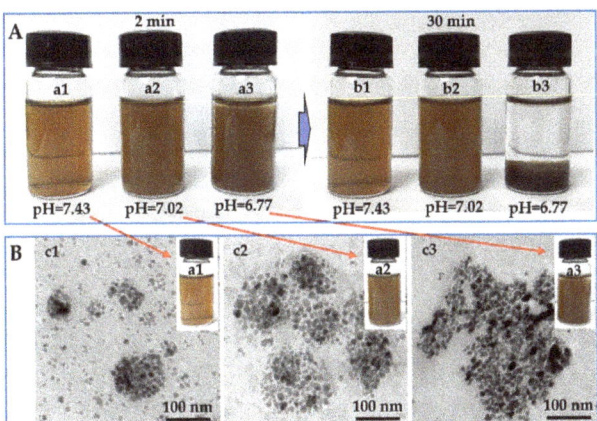

Figure 5. The macroscopic states (digital photo) and microscopic morphologies (TEM) of the tumor microenvironment-responsive MNF in different buffers (0.5 mg mL^{-1}): (**A**) digital photos of the MNF for 2 and 30 min; (**B**) TEM results of the MNF for 2 min.

Corresponding to a pK_a value of the PCL-b-pSMA, the MNF could disperse very well in the aqueous phase with a physiological pH value (pH ≈ 7.43), forming a transparent brown liquid in the macroscopic state. Furthermore, we assessed the long-term stability of the MNF (1~13 d) under a physiological pH value (≈7.43), as shown in Figure S5, which confirmed its high colloidal stability under physiological conditions. At the same time, the MNF solution with a neutral pH value (pH ≈ 7.02) became a dark-brown liquid at the macroscopic level. With the further decrease in the pH value, the MNF lost its colloidal stability in the solution with weak acidity (pH ≈ 6.77), as shown in Figure 5A; many sediments could be observed after adjusting the pH to 6.77 for 2 min. With the prolonged observation time of 30 min, in physiological and neutral conditions, the MNF maintained its original states; however, the MNF in a weak acidic environment dropped completely to the bottom of the container. In addition to the differences at the macroscopic level, the MNF solutions with corresponding pH values for 2 min also showed quite different microscopic morphologies, as shown in Figure 5B. The MNF in the aqueous phase with pH = 7.43 exhibited a similar morphology as the TEM result in Figure 4B, indicating its colloidal stability under the physiological conditions again. However, in a neutral environment, several micellar MNF formed a large Fe_3O_4 cluster, as shown in Figure 5B, resulting in the low transmittance of the sample. When the surrounding pH value was downregulated to weak acidity (pH ≈ 6.77), many Fe_3O_4 nanoparticles piled up chaotically, also shown in Figure 5B, because the surrounding pH value was lower than the pK_a of the PCL-b-pSMA. In addition to the macroscopic states and microscopic morphologies, we also quantified the diameters (Figure S6) and zeta potentials (Figure S7) of the MNF in solutions with corresponding pH values, which are shown in Figures S6 and S7. Apparently, in a neutral and weak acid solution, the MNF not only displayed larger diameters but also showed higher surface potentials (negative charge) compared to their counterparts in a physiological environment. According to these results, the MNF exhibited a similar pH responsiveness with a neutral pH value, which can be ascribed to the pK_a of the PCL-b-pSMA. Considering a tumor microenvironment pH value (7.1~6.7) [13], the tumor microenvironment-responsive MNF should possess a potential for targeted accumulation in a tumor stroma.

2.3. Advantages of Tumor Microenvironment-responsive MNF for Tumor Treatment and Diagnosis

Due to the high magnetic particle content, we studied the magnetocaloric effects of the MNF under different conditions, and the corresponding heating curves are shown in Figure 6A.

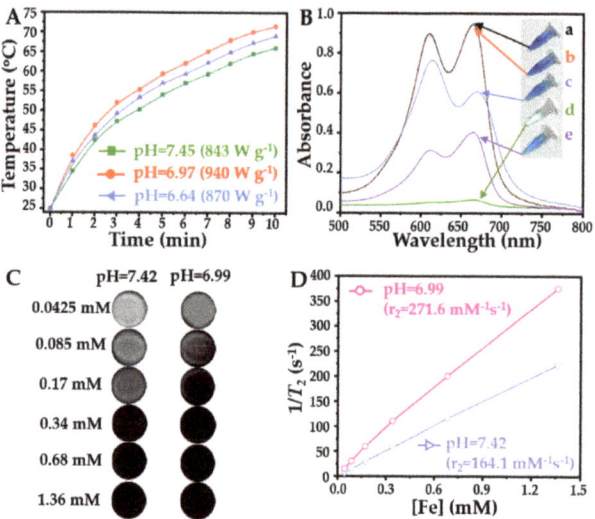

Figure 6. The effect of the tumor microenvironmental pH value on the tumor microenvironment-responsive MNF's applications, including (**A**) enhanced MH with a concentration of Fe at 100 µg mL^{-1}; (**B**) increased ROS generation with the concentration of the MNF at 250 µg mL^{-1}; (**C,D**) improved T_2 relaxivity of the MRI with varied Fe concentrations from 1.36 to 0.0425 mM.

Under the same concentration of Fe (100 µg mL^{-1}), the MNF could increase the surrounding temperature rapidly in solutions with different pH values; however, the fastest heating rate and highest heating temperature occurred in neutral conditions simultaneously. Additionally, the initial heating rate and final heating temperature of the MNF in a weak acid environment were also higher than its counterpart in physiological conditions. Therefore, the ranking of the MNF's SAR in the different buffers is neutral condition > weak acid > physiological condition, which is also shown in Figure 6A. This is an interesting phenomenon, because environmental factors of MH are rarely reported. According to the mechanism of MH, the monodispersed SPIO nanoparticles with a small diameter (≤10 nm), as used in this study, induced a magnetocaloric effect under AMF mostly by Néel relaxation, which is associated with magnetic moment [4]. Therefore, many previous studies have focused on material factors for enhancement of the magnetic moment of SPIO, including composition [30], shape [31], and structure [32]. However, in the past decade, many relevant studies also found that the micellar MNF with a large diameter exhibited high efficiency in producing thermal energy by Néel relaxation [23,33], because the effective magnetic moment of the SPIO could be improved by increasing the diameter of the magnetic nanocluster. In this study, due to the results shown in Figure 5B and Figure S6, the tumor microenvironment-responsive MNF in neutral and weak acid conditions displayed a larger diameter by the aggregation of multi-magnetic micelles, compared to its counterpart in a physiological environment. Consequently, the magnetocaloric effect of the MNF could be enhanced specifically in tumor stroma, which should benefit the application of tumor microenvironment-responsive MNF for clinical MH. However, it is worth noting that the tumor microenvironment-responsive MNF showed the highest SAR value under neutral conditions. This should be attributed to the Brownian relaxation of the MNF under AMF, because the agglomerated MNF could maintain dispersibility in the neutral solution, as shown in Figure 5, leading to their free rotation under AMF. Therefore, the tumor microenvironment-responsive MNFs could generate thermal energy efficiently in the neutral solution by integrating Brownian relaxation and Néel relaxation. On the contrary, in a weak acid environment, the MNF could not undergo Brownian motion easily, because it formed precipitates rapidly. Consequently, the MH of the MNF in the weak acid solution could be induced by Néel relaxation alone.

In addition to MH, the neutral condition could also improve the catalytic performance of the MNF to generate •OH, as shown in Figure 6B. It is well known that Fe^{2+} can decompose low toxic H_2O_2 to form high toxic •OH by FR efficiently [34,35], inducing the application of the SPIO nanoparticles for CDT in many previous studies [36]. Therefore, in this study, we evaluated the •OH-generating ability of the MNF in solutions with different pH values using methylene blue (MB) as a detection probe, since the MB could be decomposed by •OH. Obviously, H_2O_2 could not break the structure of the MB, as the UV spectrum of the MB alone (a) coincided with that of the mixture of MB and H_2O_2 (b). However, by incubating with H_2O_2 and the MNF (c~e) simultaneously, the UV absorbance of the MB declined, indicating its degradation. Moreover, the surrounding pH value influenced the degradation of the MB significantly, also shown in Figure 6B, in which a neutral environment (d) was the best condition for the catalytic performance of the tumor microenvironment-responsive MNF. This was an unexpected result, because most previous studies showed that an acidic environment (pH $\leq$ 6.0) could improve the efficiency of FR [34,37]. However, in these studies, the corresponding iron-based nanocatalysts maintained a high colloidal stability in a neutral environment, which reduced the interaction between the naked SPIO nanoparticles and H_2O_2. In our study, due to the phase transition of the PCL-b-pSMA, the interactions between H_2O_2 and the naked SPIO increased. More importantly, as shown in Figure 5, the agglomerated MNF could maintain the dispersed state in the aqueous phase for long time in a neutral environment; meanwhile, its counterpart under weak acidic conditions precipitated rapidly. This phenomenon indicated that the tumor microenvironment-responsive MNF presented a state of transition in a neutral environment, which increased the probability of an interfacial reaction between the Fe_3O_4 nanoparticles and H_2O_2 dramatically. Considering a neutral or weak acidic microenvironment of a tumor stroma, the tumor microenvironment-responsive MNF possesses a unique advantage for tumor microenvironment-responsive CDT.

The agglomerated MNF in a neutral environment not only presented an excellent catalytic performance but also enhanced the T_2 relaxivity in the MRI, which is shown in Figure 6C,D. For a given Fe concentration, the T_2 imaging of the MNF under neutral conditions (pH $\approx$ 6.99) was significantly darker than its counterpart in a physiological environment, as shown in Figure 6C. As the T_2 imaging of the MRI represented a negative signal contrast, the darker imaging MNF in neutral conditions indicated the enhancement of the T_2 imaging. Based on the results in Figure 6C, we quantified the T_2 relaxivities of the MNF under different conditions, as shown in Figure 6D. The MNF in neutral conditions possessed a steeper slope (r_2 = 271.6 mM^{-1}s^{-1}) compared to its counterpart in physiological conditions (r_2 = 164.1 mM^{-1}s^{-1}). The results of the T_2 imaging enhancement correspond to many relevant studies [22,38–40]; all of them confirmed that the T_2 relaxation rate of the MRI could be enhanced by forming SPIO clusters and increasing the diameter of these clusters. Although the MNF was a micellar cluster of SPIO nanoparticles in a physiological environment, as shown in Figure 5, the particle size of the SPIO clusters could be increased further in neutral conditions. Therefore, the T_2 imaging of the MNF could be enhanced by a neutral environment, indicating its application for tumor detection by MRI.

2.4. MH-Induced Apoptosis and Intracellular •OH Generation In Vitro

As it is hard to distinguish the pH value of a physiological condition (pH $\approx$ 7.35–7.45) and a neutral condition (pH $\approx$ 7.0) by RPMI-1640 medium, the effect of the pH value was not considered in the cell experiment.

The Cytotoxicity experiments were studied using 4T1. Firstly, we assessed the biocompatibilities of the pH-responsive micelles and MNF, as shown in Figure 7A. It was clear that under a physiological condition (pH ≈ 7.35–7.45), the pH-responsive micelles displayed biocompatibility, as its cell survival rates at all concentrations (0.025–1 mg mL^{-1}) ranged from 100% to 90%. Compared to the pH-responsive micelles, the pH-responsive MNF showed a higher cell survival rate under same the concentration, also shown in Figure 7A, indicating the excellent biocompatibility of the MNF under physiological conditions.

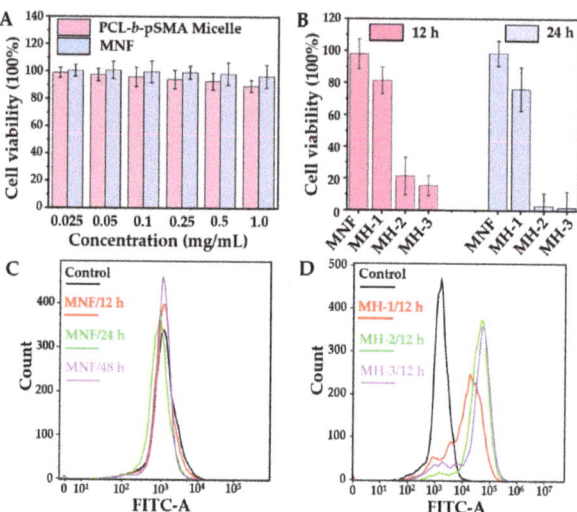

Figure 7. Cellular experiments on the biological effect of the MNF and MH, including the (**A**) biocompatibility of the PCL-*b*-pSMA micelles and MNF; (**B**) MH-induced cell death; intercellular ROS generation by (**C**) MNF (**D**) and MH.

Apparently, the MNF showed excellent biocompatibility; however, the MNF-based MH could also inhibit cell proliferation efficiently, as shown in Figure 7B. For these studies, the concentration of the MNF was fixed at 0.2 mg mL^{-1}. After incubation with the MNF alone for 12 and 24 h, the 4T1 still displayed a high cell viability, which was similar as the result in Figure 7A. Nevertheless, after exposure to AMF with different $H_{applied}$ for 10 min, the cell viabilities decreased obviously. Moreover, the inhibition rate of the 4T1's proliferation under AMF exhibited a $H_{applied}$-dependent tendency. When the $H_{applied}$ of the AMF was fixed at 21.2 kA m^{-1}, 4T1's viabilities decreased to 81.2% at 12 h and 76% at 24 h after MH for 10 min. When the $H_{applied}$ of the AMF was increased to 31.8 kA m^{-1}, 4T1's viabilities were suppressed exponentially, which was 21.4% for 12 h and 2.8% for 24 h. Therefore, the survival of the 4T1 under the AMF with the highest $H_{applied}$ (42.4 kA m^{-1}) decreased to 1.7% at 24 h after MH. To determine the relationship between the $H_{applied}$ of the MH and the cell survival rate, we recorded the heating curves of the MNF under AMF with the same condition as described in the cell experiment, and the results are shown in Figure S8. Apparently, under the AMF with the given $H_{applied}$ in this study, MH could not induce a sufficient temperature (>45 °C) to suppress cell death efficiently. Therefore, we evaluated the intercellular ROS level, another possible mechanism related to cell death, after different treatments.

As 2′,7′-dichlorodihydrofluorescin diacetate (DCFH-DA) can be metabolized within the cell by intercellular ROS, forming a fluorescent compound, 2′,7′-dichlorofluorescein (DCF), flow cytometry was utilized to quantify the intercellular ROS level by detecting the fluorescent intensity of the DCF. In order to correspond to the cytotoxicity of the MNF for different culture times, we studied the intercellular ROS level after incubating with MNFs for 12, 24 and 48 h. The result confirmed the excellent biocompatibility of the MNF, again, as shown in Figure 7C. The fluorescent intensities of the DCF for all predetermined times overlapped with that of 4T1 under standard culture conditions for

48 h. Although the MNF showed a high biocompatibility, MNF-mediated MH could boost the intercellular ROS level, as shown in Figure 7D. Further, the intercellular ROS level under MH presented a similar trend as that of its counterpart for the cell inhibition rate. For the group of MH-1, the low $H_{applied}$ (21.2 kA m^{-1}) limited the increase in the DCF fluorescent intensity, resulting in a high cell viability, as shown in the biocompatibility for the MNF. For the groups of MH-2 (31.8 kA m^{-1}) and MH-3 (42.2 kA m^{-1}), they showed similar intercellular ROS levels, corresponding to their cell mortality rate efficiencies on inhibiting 4T1 proliferation. Therefore, the SPIO biocompatibility did not conflict with the SPIO-mediated CDT. The occurrence of CDT should be triggered by a certain stimulation, such as MH [41], photothermal treatment [42], photodynamic therapy [43], and tumor microenvironment [44]. On the basis of the pH responsiveness under neutral conditions, the MNF possessed many advantages for tumor microenvironment-enhanced MH, catalytic activity and MRI. This novel MNF should be a competitive candidate for tumor diagnosis and treatment.

3. Materials and Methods

3.1. Materials

The Sn(Oct)$_2$ (92.5–100%), 4,4′-Azobis(4-cyanovaleric acid) (V501, 98%), 1,2-hexadecanediol (97%) and Oleylamine (>70%) were purchased from Sigma Aldrich (Steinheim, Germany). ε-Caprolactone (ε-CL, 99%), N,N′-dicyclohexylcarbodiimide (DCC, 98%), 4-dimethylaminopyridine (DMAP, 99%) and sulfadimethoxine (SM, 98%) were purchased from Tokyo Chemical Industry (TCI, Tokyo, Japan). Iron(III) acetylacetonate [Fe(acac)$_3$], benzyl ether (99%) and oleic acid (90%) were purchased from Alfa-Aesar (Heysham, England). Benzyl alcohol (BaOH, 99%, safe dry), acryloyl chloride (98%), tetrahydrofuran (THF, 99%) and MB (95%) were purchased from Admas (Shanghai, China). The dialysis tubing (8000–14,000 Da), dichloromethane (DCM, 99.9%), dioxane (99%), ethyl ether (99.5%), methanol (99.5%) and H$_2$O$_2$ (30%) were purchased from Sinopharm Chemical Reagent Co., Ltd. (Shanghai, China). 3-(4,5-Dimethyl-thiazol-2-yl)-2,5-diphenyl tetrazoliumbromide (MTT) was purchased from Beyotime Biotech. Co., Ltd. (Shanghai, China).

The SMA was synthesized by the procedure described in the relevant literature [45]. The DDMAT was synthesized according to [27], and the monodisperse superparamagnetic Fe$_3$O$_4$ nanoparticles were synthesized according to [46], with minor modifications. The typical synthetic procedure is described as follows: A certain amount of Fe(acac)$_3$, 1,2-hexadecanediol, oleic acid and oleylamine with molar numbers of 2, 10, 2 and 2 mmol were dispersed successively in benzyl ether (20 mL). After deoxidizing by argon at 50 °C for 30 min, the mixture was heated to 200 °C for 2 h under an argon atmosphere and then heated further to reflux (≈300 °C) for two and a half hours. The product, monodispersed Fe$_3$O$_4$ nanoparticles, was precipitated by excess ethanol and then collected by centrifugation. The purified process was repeated three times. The purified Fe$_3$O$_4$ nanoparticles were dried by a high-purity argon flow. Finally, the magnetic nanoparticles were dispersed in THF with a concentration of 10 mg mL^{-1} for storage under −20 °C.

The other reagents were used as received. The water used in all experiments was deionized with a Millipore Milli-Q system (Billerica, USA).

3.2. Synthesis of the pH-Responsive Amphiphilic Copolymer

The pH-responsive amphiphilic copolymer, PCL-b-pSMA, was synthesized by the reaction procedure, as shown in Figure S1, which was described as follows.

In the first step, the PCL was synthesized by ROP using BaOH as an initiator and ε-CL as monomers with a corresponding molar ratio of 1:50. The reaction was heated to 110 °C under an argon (Ar$_2$) atmosphere for 24 h. The product, PCL, was purified by precipitating in excess ethyl ether three times from its DCM solution. Finally, the PCL was dried until reaching a constant weight in a vacuum oven at an ambient temperature.

The second reaction was to prepare the macro-CTA, PCL-DDMAT, by esterification between the PCL and DDMAT, according to the established method [25]. In the reaction, a certain amount of PCL, DDMAT, DCC and DMAP with a corresponding molar ratio of 1:5:5:1 was weighted accurately and dissolved in anhydrous DCM by magnetic stirring. The esterification was carried out under an Ar_2 atmosphere for 48 h. To purify the PCL-DDMAT, the supernatant of the reaction was collected and successively precipitated in excess cold ethyl ether. The process for the purification was repeated several times until the supernatant was without any DDMAT. Finally, the purified PCL-DDMAT was dried in a vacuum oven at an ambient temperature and preserved in Ar_2 under a low temperature (−20 °C).

The third reaction was the synthesis of the PCL-b-pSMA by a RAFT reaction. In the reaction, the PCL-DDMAT (0.02 mmol, 110 mg), SMA (2 mmol, 728 mg) and V501 (0.004 mmol, 1.1 mg) were dissolved in dioxane of 5 mL under magnetic stirring. Then, the mixture was thoroughly degassed by three freeze–pump–thaw cycles. The reaction was carried out at 70 °C for 10 h. The final product, PCL-b-pSMA, was purified by repeated precipitation in excess methanol, followed by freeze-dried treatment and also preserved in Ar_2 under a low temperature (−20 °C).

3.3. Characterization of the pH-Responsive Amphiphilic Copolymer

All products were characterized by their ^{1}H NMR spectrum, with $CDCl_3$ or DMSO-d_6 as the solvent, and their chemical shifts relative to tetramethylsilane (TMS) were identified. In order to identify the pH responsiveness of the PCL-b-pSMA, we prepared micelles of the PCL-b-pSMA first, where the THF solution of the PCL-b-pSMA (20 mg mL^{-1}) was dialyzed against an alkaline solution (pH = 9.13) for 48 h. After, the obtained micelle solution of the PCL-b-pSMA with a high concentration (>3 mg mL^{-1}) downregulated its pH value by the gradual addition of a small amount of hydrochloric acid solution (1 M). By using a UV-Vis spectrophotometer (Shimadzu, UV2600, Tokyo, Japan), we recorded its light transmittance at different pH values (9.13~5.18). The pK_a value of the PCL-b-pSMA was defined as the surrounding pH value, producing a 50% decrease in the optical transmittance at 500 nm [29]. At the same time, the pK_a value of the PCL-b-pSMA was also identified by DLS (Malvern, Nano ZS90, Worcestershire, UK), which measured the size distribution of the dilute PCL-b-pSMA micelles (0.3 mg mL^{-1}) with varied surrounding pH values. Moreover, the morphologies of the PCL-b-pSMA micelles at pH values under physiological and neutral conditions were observed directly by TEM (Hitachi, HT-7800, Tokyo, Japan), in which the samples were stained by phosphotungstic acid (2%).

3.4. Preparation of the Tumor Microenvironment-responsive MNF

The tumor microenvironment-responsive MNF was prepared by ultrasound-assisted self-assembly. In a typical procedure, the PCL-b-pSMA (210 mg) and Fe_3O_4 (90 mg) were dissolved in THF (10 mL) completely by oscillation. The mixed solution was then slowly added into an excess alkaline solution (pH ≈ 9, 50 mL) under sonication, followed by dialyzing against the same alkaline solution for 48 h. The dialysis solution was purified by centrifugation (2000 RPM, 10 min), and the supernatant was collected. Finally, the tumor microenvironment-responsive MNF was purified from the supernatant by high-speed centrifugation (100,000× g, 20 min). The obtained sediment was collected by lyophilization and stored at 4 °C.

3.5. Physicochemical Properties of the Tumor Microenvironment-responsive MNF

First, the morphologies of the Fe_3O_4 nanoparticles and MNF were characterized by TEM (Hitachi, HT-7800, Tokyo, Japan) directly, in which the MNF was dispersed into an alkaline solution (pH ≈ 9). Their particle sizes were measured by DLS (Malvern, Nano ZS90, Worcestershire, UK) under an ambient condition. In order to confirm the pH responsiveness of the MNF, we dissolved the MNF into an alkaline solution (pH ≈ 9) and downregulated the surrounding pH value to physiological (pH ≈ 7.43), neutral (pH ≈ 7.02) and weak acidic (pH ≈ 6.67) conditions. Then, we studied their colloidal stability by qualitative observation (digital imaging and TEM) and quantitative analysis (DLS). In addition, the zeta potentials of the MNF in the corresponding buffers (pH ≈ 7.43, pH ≈ 7.02 and pH ≈ 6.67) were characterized simultaneously by DLS. The long colloidal stability of the MNF was also assessed by DLS from 1 to 13 d. The content of the Fe_3O_4 in the tumor microenvironment-responsive MNF was measured by TGA (NETZSCH STA 449 F3, Weimar, Germany).

3.6. Enhancements of the MNF for MH, FR and MRI under a Neutral Condition

In order to determine the magnetocaloric effect of the MNF, the concentration of Fe ([Fe]) was fixed at 100 μg mL^{-1}, which was identified by an inductively coupled plasma mass spectrometer (ICP-MS, Thermo scientific, Xseries II, Waltham, USA). Then, the heating curves of the MNF under physiological (pH ≈ 7.45), neutral (pH ≈ 6.97) and weak acidic (pH ≈ 6.64) conditions were plotted. In this study, an AMF generator (SPG-20AB, ShuangPing Tech. Ltd., Shenzhen, China) with the corresponding frequency (f, 114 kHz) and strength ($H_{applied}$, 89.9 kA m^{-1}) was employed. The inner diameter of the heating coil was 28 mm. The increasing temperature was recorded by a computer-attached fiber optic temperature sensor (FISO, FOT-M, Québec, Canada). Finally, the SAR was calculated by the formula described in a relative study [23].

In addition to the MH, the catalytic potential of MNF under physiological (pH ≈ 7.45), neutral (pH ≈ 6.97) and weak acidic (pH ≈ 6.64) conditions was also studied by detecting the generation of •OH. As the •OH can induce the degradation of MB [47], the study was divided into five groups: MB, MB + H_2O_2, MB + H_2O_2 + MNF (pH = 7.45), MB + H_2O_2 + MNF (pH = 6.97) and MB + H_2O_2 + MNF (pH ≈ 6.64). In this study, the concentrations of MB, H_2O_2 and MNF were 50 μg mL^{-1}, 1 mM and 250 μg mL^{-1}. Then, the degradation of MB was observed using digital imaging and monitored using a UV-Vis spectrophotometer (Shimadzu, UV2600, Tokyo, Japan) 2 h later.

The MRI studies were performed with a 3.0-T clinic MRI imaging system (Siemens Trio 3T MRI Scanner, Erlangen, Germany), which was equipped by a micro coil for the transmission and reception of the signal. After dissolving the MNF in an alkaline solution (pH ≈ 8.45), the concentrations of Fe ([Fe]) were identified by ICP-MS first. Then, the study was divided into two groups: physiological condition (pH ≈ 7.42) and neutral condition (pH ≈ 6.99). All groups possessed identifiable [Fe] from 1360 to 42.5 μM.

For the T_2-weighted images, two groups with a series of [Fe] gradients were scanned under these conditions, listed as the following: TR = 5000 ms, TE = 10–90 ms, slice thickness = 3 mm and flip angle = 150°.

3.7. Cellular Studies on MH and MH-Induced ROS Generation

In this study, we used a mouse-derived breast cancer cell line, 4T1, purchased from the Chinese Academy of Sciences (Shanghai, China). The 4T1 was cultured using RPMI-1640 medium (Hyclone) containing 10% fetal bovine serum (FBS, every green, Hangzhou, China) and then placed in an incubator at 37 °C with 5% CO_2 and humidified conditions. The cytotoxicity in vitro was performed by the standard MTT assay. In the research, the biocompatibilities of the PCL-b-pSMA and MNF with varied concentrations from 0.25–1 mg mL^{-1} under physiological conditions for 48 h were studied.

To evaluate the efficiency of the MH in vitro, the MNF was dissolved in RPMI-1640 medium (containing 10% FBS and 1% penicillin–streptomycin) at a concentration of 0.2 mg mL^{-1}. Considering the effect of $H_{applied}$ on the MH, the study was divided into three group, MH-1, MH-2 and MH-3, which were operated under the corresponding $H_{applied}$ as 21.2, 31.8 and 42.4 kA m^{-1}, respectively. The 4T1 was incubated in a culture dish (35 mm) at a density of 4 × 10^5 cells per dish in 2 mL of corresponding medium. After incubating for 24 h, the culture medium was replaced by the corresponding medium containing MNF (0.2 mg mL^{-1}). Then, the 4T1 was placed in a heating coil with an inner diameter of approximately 38 mm. The applied AMF possessed a constant frequency (f = 114 kHz) and varied $H_{applied}$ (21.2, 31.8 and 42.4 kA m^{-1}). The exposure time under AMF was fixed at 10 min. After MH, the cells were cultured for a prolonged 12 or 24 h.

Finally, the cell viabilities were quantified by MTT. After the cell experiment, the heating curves of the MNF (dissolved in RPMI-1640 medium) were recorded in a culture dish (35 mm) under AMF with the same conditions as described for the MH study.

For detecting the ROS generation, DCFH-DA was used following the instructions of the ROS Assay Kit (Beyotime Biotech. Co., Ltd., Shanghai, China). Prior to treatment of the DCFH-DA, 4T1 was incubated in a culture dish (35 mm) at a density of 2×10^5 cells per dish in 2 mL of corresponding medium. Then, the 4T1 was treated by the MNF (0.2 mg mL^{-1}) alone for different culture times (12, 24 and 48 h) or MH for 12 h under the established conditions, as described in the MH study. After pretreatment, the culture medium of the 4T1 was replaced by serum-free medium containing DCFH-DA (10 μM) for 40 min. Finally, 4T1 was collected and analyzed by flow cytometry.

4. Conclusions

We successfully prepared tumor microenvironment-responsive MNFs by the self-assembly of pH-responsive PCL-*b*-pSMA and superparamagnetic hydrophobic Fe_3O_4 nanoparticles for targeted tumor theranostics. As the PCL-*b*-pSMA possessed a pK_a within a pH range of the tumor microenvironment, the MNF exhibited a great potential for tumor targeting, by maintaining a high colloidal stability in a physiological environment for a long time, forming large, agglomerated clusters in the tumor microenvironment rapidly. Because the tumor microenvironment-responsive MNF showed larger agglomerated clusters in a tumor microenvironment, the close-packed multiple SPIOs with a larger diameter exhibited better performance in reducing the T_2 and increasing SAR simultaneously. Meanwhile, due to the agglomeration of the MNF in the tumor tissue, the encapsulated Fe_3O_4 nanoparticles could be exposed from the inner core of the micellar MNF, which induced efficient ER by the interaction between Fe^{2+} and endogenous H_2O_2. The further cell experiments confirmed that the tumor microenvironment-responsive MNF displayed excellent biocompatibility, corresponding to its high stability in a physiological environment. However, after applying AMF, the tumor microenvironment-responsive MNF exhibited high efficiency in inhibiting cell proliferation, because of the MH-induced CDT. According to these results, the tumor microenvironment-responsive MNF not only showed high safety in medical areas but also showed itself as a powerful tool to enhance tumor contrast by MRI and improve tumor treatment by combing MH and CDT specifically.

Supplementary Materials: The following supporting information can be downloaded at: https://www.mdpi.com/article/10.3390/ph16020166/s1, Figure S1: Synthetic scheme of PCL-*b*-pSMA; Figure S2: ^{1}H NMR spectrum of PCL; Figure S3: ^{1}H NMR spectrum of PCL-DDMAT; Figure S4: Content of Fe_3O_4 in the tumor microenvironment-responsive MNF; Figure S5: Time-dependent hydrodynamic diameters of the tumor microenvironment-responsive MNF in physiological conditions; Figure S6: Particle sizes of the tumor microenvironment-responsive MNF in solutions with different pH values; Figure S7: Zeta potentials of the tumor microenvironment-responsive MNF in solutions with different pH values; Figure S8: Time-dependent temperature curves of the tumor microenvironment-responsive MNs under AMF with different $H_{applied}$.

Author Contributions: Conceptualization, Y.L.; methodology, Y.X.; software, Y.Y.; validation, M.S.; formal analysis, Y.L. and Y.X.; investigation, L.S. and X.Z.; resources, Y.L. and Y.X.; data curation, Z.L. and M.S.; writing—original draft preparation, L.S. and X.Z.; writing—review and editing, Y.L. and Y.X.; supervision, Y.L. and Y.X. All authors have read and agreed to the published version of the manuscript.

Funding: This research was funded by the National Natural Science Foundation of China, grant numbers: 81871343 and 51703086; China Postdoctoral Science Foundation, grant number: 2019M651730; Nature Science Foundation of Jiangsu Province, grant number: BK 20160496; Key Research and Development Project of Jiangsu Province, grant number: BE2021693; Postdoctoral Science Foundation of Jiangsu Province, grant number: 2018K057C.

Institutional Review Board Statement: Not applicable.

Informed Consent Statement: Not applicable.

Data Availability Statement: Data is contained within the article and supplementary material.

Acknowledgments: The authors would like to thank Mengji Rui, who donated the 4T1 cell line.

Conflicts of Interest: The authors declare no conflict of interest.

References

1. Qu, Y.; Wang, Z.; Sun, M.; Zhao, T.; Zhu, X.; Deng, X.; Zhang, M.; Xu, Y.; Liu, H. A Theranostic Nanocomplex Combining with Magnetic Hyperthermia for Enhanced Accumulation and Efficacy of pH-Triggering Polymeric Cisplatin (IV) Prodrugs. *Pharmaceuticals* **2022**, *15*, 480. [CrossRef] [PubMed]
2. Yallapu, M.M.; Othman, S.F.; Curtis, E.T.; Gupta, B.K.; Jaggi, M.; Chauhan, S.C. Multi-functional magnetic nanoparticles for magnetic resonance imaging and cancer therapy. *Biomaterials* **2011**, *32*, 1890–1905. [CrossRef] [PubMed]
3. Zhou, Z.; Yang, L.; Gao, J.; Chen, X. Structure-Relaxivity Relationships of Magnetic Nanoparticles for Magnetic Resonance Imaging. *Adv. Mater.* **2019**, *31*, 1804567. [CrossRef]
4. Rosensweig, R.E. Heating magnetic fluid with alternating magnetic field. *J. Magn. Magn. Mater.* **2002**, *252*, 370–374. [CrossRef]
5. Nuñez, M.T.; Chana-Cuevas, P. New Perspectives in Iron Chelation Therapy for the Treatment of Neurodegenerative Diseases. *Pharmaceuticals* **2018**, *11*, 109. [CrossRef]
6. Belleperche, M.; DeRosa, M.C. pH-Control in Aptamer-Based Diagnostics, Therapeutics, and Analytical Applications. *Pharmaceuticals* **2018**, *11*, 80. [CrossRef] [PubMed]
7. Castelli, R.; Ibarra, M.; Faccio, R.; Miraballes, I.; Fernández, M.; Moglioni, A.; Cabral, P.; Cerecetto, H.; Glisoni, R.J.; Calzada, V. T908 Polymeric Micelles Improved the Uptake of Sgc8-c Aptamer Probe in Tumor-Bearing Mice: A Co-Association Study between the Probe and Preformed Nanostructures. *Pharmaceuticals* **2021**, *15*, 15. [CrossRef] [PubMed]
8. Shi, J.; Kantoff, P.W.; Wooster, R.; Farokhzad, O.C. Cancer nanomedicine: Progress, challenges and opportunities. *Nat. Rev. Cancer* **2017**, *17*, 20–37. [CrossRef] [PubMed]
9. Kamaly, N.; Yameen, B.; Wu, J.; Farokhzad, O.C. Degradable Controlled-Release Polymers and Polymeric Nanoparticles: Mechanisms of Controlling Drug Release. *Chem. Rev.* **2016**, *116*, 2602–2663. [CrossRef]
10. Xu, X.; Wu, J.; Liu, Y.; Yu, M.; Zhao, L.; Zhu, X.; Bhasin, S.; Li, Q.; Ha, E.; Shi, J.; et al. Ultra-pH-Responsive and Tumor-Penetrating Nanoplatform for Targeted siRNA Delivery with Robust Anti-Cancer Efficacy. *Angew. Chem. Int. Ed.* **2016**, *55*, 7091–7094. [CrossRef]
11. Kanamala, M.; Wilson, W.R.; Yang, M.; Palmer, B.D.; Wu, Z. Mechanisms and biomaterials in pH-responsive tumour targeted drug delivery: A review. *Biomaterials* **2016**, *85*, 152–167. [CrossRef] [PubMed]
12. Wang, Z.; Deng, X.; Ding, J.; Zhou, W.; Zheng, X.; Tang, G. Mechanisms of drug release in pH-sensitive micelles for tumour targeted drug delivery system: A review. *Int. J. Pharmaceut.* **2017**, *535*, 253–260. [CrossRef] [PubMed]
13. Webb, B.A.; Chimenti, M.; Jacobson, M.P.; Barber, D.L. Dysregulated pH: A perfect storm for cancer progression. *Nat. Rev. Cancer* **2011**, *11*, 671–677. [CrossRef] [PubMed]
14. Larroque-Lombard, A.L.; Chatelut, E.; Delord, J.P.; Imbs, D.C.; Rochaix, P.; Jean-Claude, B.; Allal, B. Design and Mechanism of Action of a New Prototype of Combi-Molecule "Programed" to Release Bioactive Species at a pH Range Akin to That of the Tumor Microenvironment. *Pharmaceuticals* **2021**, *14*, 160. [CrossRef]
15. Ma, X.; Wang, Y.; Zhao, T.; Li, Y.; Su, L.C.; Wang, Z.; Huang, G.; Sumer, B.D.; Gao, J. Ultra-pH-sensitive nanoprobe library with broad pH tunability and fluorescence emissions. *J. Am. Chem. Soc.* **2014**, *136*, 11085–11092. [CrossRef]
16. Bersani, S.; Vila-Caballer, M.; Brazzale, C.; Barattin, M.; Salmaso, S. pH-sensitive stearoyl-PEG-poly (methacryloyl sulfadimethoxine) decorated liposomes for the delivery of gemcitabine to cancer cells. *Eur. J. Pharm. Biopharm.* **2014**, *88*, 670–682. [CrossRef]
17. Sethuraman, V.A.; Lee, M.C.; Bae, Y.H. A biodegradable pH-sensitive micelle system for targeting acidic solid tumors. *Pharm. Res.* **2008**, *25*, 657–666. [CrossRef]
18. Gao, G.H.; Im, G.H.; Kim, M.S.; Lee, J.W.; Yang, J.; Jeon, H.; Lee, J.H.; Lee, D.S. Magnetite-nanoparticle-encapsulated pH-responsive polymeric micelle as an MRI probe for detecting acidic pathologic areas. *Small* **2010**, *6*, 1201–1204. [CrossRef]
19. Wang, Y.; Zhou, K.; Huang, G.; Hensley, C.; Huang, X.; Ma, X.; Zhao, T.; Sumer, B.D.; DeBerardinis, R.J.; Gao, J. A nanoparticle-based strategy for the imaging of a broad range of tumours by nonlinear amplification of microenvironment signals. *Nat. Mater.* **2014**, *13*, 204–212. [CrossRef]
20. Lee, E.S.; Na, K.; Bae, Y.H. Super pH-sensitive multifunctional polymeric micelle. *Nano Lett.* **2005**, *5*, 325–329. [CrossRef]
21. Lin, H.P.; Akimoto, J.; Li, Y.K.; Ito, Y. Selective Control of Cell Activity with Hydrophilic Polymer-Covered Cationic Nanoparticles. *Macromol. Biosci.* **2020**, *20*, 2000049. [CrossRef] [PubMed]
22. Lu, H.; Xu, Y.; Qiao, R.; Lu, Z.; Wang, P.; Zhang, X.; Chen, A.; Zou, L.; Wang, Z. A novel clustered SPIO nanoplatform with enhanced magnetic resonance T_2 relaxation rate for micro-tumor detection and photothermal synergistic therapy. *Nano Res.* **2020**, *13*, 2216–2225. [CrossRef]
23. Qu, Y.; Li, J.; Ren, J.; Leng, J.; Lin, C.; Shi, D. Enhanced magnetic fluid hyperthermia by micellar magnetic nanoclusters composed of Mn x Zn1−x Fe2O4 nanoparticles for induced tumor cell apoptosis. *ACS Appl. Mater. Interfaces* **2014**, *6*, 16867–16879. [CrossRef]
24. Abel, B.A.; Sims, M.B.; McCormick, C.L. Tunable pH-and CO_2-responsive sulfonamide-containing polymers by RAFT polymerization. *Macromolecules* **2015**, *48*, 5487–5495. [CrossRef]

25. Bian, Q.; Xiao, Y.; Lang, M. Thermoresponsive biotinylated star amphiphilic block copolymer: Synthesis, self-assembly, and specific target recognition. *Polymer* **2012**, *53*, 1684–1693. [CrossRef]
26. Kuo, C.Y.; Don, T.M.; Lin, Y.T.; Hsu, S.C.; Chiu, W.Y. Synthesis of pH-sensitive sulfonamide-based hydrogels with controllable crosslinking density by post thermo-curing. *J. Polym. Res.* **2019**, *26*, 18. [CrossRef]
27. Lai, J.T.; Filla, D.; Shea, R. Functional Polymers from Novel Carboxyl-Terminated Trithiocarbonates as Highly Efficient RAFT Agents. *Macromolecules* **2002**, *35*, 6754–6756. [CrossRef]
28. Kang, S.I.; Bae, Y.H. pH-induced solubility transition of sulfonamide-based polymers. *J. Control. Release* **2002**, *80*, 145–155. [CrossRef]
29. Park, S.Y.; Bae, Y.H. Novel pH-sensitive polymers containing sulfonamide groups. *Macromol. Rapid Comm.* **1999**, *20*, 269–273. [CrossRef]
30. Jang, J.t.; Nah, H.; Lee, J.H.; Moon, S.H.; Kim, M.G.; Cheon, J. Critical enhancements of MRI contrast and hyperthermic effects by dopant-controlled magnetic nanoparticles. *Angew. Chem. Int. Ed.* **2009**, *48*, 1234–1238. [CrossRef]
31. Guardia, P.; Di Corato, R.; Lartigue, L.; Wilhelm, C.; Espinosa, A.; Garcia-Hernandez, M.; Gazeau, F.; Manna, L.; Pellegrino, T. Water-Soluble Iron Oxide Nanocubes with High Values of Specific Absorption Rate for Cancer Cell Hyperthermia Treatment. *ACS Nano* **2012**, *6*, 3080–3091. [CrossRef] [PubMed]
32. Lartigue, L.; Hugounenq, P.; Alloyeau, D.; Clarke, S.P.; Levy, M.; Bacri, J.C.; Bazzi, R.; Brougham, D.F.; Wilhelm, C.; Gazeau, F. Cooperative organization in iron oxide multi-core nanoparticles potentiates their efficiency as heating mediators and MRI contrast agents. *ACS Nano* **2012**, *6*, 10935–10949. [CrossRef] [PubMed]
33. Saville, S.L.; Qi, B.; Baker, J.; Stone, R.; Camley, R.E.; Livesey, K.L.; Ye, L.; Crawford, T.M.; Mefford, O.T. The formation of linear aggregates in magnetic hyperthermia: Implications on specific absorption rate and magnetic anisotropy. *J. Colloid Interf. Sci.* **2014**, *424*, 141–151. [CrossRef] [PubMed]
34. Yang, B.; Chen, Y.; Shi, J. Reactive Oxygen Species (ROS)-Based Nanomedicine. *Chem. Rev.* **2019**, *119*, 4881–4985. [CrossRef] [PubMed]
35. Zhang, S.; Cao, C.; Lv, X.; Dai, H.; Zhong, Z.; Liang, C.; Wang, W.; Huang, W.; Song, X.; Dong, X. A H_2O_2 self-sufficient nanoplatform with domino effects for thermal-responsive enhanced chemodynamic therapy. *Chem. Sci.* **2020**, *11*, 1926–1934. [CrossRef] [PubMed]
36. Qian, X.; Zhang, J.; Gu, Z.; Chen, Y. Nanocatalysts-augmented Fenton chemical reaction for nanocatalytic tumor therapy. *Biomaterials* **2019**, *211*, 1–13. [CrossRef]
37. Xu, L.; Wang, J.; Wang, J.; Lu, S.Y.; Yang, Q.; Chen, C.; Yang, H.; Hong, F.; Wu, C.; Zhao, Q.; et al. Polypyrrole-iron phosphate-glucose oxidase-based nanocomposite with cascade catalytic capacity for tumor synergistic apoptosis-ferroptosis therapy. *Chem. Eng. J.* **2022**, *427*, 131671. [CrossRef]
38. Ai, H.; Flask, C.; Weinberg, B.; Shuai, X.-T.; Pagel, M.D.; Farrell, D.; Duerk, J.; Gao, J. Magnetite-Loaded Polymeric Micelles as Ultrasensitive Magnetic-Resonance Probes. *Adv. Mater.* **2005**, *17*, 1949–1952. [CrossRef]
39. Lu, J.; Ma, S.; Sun, J.; Xia, C.; Liu, C.; Wang, Z.; Zhao, X.; Gao, F.; Gong, Q.; Song, B.; et al. Manganese ferrite nanoparticle micellar nanocomposites as MRI contrast agent for liver imaging. *Biomaterials* **2009**, *30*, 2919–2928. [CrossRef]
40. Zhang, B.; Li, Q.; Yin, P.; Rui, Y.; Qiu, Y.; Wang, Y.; Shi, D. Ultrasound-Triggered BSA/SPION Hybrid Nanoclusters for Liver-Specific Magnetic Resonance Imaging. *ACS Appl. Mater. Interfaces* **2012**, *4*, 6479–6486. [CrossRef]
41. Zhang, Y.; Wang, X.; Chu, C.; Zhou, Z.; Chen, B.; Pang, X.; Lin, G.; Lin, H.; Guo, Y.; Ren, E.; et al. Genetically engineered magnetic nanocages for cancer magneto-catalytic theranostics. *Nat. Commun.* **2020**, *11*, 5421. [CrossRef] [PubMed]
42. Chen, F.; An, P.; Liu, L.; Gao, Z.; Li, Y.; Zhang, Y.; Sun, B.; Zhou, J. A polydopamine-gated biodegradable cascade nanoreactor for pH-triggered and photothermal-enhanced tumor-specific nanocatalytic therapy. *Nanoscale* **2021**, *13*, 15677–15688. [CrossRef] [PubMed]
43. Chen, Q.; Ma, Y.; Bai, P.; Li, Q.; Canup, B.S.B.; Long, D.; Ke, B.; Dai, F.; Xiao, B.; Li, C. Tumor Microenvironment-Responsive Nanocktails for Synergistic Enhancement of Cancer Treatment via Cascade Reactions. *ACS Appl. Mater. Interfaces* **2021**, *13*, 4861–4873. [CrossRef] [PubMed]
44. Feng, L.; Xie, R.; Wang, C.; Gai, S.; He, F.; Yang, D.; Yang, P.; Lin, J. Magnetic Targeting, Tumor Microenvironment-Responsive Intelligent Nanocatalysts for Enhanced Tumor Ablation. *ACS Nano* **2018**, *12*, 11000–11012. [CrossRef]
45. Kim, D.H.; Seo, Y.K.; Thambi, T.; Moon, G.J.; Son, J.P.; Li, G.; Park, J.H.; Lee, J.H.; Kim, H.H.; Lee, D.S.; et al. Enhancing neurogenesis and angiogenesis with target delivery of stromal cell derived factor-1α using a dual ionic pH-sensitive copolymer. *Biomaterials* **2015**, *61*, 115–125. [CrossRef]
46. Sun, S.; Zeng, H.; Robinson, D.B.; Raoux, S.; Rice, P.M.; Wang, S.X.; Li, G. Monodisperse MFe_2O_4 (M = Fe, Co, Mn) Nanoparticles. *J. Am. Chem. Soc.* **2004**, *126*, 273–279. [CrossRef]
47. Duan, H.; Guo, H.; Zhang, R.; Wang, F.; Liu, Z.; Ge, M.; Yu, L.; Lin, H.; Chen, Y. Two-dimensional silicene composite nanosheets enable exogenous/endogenous-responsive and synergistic hyperthermia-augmented catalytic tumor theranostics. *Biomaterials* **2020**, *256*, 120206. [CrossRef]

Disclaimer/Publisher's Note: The statements, opinions and data contained in all publications are solely those of the individual author(s) and contributor(s) and not of MDPI and/or the editor(s). MDPI and/or the editor(s) disclaim responsibility for any injury to people or property resulting from any ideas, methods, instructions or products referred to in the content.

Recent Development of LDL-Based Nanoparticles for Cancer Therapy

Binghong He and Qiong Yang *

Beijing Key Laboratory of Gene Resource and Molecular Development, College of Life Sciences, Beijing Normal University, Beijing 100875, China
* Correspondence: yangqiong@bnu.edu.cn

Abstract: Low-density lipoprotein (LDL), a natural lipoprotein transporting cholesterol in the circulatory system, has been a possible drug carrier for targeted delivery. LDL can bind to the LDL receptor (LDLR) with its outside apolipoprotein B-100 and then enter the cell via LDLR-mediated endocytosis. This targeting function inspires researchers to modify LDL to deliver different therapeutic drugs. Drugs can be loaded in the surficial phospholipids, hydrophobic core, or apolipoprotein for the structure of LDL. In addition, LDL-like synthetic nanoparticles carrying therapeutic drugs are also under investigation for the scarcity of natural LDL. In addition to being a carrier, LDL can also be a targeting molecule, decorated to the surface of synthetic nanoparticles loaded with cytotoxic compounds. This review summarizes the properties of LDL and the different kinds of LDL-based delivery nanoparticles, their loading strategies, and the achievements of the recent anti-tumor advancement.

Keywords: low-density lipoprotein; nanoparticle; cancer therapy

1. Introduction

In recent years, cancer has become a major public health problem worldwide, and the latest cancer statistics showed that cancer is the second leading cause of death in the United States [1]. Chemotherapy is one type of cancer treatment under investigation to improve mortality [2–4]. Although chemotherapy kills fast-growing cancer cells, the fast-growing and dividing healthy cells will also be affected [5]. Nanoparticles (NPs) carrying cytotoxic agents to cancer cells help lessen the toxicity of chemotherapy and provide a new strategy for targeted cancer therapy [6,7]. Traditional NPs are enriched in the tumor through the high permeability and retention effect (EPR effect) with their sizes, for instance, polymers, micelles, microspheres, liposomes, and so on [8–10]. Some of them have been approved by the FDA and clinical studies show that the utilization of these therapeutic particles significantly prevents the spread of liver cancer [9], gastric cancer [10] and breast cancer [11], and so on. However, most of these targeted NPs are passive NPs that would not actively target cancer cells. Active targeted NPs that can specifically target specific cancer cells with particular ligands or proteins might effectively increase the enrichment of NPs and reduce side effects [12].

Low-density lipoprotein (LDL) is one kind of nanoscale molecule that could be an actively targeted NP [13]. LDL is the cholesterol transporter in the body to deliver cholesterol to the cells expressing the LDL receptor (LDLR) [14]. LDLR is overexpressed on the hyperproliferative cells, especially cancer cells such as liver cancers, glioma cancers, and lung cancers [15–18]. LDLR would recognize the apolipoprotein B-100 (ApoB-100) on the LDL and then form the LDL-LDLR complex to start the endocytosis. ApoB-100 is the apolipoprotein on the LDL that confirms the targeting characteristic of this nanoscale molecule [19]. As an endogenous molecule, LDL would not trigger an immune response and reduce unnecessary stress for the body.

2. LDL and LDL Receptors

LDL is a spherical nanoscale molecule with a diameter of 18–25 nm [20], whose outer layer is a hydrophilic phospholipid monolayer, accompanied by ApoB-100 and free cholesterol, and the inner layer is a hydrophobic core composed of esterified cholesterol and triacylglycerol (Figure 1). The component of LDL is approximately 50% cholesterol, 25% protein, 20% phospholipids, and 5% triacylglycerol. ApoB-100 on the surface of LDL recognizes and binds to LDLR during endocytosis [21].

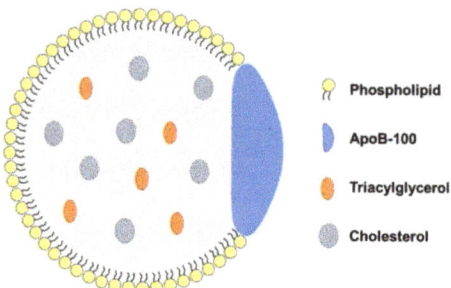

Figure 1. Schematic diagram of LDL structure. LDL is composed of phospholipid monolayers, cholesterols, triglycerides, and ApoB-100.

LDLR, a transmembrane glycoprotein consisting of 4536 amino acid residues, is one of the largest monomeric proteins [17]. LDLR is a widely expressed protein that absorbs approximately 70% of circulating LDLs via LDLR-mediated endocytosis [16]. During the endocytosis, the apoB-100 on the LDL would recognize the LDLR, and then LDL and LDLR form a complex. The complex enters the cell through the pits of the clathrin envelopes and is surrounded into a coated vesicle. Facilitated with the low pH environment of endosome and lysosome, LDL is digested to cholesterol and triglyceride while the LDLR returns to the cell membrane to restart another endocytosis [22].

LDLs, as the crucial source of exogenous cholesterol, play a crucial role in providing cholesterol for cell proliferation. LDLR is highly expressed in malignant tumors such as gastric cancer [23], liver cancer [24], breast cancer [25], and leukemia [26], indicating that the intake of LDL might accelerate oncogenic processes. Caruso et al. found that, in rapidly proliferating tumor cells, the metabolic rate of LDLR significantly accelerated [27]. Given this function, Krieger et al. combined cytotoxic drugs with LDL to form LDL-based NPs and observed more accumulation of NPs in LDLR overexpressing tumor cells [28]. The intake of LDL-based NPs is dependent on the LDLR-mediated endocytosis, and the release of drugs is facilitated with lysosome (Figure 2). The targeting function of LDL-based NPs relies on the LDLR expression level but not the EPR effect; therefore, LDL-based NPs are suitable for malignancy including leukemia and solid tumor cells.

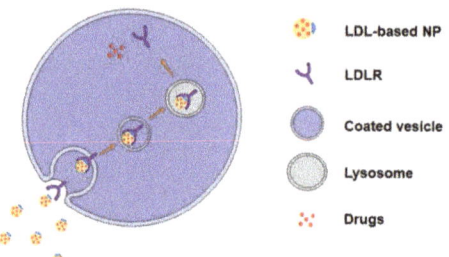

Figure 2. Schematic diagram of cellular uptake of LDL-based NPs loaded with drugs by LDLR-mediated endocytosis.

3. Categories of LDL-Based NPs

The affinity of ApoB-100 with LDLR results in the combination of LDL and LDLR, which facilitates the uptake of LDL. Thus, LDL particles containing apoB-100 can be developed as an active targeted carrier to transport therapeutic drugs. Another modification to utilize the LDL and LDLR interaction is to use the whole LDL as a wizard decorated on the surface of the NPs to target LDLR overexpressed cells. Therapeutic agents can be added to its comparatively large-load hydrophobic core, apolipoprotein, and monolayer phospholipid when LDL is used as carrier [29]. Because of the limited sources of native LDL, Nikanjam and collaborators used phosphatidylcholine, cholesterol oleic acid, ApoB-100 protein, or other synthetic peptides to develop synthesized LDL-like nanoparticles [16]. From then on, synthesized LDL-drugs nanoparticles are developed to deliver therapeutic drugs in vitro and in vivo. Here, we classify LDL-based drug-loaded particles into three types according to their source and function:

Native LDL-drug nanoparticles (nLDL-drugs) refer to nanoparticles composed of natural LDLs and cytotoxic drugs. **Synthesized LDL-drug nanoparticles (sLDL-drugs)** refer to nanoparticles that own the basic structure of LDL, coming from de novo synthesized LDL-like nanoparticles with therapeutic drugs loaded. **LDL decorated targeting nanoparticles (LDL-NPs)** refer to artificial nanoparticles formed by coupling native LDLs to the outer layer of the synthetic inorganic NPs carried therapeutic drugs.

We summarize the reconstruction methods of LDL-based nanoparticles and their recent achievements, which will provide the newest investigations of the LDL-based targeted delivery. LDL-based NPs owns the following advantages.

Firstly, LDL-based NPs are highly biologically safe. As a biological molecule, LDL has biocompatibility and good biodegradability. LDL will be degraded into recyclable units, including cholesterol, fatty acids, and amino acids in the lysosome.

Secondly, LDL-carriers can effectively avoid triggering the immune system, ensuring that the delivered drugs reach the target cells before the clearance.

Thirdly, LDL enhances the targeting function of anticancer drugs through LDLR-mediated endocytosis. The LDLR and LDL would form a complex and then enter cells through the clathrin internalization pathway. About 30–40% of LDL is cleared every day, and two-thirds of them are absorbed by receptor-mediated endocytosis.

Fourthly, LDL has a long circulation time (2–4 days), which can maintain the drug concentration in the body and prolong the residence of the drugs.

3.1. Native LDL-Drug Particles (nLDL-Drugs)

Commercial LDLs are mainly derived from native LDLs isolated from human or animal plasma. The native LDLs own the advantages of stable structure, immunogenicity-reduction, and superior targeting function. Usually, there are three strategies to form nLDL-drugs due to the structure of LDL, including phospholipid monolayer loading, protein loading, and core loading. The hydrophobic lipid core and amphiphilic phospholipids of LDLs can load with a mass of lipophilic and amphiphilic drugs, and the amino acid residues of ApoB-100 can be covalently bound to diagnostic ligands or therapeutic agents [30] (Table 1).

Table 1. Advantages and disadvantages of different modification strategies.

Strategy	Advantage	Disadvantages
Phospholipid monolayer loading	1. Simple operation 2. Larger drug load	1. Drug Amphiphile 2. Easy leakage
Apolipoprotein loading	1. Simple operation	1. ApoB-100 inactivation 2. Less drug load
Core loading	1. Large drug load 2. Less damage to the shell	1. Cumbersome operation 2. Drug hydrophobicity

Phospholipid monolayer loading This modification of the phosphate monolayer of LDL mainly relies on relatively weak interactions such as van der Waals forces or other non-covalent bonds. Usually, therapeutic drugs are inserted into the phospholipid monolayer [26] (Figure 3a). Because of the amphiphilic characteristic of the phospholipid, it is easier for therapeutic drugs with the amphiphilic structure to be inserted, while non-amphiphilic drugs require more steps to insert into the phospholipid. The nLDL-drugs from this way are relatively simple, uniform, and high-integrity.

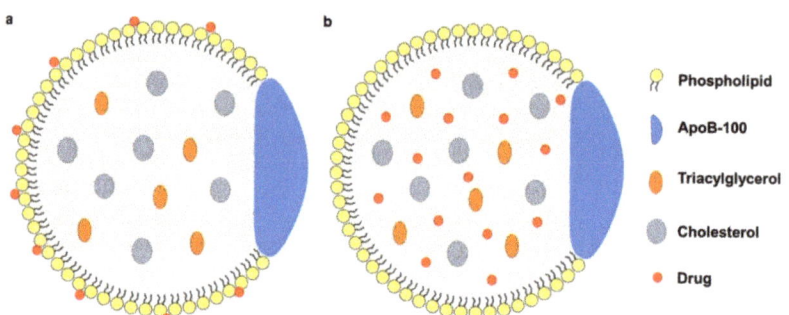

Figure 3. The modification strategy of nLDL-drugs particles. (**a**) drugs are inserted in the phospholipid monolayer; (**b**) drugs are loaded to the hydrophobic core.

Apolipoprotein loading This method involves the covalent binding of diagnostic or therapeutic drugs to ApoB-100. Lysine, arginine, tyrosine, and cysteine residues are used to couple amino acids on apolipoprotein residue [31], of which the lysine side chain is connected. To date, this method mainly delivers a contrast agent to monitor the biodistribution in the human body for its limited loading capacity. Meanwhile, the inactivation of ApoB-100 for extensive covalent modification [32] should be considered.

Core loading This method mainly refers to the reconstruction of therapeutic drugs on the core of LDL (Figure 3b). After the replacement of the non-polar core is achieved by freeze-drying or organic extraction [8], a drug/cholesterol mixture or drug-cholesterol conjugate [33] is used to form the reconstruction of the hydrophobic core. This method maintains the structure of phospholipids and apolipoprotein and ensures the binding activity of ApoB-100. Both hydrophilic and hydrophobic drugs could be delivered in this way. At the same time, sustained release and bioavailability are guaranteed.

3.2. Synthesized LDL-Drug Particles (sLDL-Drugs)

The sLDL-drugs are mainly obtained by the solvent evaporation method [16] or the solvent emulsification method [34]. In addition, sLDL-drugs are usually composed of a purified lipid emulsion with LDLR recognition functions and therapeutic drugs. Antitumor drugs are encapsulated in a hydrophobic core (Figure 4a) [16,35] with mixed alcohol oleic acid. The outer layer is a single-layer shell composed of hydrophilic phospholipids, where the ApoB-100 is embedded. Sometimes, special proteins or polypeptides would replace the apoB-100 to bind to the LDLR binding domain (Figure 4b) [16]. Compared with nLDL-drugs, the sLDL-drugs obtained by this method are more structurally stable and overcome leakage during transportation.

3.3. LDL Decorated LDLR Targeting Nanoparticles NPs (LDL-NPs)

Because of the good biocompatibility and biodegradability property of chitosan (CS) and silica nanoparticles (SLN), CS or SLN-based LDL-containing targeting nanoparticles have been constantly developed [36]. In LDL-modified NPs, LDL serves as the targeting molecule in therapy (Figure 5). Due to the large loading capacity of CS and SLN, multiple active pharmaceutical ingredients can be encapsulated in a single NP, thereby achieving synergistic therapy. LDL and synthetic nanoparticles are mainly combined with electrostatic interactions in this way.

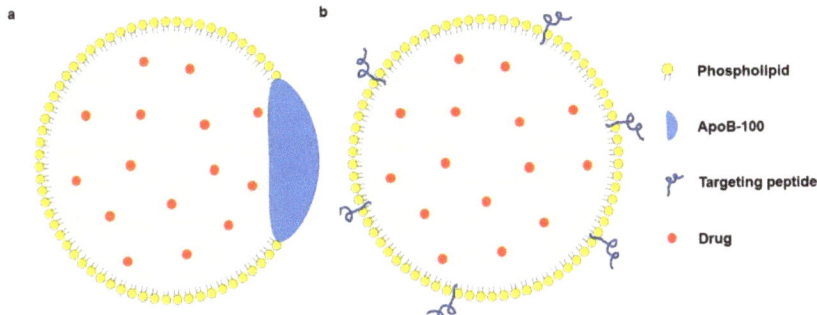

Figure 4. The modification strategy of sLDL-drugs. (**a**) targeting function is provided by ApoB-100; (**b**) targeting function is provided by biomimetic peptide.

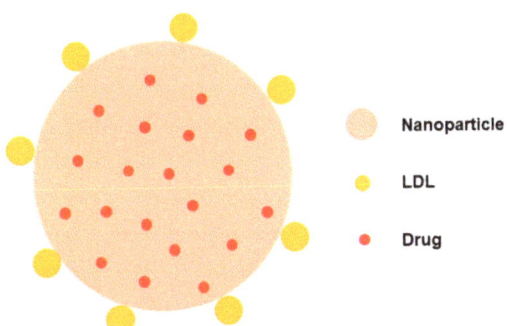

Figure 5. Model diagram of LDL-NPs. The NP core is loaded with small molecule drugs, and the LDL is attached to the outer layer of the NP as a targeting molecule.

4. Application of LDL-Based NPs in Cancer Therapy
4.1. nLDL-Drugs

Using natural LDL as a carrier to deliver therapeutic drugs has successfully inhibited the proliferation of melanoma, liver cancer, lung cancer, and so on [22,23]. There are several nLDL-drugs under investigation, and they made progress in cancer therapy (Table 2). Krieger et al. first designed r [25-HC-oleate] LDL to effectively reduce the activity of 3-hydroxy-3-methylglutaryl coenzyme A reductase in human fibroblasts, proving that constitutive LDL could selectively transport hydrophobic compounds to cells with LDLR [28]. Then, Masquelier et al. obtained an antitumor drug composed of a lipophilic derivation of doxorubicin (DNR) and LDL, termed DNR-LDL via lyophilization [26]. By investigating the in vivo fate of the complex, it was found that the DNR-LDL was quite similar to native LDL, and the high LDLR activity of the cancer cells resulted in the accumulation of DNR-LDL. Samadi-Baboli et al. confirmed that LDL-based nanoparticles were dependent on LDLR-mediated endocytosis, and the potency of lipophilic cytotoxic drugs against tumors was improved when combined with LDL [37]. Lo et al. prepared LDL-Doxorubicin (LDL-DOX) and injected it to liver cancer-bearing mice. It is found that LDL-DOX could selectively accumulate in the cancer cells, indicating that cancer cells had elevated expression of LDLR and more intake of LDL [38].

In addition, to widely incorporate cytotoxic drugs into LDL, LDL could also carry low-toxicity docosahexaenoic acid (DHA), an omega-3 polyunsaturated fatty acid, to improve cardiovascular health and prevent cancer. Reynolds et al. constructed LDL-DHA nanoparticles and found that the effective therapeutic dose of LDL-DHA on cancer cells does not influence normal cells, which may rely on the active lipid peroxidation and selective induction of reactive oxygen for cancer cells [8]. Yang et al. further evaluated the LDL-DHA on human liver cancer stem cells (CSC) and found that CSCs had a lower survival rate than normal cancer cells for the different LDLR expression [39], verifying LDL as a suitable delivery platform for drug-resistant cancer stem cells. Wen et al. achieved significant disease burden reduction by using synthetic LDL-DHA for liver cancer in situ [17]. Malik et al. combined LDL-DHA with pulsed-focused ultrasound technology to deliver LDL-DHA locally to the brain, and highly concentrated LDL-DHA in the treatment area was observed [40].

Table 2. nLDL-drugs and applications.

Category	Drugs	Indications	Reference
DNR-LDL	Doxorubicin	Leukemia cells	[26]
m-LDL	Cytotoxic compound 25	Lung fibroblasts	[41]
OL-NME-LDL	Elliptinium-oleate	B16 melanoma	[37]
Paclitaxel-LDL	Paclitaxel	Leukemia cells	[26]
LDL-DOX	Doxorubicin	HepG2 cells	[42]
LDL-DOX	Doxorubicin	R-HepG2 cells	[38]
r-Pc-LDL-FA	Tetra-t-butyl-silicon phthalocyanine	KB cells, HT-1080 cells, and HepG2 cells	[30]
Hyp-LDL	Hypericin	U87-MG cells	[43]
LDL-DHA	Docosahexaenoic acid	Hepatoma cells (H4IIE)	[15]
LDL-DNA	Docosahexaenoic acid	Fibroblasts	[44]
CaP@LDL	STAT3-decoyodns	HepG2 and PLC/PRF/5 cells	[45]
DOX-LDL	Doxorubicin	A549 cells	[18]
LDL-DHA	Docosahexaenoic acid	HuH-7 and HepG2 cells	[39]
LDL-DHA	Docosahexaenoic acid	TIB-75 cells	[8]

4.2. sLDL-Drugs

Since LDL source is scarce, synthetic LDL-like particles gradually become prevalent in reconstructed LDL-based NPs. The research on the combination of synthetic LDL (sLDL) and their different therapeutic preparations develop rapidly and achieve superior therapeutic effects (Table 3).

Baillie et al. prepared sLDL by combining lipid microemulsion with amphiphilic peptides containing apolipoprotein B receptor domain. This sLDL was taken up via LDLR-mediated endocytosis and could support the proliferation of U937 in culture [46]. Nikanjam et al. synthesized a new nanoparticle composed of an LDL-like shell with Paclitaxel oleate (PO) loaded, which was termed nLDL-PO, and demonstrated that only 6 h was needed for nLDL-PO to deliver Paclitaxel (PTX) to glioma cells via LDLR-mediated endocytosis [17]. Kim et al. developed biocompatible anti-cancer paclitaxel therapeutic solid lipid nanoparticles (PtSLNs) by containing paclitaxel in the core and modifying PEG on the surface to connect the tumor-targeting ligand [47]. As excepted, PtSLNs demonstrated a better targeting effect than the clinically free Taxol. Su et al. prepared sLDL to encapsulate paclitaxel-alpha linolenic acid (PALA) for tumor therapy. PTX-loaded nano-drug PALA-sLDL had a suitable size (approximately 66 nm) and high loading efficiency, and a good tumor growth inhibitory effect in U87 MG mice [48]. Qian et al. connected the lipid binding motif of apoB-100 to one end of PEG and introduced folate acid (FA) as a tumor-targeting moiety to the other end of PEG, constructing targeted folate receptor (FR) LDL bionic nanoparticles [34]. The uptake of these nanoparticles in FR-overexpressing tumor cells (HeLa cells) was much higher than that of FR-deficient tumor cells (A549 cells), at the same time producing a very significant anti-tumor efficiency in M109 tumor-bearing mice. Similar folic acid functionalized LDL biomimetic particles achieved co-delivery of anticancer drugs and superparamagnetic nanocrystals in MCF cells [25].

Table 3. sLDL-drugs and applications.

Category	Drugs	Indications	Reference
nLDL-PO	Paclitaxel oleate	GBM cells	[17]
siRNA-PEG/SLN	siRNA	PC3 cells	[49]
Targeted PtSLNs	Paclitaxel	NCI-H1975, NCI-H1650, NCI-H520, PC9	[47]
FA-mpLNPs	Iron oxide nanocrystals	MCF-7	[25]
PALA-sLDL	Paclitaxel-alpha linolenic acid	U87 MG, HepG2	[48]
FPLM NPs	Paclitaxel	HeLa, A549	[34]
AODN	Pro-doxorubicin	4T1	[35]
Lf-mNLC	Curcumin	BCECs	[50]

4.3. LDL-NPs

LDL-modified NPs are prepared using chitosan (CS) or solid lipid nanoparticles (SLN) as the carriers and LDL molecules as targeting ligands. This nanoparticle has a better targeting capacity to LDLR overexpressed cells and higher loading ability (Table 4). Currently, LDL-NPs are applied in the treatment of liver and breast cancer. Zhang et al. first synthesized N-succinyl-chitosan (NSC) as the center part of NPs and then loaded osthole to obtain Ost/LDL-NSC-NPs. Excellent proliferation inhibition could be observed when applying these NPs to HepG2 cells [36]. Based on this, Zhu et al. used LDL-SCS-NPs to deliver siRNA and doxorubicin to liver cancers, providing a novel and effective way for the co-delivery of genes and chemotherapeutic drugs [51]. Ao et al. developed the SLN-based docetaxel (DTX) and thalidomide (TDD) co-delivery system and found that these NPs had strong targeting properties [52]. Ye et al. used SLN-based LDL-containing NPs to co-deliver sorafenib (Sor) and doxorubicin (Dox). Obvious tumor inhibition was observed in vitro and in vivo [53]. Wang et al. developed co-drug lipid nanoparticles LD-SDN to transport sorafenib and dihydroartemisinin to liver cancer cells, revealing excellent apoptosis induction [24].

Yang et al. developed a binary copolymer system based on N-succinyl chitosan lipoic acid micelles to co-deliver the siRNA and paclitaxel [54] to inhibit the growth of breast cancer cells in vitro and in vivo. Zhu et al. prepared PTX and siRNA co-loading drug siRNA-PTX/LDL-NSC-SS-UA and made significant progress in overcoming multidrug resistance [55]. Pan et al. used the SLN-designed and synthesized indocyanine green multifunctional platform (LDL/SLN) to target breast cancer cells, which provided new ideas for the development of photothermal therapy for breast cancer [56].

Table 4. LDL-NPs and applications.

Category	Drugs	Indications	Reference
Ost/LDL-NSC-NPs	Osthole	HepG2 cells	[36]
Dox-siRNA/LDL-SCS-NPs	Dox siRNA	HepG2, H22	[51]
PTX-siRNA/LDL-NSC-LA micelles	MDR1 siRNA and paclitaxel	MCF-7 cells	[54]
LDL/SLN/DTX/TDD	Docetaxel (DTX), Thalidomide (TDD)	HepG2 cells	[52]
LDL/SLN/Adr	Adriamycin	Colorectal cancer	[57]
LDL-SLN/Sor/Dox	Sorafenib, Doxorubicin	HepG2 cells	[53]
LD-SDN	Sorafenib, Dihydroartemisinin	HepG2 cells	[24]
LDL/SLN/ICG	Sorafenib, Dihydroartemisinin	MCF-7 cells	[56]

Nowadays, more and more studies are focused on bionic nanoparticles. Compared with the modification of nLDL-drugs particles, LDL-NPs can further save costs, improve plasticity, and provide more modification methods and materials. These biomimetic materials have larger particle sizes and more target candidates to interact with cancer cells. Although the nLDL-drugs have been investigated for a long time, and the experimental protocols are experienced, there are still some challenges to uniformity and integrity. Therefore, more and more investigation of sLDL-drugs and LDL-NPs is prevalent. Here, we compare the advantages and disadvantages of these three particles (Table 5).

Table 5. Comparison of LDL-based NPs.

Strategy	Advantages	Disadvantages
nLDL-drugs	1. Biocompatibility, biodegradability 2. Targeting 3. Long half-life	1. Scarce raw materials and high cost [18] 2. Poor stability, harsh storage conditions [8]
sLDL-drugs	1. Low cost 2. High loading capacity 3. Targeting peptides to further improve targeting	1. Complex process requirements [17] 2. Not very targeting capacity [58]
LDL-NPs	1. Low cost 2. Simple protocol 3. Diversity targeting moiety	1. Large size [24] 2. Exogenous material [56]

5. Conclusions and Future Prospects

LDL has the characteristics of small size, amphiphilic molecular surface, receptor-mediated internalization, and long circulation time. With these functions, therapeutic drugs can be combined with LDL to target LDLR-overexpressed tumor cells. As an ideal carrier and effective ligand for targeted therapy, LDL-based drug-loaded nanoparticles further promote the development of targeted delivery and expand the application of LDL in cancer therapy. Most targeting NPs are designed for solid tumors but not hematological malignancies. This is because hematological oncology is different from solid ones in that leukemia cells might be all around the body, while solid tumor cells usually locate in a particular tissue. LDL-based NPs depend on LDLR-endocytosis to effectively target cancer cells and thus can be utilized in leukemia and solid tumors. By comparing the degradation efficiency of monocyte 125I-LDL isolated from healthy individuals and leukemia patients, Viitols et al. found that primary leukemia cells had a higher degradation rate of 125I-LDL [59]. Then, Zhou et al. found that the intake of sLDL was inversely proportional to the degree of cell differentiation by using synthetic LDL particles to target leukemia cell lines and CML patient stem/progenitor cells [60]. Hence, LDL could be a potential drug delivery carrier for leukemia disease.

Although the research on LDL-based NPs has made many achievements, there are still limitations to clinical advancement. The limits are the sources of LDL, the complex processing requirements, and the trigger of atherosclerosis in the body. sLDL-drugs and LDL-NPs are derived from non-plasma-separated LDL, overcoming the problem of resource limitations. In addition, they still restore the targeting characteristics of LDL and keep the simple and controllable synthesis process. Due to the larger particle diameter, the loading capacity also increases. Meanwhile, LDL-based targeting NPs not only target solid tumors but also hematological malignancy. More importantly, these NPs have stronger targeting function to cancer stem cells or drug-resistant cells for these cells overexpressing LDLR. In short, LDL-based nanoparticles have good application prospects in cancer-targeted therapy.

Author Contributions: B.H. wrote the manuscript and Q.Y. revised the manuscript. All authors have read and agreed to the published version of the manuscript.

Funding: This work is supported by the Natural Science Foundation of Beijing Municipality (2202021) and the National Natural Science Foundation of China (22072005, 21773015).

Institutional Review Board Statement: Not applicable.

Informed Consent Statement: Not applicable.

Data Availability Statement: Data sharing not applicable.

Conflicts of Interest: The authors declare no conflict of interest.

References

1. Siegel, R.L.; Miller, K.D.; Fuchs, H.E.; Jemal, A. Cancer Statistics, 2022. *CA. Cancer J. Clin.* **2022**, *72*, 7–33. [CrossRef] [PubMed]
2. Sparano, J.A.; Gray, R.J.; Makower, D.F.; Albain, K.S.; Saphner, T.J.; Badve, S.S.; Wagner, L.I.; Kaklamani, V.G.; Keane, M.M.; Gomez, H.L.; et al. Clinical Outcomes in Early Breast Cancer With a High 21-Gene Recurrence Score of 26 to 100 Assigned to Adjuvant Chemotherapy Plus Endocrine Therapy: A Secondary Analysis of the TAILORx Randomized Clinical Trial. *JAMA Oncol.* **2020**, *6*, 367–374. [CrossRef] [PubMed]
3. Moy, B.; Rumble, R.B.; Come, S.E.; Davidson, N.E.; Di Leo, A.; Gralow, J.R.; Hortobagyi, G.N.; Yee, D.; Smith, I.E.; Chavez-MacGregor, M.; et al. Chemotherapy and Targeted Therapy for Patients With Human Epidermal Growth Factor Receptor 2-Negative Metastatic Breast Cancer That Is Either Endocrine-Pretreated or Hormone Receptor-Negative: ASCO Guideline Update. *J. Clin. Oncol.* **2021**, *39*, 3938–3958. [CrossRef]
4. Lu, S.; Wu, L.; Jian, H.; Chen, Y.; Wang, Q.; Fang, J.; Wang, Z.; Hu, Y.; Sun, M.; Han, L.; et al. Sintilimab plus Bevacizumab Biosimilar IBI305 and Chemotherapy for Patients with EGFR-Mutated Non-Squamous Non-Small-Cell Lung Cancer Who Progressed on EGFR Tyrosine-Kinase Inhibitor Therapy (ORIENT-31): First Interim Results from a Randomised, Double-Blind, Multicentre, Phase 3 Trial. *Lancet. Oncol.* **2022**, *23*, 1167–1179. [PubMed]
5. Schwartzberg, L.S.; Modiano, M.R.; Rapoport, B.L.; Chasen, M.R.; Gridelli, C.; Urban, L.; Poma, A.; Arora, S.; Navari, R.M.; Schnadig, I.D. Safety and Efficacy of Rolapitant for Prevention of Chemotherapy-Induced Nausea and Vomiting after Administration of Moderately Emetogenic Chemotherapy or Anthracycline and Cyclophosphamide Regimens in Patients with Cancer: A Randomised, Active-Controlled, Double-Blind, Phase 3 Trial. *Lancet. Oncol.* **2015**, *16*, 1071–1078.
6. An, X.; Zhu, A.; Luo, H.; Ke, H.; Chen, H.; Zhao, Y. Rational Design of Multi-Stimuli-Responsive Nanoparticles for Precise Cancer Therapy. *ACS Nano* **2016**, *10*, 5947–5958. [CrossRef]
7. Aikins, M.E.; Xu, C.; Moon, J.J. Engineered Nanoparticles for Cancer Vaccination and Immunotherapy. *Acc. Chem. Res.* **2020**, *53*, 2094–2105. [CrossRef]
8. Reynolds, L.; Mulik, R.S.; Wen, X.; Dilip, A.; Corbin, I.R. Low-Density Lipoprotein-Mediated Delivery of Docosahexaenoic Acid Selectively Kills Murine Liver Cancer Cells. *Nanomedicine* **2014**, *9*, 2123–2141. [CrossRef]
9. Tabernero, J.; Shapiro, G.I.; LoRusso, P.M.; Cervantes, A.; Schwartz, G.K.; Weiss, G.J.; Paz-Ares, L.; Cho, D.C.; Infante, J.R.; Alsina, M.; et al. First-in-Humans Trial of an RNA Interference Therapeutic Targeting VEGF and KSP in Cancer Patients with Liver Involvement. *Cancer Discov.* **2013**, *3*, 406–417. [CrossRef]
10. Xu, X.; Wang, L.; Xu, H.Q.; Huang, X.E.; Qian, Y.D.; Xiang, J. Clinical Comparison between Paclitaxel Liposome (Lipusu®) and Paclitaxel for Treatment of Patients with Metastatic Gastric Cancer. *Asian Pac. J. Cancer Prev.* **2013**, *14*, 2591–2594. [CrossRef]
11. Awada, A.; Garcia, A.A.; Chan, S.; Jerusalem, G.H.M.; Coleman, R.E.; Huizing, M.T.; Mehdi, A.; O'Reilly, S.M.; Hamm, J.T.; Barrett-Lee, P.J.; et al. Two Schedules of Etirinotecan Pegol (NKTR-102) in Patients with Previously Treated Metastatic Breast Cancer: A Randomised Phase 2 Study. *Lancet. Oncol.* **2013**, *14*, 1216–1225. [CrossRef] [PubMed]
12. Wicki, A.; Witzigmann, D.; Balasubramanian, V.; Huwyler, J. Nanomedicine in Cancer Therapy: Challenges, Opportunities, and Clinical Applications. *J. Control. Release* **2015**, *200*, 138–157. [CrossRef] [PubMed]
13. McConathy, W.J.; Paranjape, S.; Mooberry, L.; Buttreddy, S.; Nair, M.; Lacko, A.G. Validation of the Reconstituted High-Density Lipoprotein (RHDL) Drug Delivery Platform Using Dilauryl Fluorescein (DLF). *Drug Deliv. Transl. Res.* **2011**, *1*, 113–120. [CrossRef] [PubMed]
14. Taskinen, M.R. LDL-Cholesterol, HDL-Cholesterol or Triglycerides - Which Is the Culprit? *Diabetes Res. Clin. Pract.* **2003**, *61*, S19–S26. [CrossRef]
15. Wen, X.; Reynolds, L.; Mulik, R.S.; Kim, S.Y.; Van Treuren, T.; Nguyen, L.H.; Zhu, H.; Corbin, I.R. Hepatic Arterial Infusion of Low-Density Lipoprotein Docosahexaenoic Acid Nanoparticles Selectively Disrupts Redox Balance in Hepatoma Cells and Reduces Growth of Orthotopic Liver Tumors in Rats. *Gastroenterology* **2016**, *150*, 488. [CrossRef]
16. Nikanjam, M.; Blakely, E.A.; Bjornstad, K.A.; Shu, X.; Budinger, T.F.; Forte, T.M. Synthetic Nano-Low Density Lipoprotein as Targeted Drug Delivery Vehicle for Glioblastoma Multiforme. *Int. J. Pharm.* **2007**, *328*, 86–94. [CrossRef]
17. Nikanjam, M.; Gibbs, A.R.; Hunt, C.A.; Budinger, T.F.; Forte, T.M. Synthetic Nano-LDL with Paclitaxel Oleate as a Targeted Drug Delivery Vehicle for Glioblastoma Multiforme. *J. Control. Release* **2007**, *124*, 163–171. [CrossRef]
18. Zhu, C.; Pradhan, P.; Huo, D.; Xue, J.; Shen, S.; Roy, K.; Xia, Y. Reconstitution of Low-Density Lipoproteins with Fatty Acids for the Targeted Delivery of Drugs into Cancer Cells. *Angew. Chem. Int. Ed. Engl.* **2017**, *56*, 10399–10402. [CrossRef]
19. Young, S.G. Recent Progress in Understanding Apolipoprotein B. *Circulation* **1990**, *82*, 1574–1594. [CrossRef]
20. Zhang, Y.; Sun, T.; Jiang, C. Biomacromolecules as Carriers in Drug Delivery and Tissue Engineering. *Acta Pharm. Sin. B* **2018**, *8*, 34–50. [CrossRef]
21. Damiano, M.G.; Mutharasan, R.K.; Tripathy, S.; McMahon, K.M.; Thaxton, C.S. Templated High Density Lipoprotein Nanoparticles as Potential Therapies and for Molecular Delivery. *Adv. Drug Deliv. Rev.* **2013**, *65*, 649–662. [CrossRef] [PubMed]
22. Jeon, H.; Blacklow, S.C. Structure and Physiologic Function of the Low-Density Lipoprotein Receptor. *Annu. Rev. Biochem.* **2005**, *74*, 535–562. [CrossRef] [PubMed]

23. Li, C.; Zhang, J.; Wu, H.; Li, L.; Yang, C.; Song, S.; Peng, P.; Shao, M.; Zhang, M.; Zhao, J.; et al. Lectin-like Oxidized Low-Density Lipoprotein Receptor-1 Facilitates Metastasis of Gastric Cancer through Driving Epithelial-Mesenchymal Transition and PI3K/Akt/GSK3β Activation. *Sci. Rep.* **2017**, *7*, 45275. [CrossRef] [PubMed]
24. Wang, Z.; Duan, X.; Lv, Y.; Zhao, Y. Low Density Lipoprotein Receptor (LDLR)-Targeted Lipid Nanoparticles for the Delivery of Sorafenib and Dihydroartemisinin in Liver Cancers. *Life Sci.* **2019**, *239*, 117013. [CrossRef] [PubMed]
25. Lee, J.Y.; Kim, J.H.; Bae, K.H.; Oh, M.H.; Kim, Y.; Kim, J.S.; Park, T.G.; Park, K.; Lee, J.H.; Nam, Y.S. Low-Density Lipoprotein-Mimicking Nanoparticles for Tumor-Targeted Theranostic Applications. *Small* **2015**, *11*, 222–231. [CrossRef]
26. Masquelier, M.; Vitols, S.; Palsson, M.; Mars, U.; Larsson, B.S.; Peterson, C.O. Low density lipoprotein as a carrier of cytostatics in cancer chemotherapy: Study of stability of drug-carrier complexes in blood. *J. Drug Target.* **2000**, *8*, 155–164. [CrossRef]
27. Caruso, M.G.; Notarnicola, M.; Cavallini, A.; Guerra, V.; Misciagna, G.; Di Leo, A. Demonstration of Low Density Lipoprotein Receptor in Human Colonic Carcinoma and Surrounding Mucosa by Immunoenzymatic Assay. *Ital. J. Gastroenterol.* **1993**, *25*, 361–367.
28. Krieger, M.; Goldstein, J.L.; Brown, M.S. Receptor-Mediated Uptake of Low Density Lipoprotein Reconstituted with 25-Hydroxycholesteryl Oleate Suppresses 3-Hydroxy-3-Methylglutaryl-Coenzyme A Reductase and Inhibits Growth of Human Fibroblasts. *Proc. Natl. Acad. Sci. USA* **1978**, *75*, 5052–5056. [CrossRef]
29. Chu, H.L.; Cheng, T.M.; Chen, H.W.; Chou, F.H.; Chang, Y.C.; Lin, H.Y.; Liu, S.Y.; Liang, Y.C.; Hsu, M.H.; Wu, D.S.; et al. Synthesis of Apolipoprotein B Lipoparticles to Deliver Hydrophobic/Amphiphilic Materials. *ACS Appl. Mater. Interfaces* **2013**, *5*, 7509–7516. [CrossRef]
30. Zheng, G.; Chen, J.; Li, H.; Glickson, J.D. Rerouting Lipoprotein Nanoparticles to Selected Alternate Receptors for the Targeted Delivery of Cancer Diagnostic and Therapeutic Agents. *Proc. Natl. Acad. Sci. USA* **2005**, *102*, 17757–17762. [CrossRef]
31. Bergt, C.; Fu, X.; Huq, N.P.; Kao, J.; Heinecke, J.W. Lysine Residues Direct the Chlorination of Tyrosines in YXXK Motifs of Apolipoprotein A-I When Hypochlorous Acid Oxidizes High Density Lipoprotein. *J. Biol. Chem.* **2004**, *279*, 7856–7866. [CrossRef] [PubMed]
32. Versluis, A.J.; Van Geel, P.J.; Oppelaar, H.; Van Berkel, T.J.C.; Bijsterbosch, M.K. Receptor-Mediated Uptake of Low-Density Lipoprotein by B16 Melanoma Cells in Vitro and in Vivo in Mice. *Br. J. Cancer* **1996**, *74*, 525–532. [CrossRef] [PubMed]
33. Jin, H.; Lovell, J.F.; Chen, J.; Ng, K.; Cao, W.; Ding, L.; Zhang, Z.; Zheng, G. Cytosolic Delivery of LDL Nanoparticle Cargo Using Photochemical Internalization. *Photochem. Photobiol. Sci.* **2011**, *10*, 810–816. [CrossRef] [PubMed]
34. Qian, J.; Xu, N.; Zhou, X.; Shi, K.; Du, Q.; Yin, X.; Zhao, Z. Low Density Lipoprotein Mimic Nanoparticles Composed of Amphipathic Hybrid Peptides and Lipids for Tumor-Targeted Delivery of Paclitaxel. *Int. J. Nanomedicine* **2019**, *14*, 7431–7446. [CrossRef]
35. Li, W.; Fu, J.; Ding, Y.; Liu, D.; Jia, N.; Chen, D.; Hu, H. Low Density Lipoprotein-Inspired Nanostructured Lipid Nanoparticles Containing pro-Doxorubicin to Enhance Tumor-Targeted Therapeutic Efficiency. *Acta Biomater.* **2019**, *96*, 456–467. [CrossRef]
36. Zhang, C.G.; Zhu, Q.L.; Zhou, Y.; Liu, Y.; Chen, W.L.; Yuan, Z.Q.; Yang, S.D.; Zhou, X.F.; Zhu, A.J.; Zhang, X.N.; et al. N-Succinyl-Chitosan Nanoparticles Coupled with Low-Density Lipoprotein for Targeted Osthole-Loaded Delivery to Low-Density Lipoprotein Receptor-Rich Tumors. *Int. J. Nanomedicine* **2014**, *9*, 2919–2932. [CrossRef]
37. Samadi-Baboli, M.; Favre, G.; Canal, P.; Soula, G. Low Density Lipoprotein for Cytotoxic Drug Targeting: Improved Activity of Ellipticinium Derivative against B16 Melanoma in Mice. *Br. J. Cancer* **1993**, *68*, 319–326. [CrossRef]
38. Lo, E.H.K.; Ooi, V.E.L.; Fung, K.P. Circumvention of Multidrug Resistance and Reduction of Cardiotoxicity of Doxorubicin in Vivo by Coupling It with Low Density Lipoprotein. *Life Sci.* **2002**, *72*, 677–687. [CrossRef]
39. Yang, J.; Gong, Y.; Sontag, D.P.; Corbin, I.; Minuk, G.Y. Effects of Low-Density Lipoprotein Docosahexaenoic Acid Nanoparticles on Cancer Stem Cells Isolated from Human Hepatoma Cell Lines. *Mol. Biol. Rep.* **2018**, *45*, 1023–1036. [CrossRef]
40. Mulik, R.S.; Bing, C.; Ladouceur-Wodzak, M.; Munaweera, I.; Chopra, R.; Corbin, I.R. Localized Delivery of Low-Density Lipoprotein Docosahexaenoic Acid Nanoparticles to the Rat Brain Using Focused Ultrasound. *Biomaterials* **2016**, *83*, 257–268. [CrossRef]
41. Lundberg, B. Preparation of Drug-Low Density Lipoprotein Complexes for Delivery of Antitumoral Drugs via the Low Density Lipoprotein Pathway. *Cancer Res.* **1987**, *47*, 4105–4108. [PubMed]
42. Chu, A.C.Y.; Tsang, S.Y.; Lo, E.H.K.; Fung, K.P. Low Density Lipoprotein as a Targeted Carrier for Doxorubicin in Nude Mice Bearing Human Hepatoma HepG2 Cells. *Life Sci.* **2001**, *70*, 591–601. [CrossRef] [PubMed]
43. Huntosova, V.; Buzova, D.; Petrovajova, D.; Kasak, P.; Nadova, Z.; Jancura, D.; Sureau, F.; Miskovsky, P. Development of a New LDL-Based Transport System for Hydrophobic/Amphiphilic Drug Delivery to Cancer Cells. *Int. J. Pharm.* **2012**, *436*, 463–471. [CrossRef]
44. Khan, Z.; Hawtrey, A.O.; Ariatti, M. New Cationized LDL-DNA Complexes: Their Targeted Delivery to Fibroblasts in Culture. *Drug Deliv. J. Deliv. Target. Ther. Agents* **2003**, *10*, 213–220. [CrossRef] [PubMed]
45. Shi, K.; Xue, J.; Fang, Y.; Bi, H.; Gao, S.; Yang, D.; Lu, A.; Li, Y.; Chen, Y.; Ke, L. Inorganic Kernel-Reconstituted Lipoprotein Biomimetic Nanovehicles Enable Efficient Targeting "Trojan Horse" Delivery of STAT3-Decoy Oligonucleotide for Overcoming TRAIL Resistance. *Theranostics* **2017**, *7*, 4480–4497. [CrossRef] [PubMed]
46. Baillie, G.; Owens, M.D.; Halbert, G.W. A Synthetic Low Density Lipoprotein Particle Capable of Supporting U937 Proliferation in Vitro. *J. Lipid Res.* **2002**, *43*, 69–73. [CrossRef]

47. Kim, J.H.; Kim, Y.; Bae, K.H.; Park, T.G.; Lee, J.H.; Park, K. Tumor-Targeted Delivery of Paclitaxel Using Low Density Lipoprotein-Mimetic Solid Lipid Nanoparticles. *Mol. Pharm.* **2015**, *12*, 1230–1241. [CrossRef]
48. Su, H.T.; Li, X.; Liang, D.S.; Qi, X.R. Synthetic Low-Density Lipoprotein (SLDL) Selectively Delivers Paclitaxel to Tumor with Low Systemic Toxicity. *Oncotarget* **2016**, *7*, 51535. [CrossRef]
49. Kim, H.R.; Kim, I.K.; Bae, K.H.; Lee, S.H.; Lee, Y.; Park, T.G. Cationic Solid Lipid Nanoparticles Reconstituted from Low Density Lipoprotein Components for Delivery of SiRNA. *Mol. Pharm.* **2008**, *5*, 622–631. [CrossRef]
50. Meng, F.; Asghar, S.; Gao, S.; Su, Z.; Song, J.; Huo, M.; Meng, W.; Ping, Q.; Xiao, Y. A Novel LDL-Mimic Nanocarrier for the Targeted Delivery of Curcumin into the Brain to Treat Alzheimer's Disease. *Colloids Surf. B Biointerfaces* **2015**, *134*, 88–97. [CrossRef] [PubMed]
51. Zhu, Q.L.; Zhou, Y.; Guan, M.; Zhou, X.F.; Yang, S.D.; Liu, Y.; Chen, W.L.; Zhang, C.G.; Yuan, Z.Q.; Liu, C.; et al. Low-Density Lipoprotein-Coupled N-Succinyl Chitosan Nanoparticles Co-Delivering SiRNA and Doxorubicin for Hepatocyte-Targeted Therapy. *Biomaterials* **2014**, *35*, 5965–5976. [CrossRef] [PubMed]
52. Ao, M.; Xiao, X.; Ao, Y. Low density lipoprotein modified silica nanoparticles loaded with docetaxel and thalidomide for effective chemotherapy of liver cancer. *Braz. J. Med. Biol. Res. Rev. Bras. Pesqui. Med. E Biol.* **2018**, *51*, 1–10. [CrossRef] [PubMed]
53. Ye, J.; Zhang, R.; Chai, W.; Du, X. Low-Density Lipoprotein Decorated Silica Nanoparticles Co-Delivering Sorafenib and Doxorubicin for Effective Treatment of Hepatocellular Carcinoma. *Drug Deliv.* **2018**, *25*, 2016–2023. [CrossRef]
54. Yang, S.D.; Zhu, W.J.; Zhu, Q.L.; Chen, W.L.; Ren, Z.X.; Li, F.; Yuan, Z.Q.; Li, J.Z.; Liu, Y.; Zhou, X.F.; et al. Binary-Copolymer System Base on Low-Density Lipoprotein-Coupled N-Succinyl Chitosan Lipoic Acid Micelles for Co-Delivery MDR1 SiRNA and Paclitaxel, Enhances Antitumor Effects via Reducing Drug. *J. Biomed. Mater. Res. B Appl. Biomater.* **2017**, *105*, 1114–1125. [CrossRef]
55. Zhu, W.J.; Yang, S.D.; Qu, C.X.; Zhu, Q.L.; Chen, W.L.; Li, F.; Yuan, Z.Q.; Liu, Y.; You, B.G.; Zhang, X.N. Low-Density Lipoprotein-Coupled Micelles with Reduction and PH Dual Sensitivity for Intelligent Co-Delivery of Paclitaxel and SiRNA to Breast Tumor. *Int. J. Nanomedicine* **2017**, *12*, 3375–3393. [CrossRef]
56. Pan, H.; Sun, Y.; Cao, D.; Wang, L. Low-Density Lipoprotein Decorated and Indocyanine Green Loaded Silica Nanoparticles for Tumor-Targeted Photothermal Therapy of Breast Cancer. *Pharm. Dev. Technol.* **2020**, *25*, 308–315. [CrossRef]
57. Shi, G.; Li, J.; Yan, X.; Jin, K.; Li, W.; Liu, X.; Zhao, J.; Shang, W.; Zhang, R. Low-Density Lipoprotein-Decorated and Adriamycin-Loaded Silica Nanoparticles for Tumor-Targeted Chemotherapy of Colorectal Cancer. *Adv. Clin. Exp. Med.* **2019**, *28*, 479–487. [CrossRef]
58. Liu, M.; Li, W.; Larregieu, C.A.; Cheng, M.; Yan, B.; Chu, T.; Li, H.; Mao, S.J. Development of Synthetic Peptide-Modified Liposomes with LDL Receptor Targeting Capacity and Improved Anticancer Activity. *Mol. Pharm.* **2014**, *11*, 2305–2312. [CrossRef]
59. Vitols, S.; Gahrton, G.; Ost, A.; Peterson, C. Elevated Low Density Lipoprotein Receptor Activity in Leukemic Cells With Monocytic Differentiation. *Blood* **1984**, *63*, 1186–1193. [CrossRef]
60. Zhou, P.; Hatziieremia, S.; Elliott, M.A.; Scobie, L.; Crossan, C.; Michie, A.M.; Holyoake, T.L.; Halbert, G.W.; Jørgensen, H.G. Uptake of Synthetic Low Density Lipoprotein by Leukemic Stem Cells—A Potential Stem Cell Targeted Drug Delivery Strategy. *J. Control. Release* **2010**, *148*, 380–387. [CrossRef] [PubMed]

Disclaimer/Publisher's Note: The statements, opinions and data contained in all publications are solely those of the individual author(s) and contributor(s) and not of MDPI and/or the editor(s). MDPI and/or the editor(s) disclaim responsibility for any injury to people or property resulting from any ideas, methods, instructions or products referred to in the content.

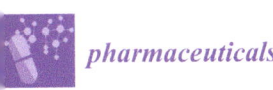

Review

Tumor-Derived Membrane Vesicles: A Promising Tool for Personalized Immunotherapy

Jiabin Xu [1,2], Wenqiang Cao [3], Penglai Wang [1,2] and Hong Liu [3,*]

1. School of Stomatology, Xuzhou Medical University, Xuzhou 221004, China; jabbyxu@foxmail.com (J.X.); wpl0771@163.com (P.W.)
2. Affiliated Stomatological Hospital of Xuzhou Medical University, Xuzhou 221004, China
3. Zhuhai Jinan Selenium Source Nanotechnology Co., Ltd., Jinan University, Zhuhai 519000, China; sesource_cwq@163.com
* Correspondence: liuhong@jnu.edu.cn

Abstract: Tumor-derived membrane vesicles (TDMVs) are non-invasive, chemotactic, easily obtained characteristics and contain various tumor-borne substances, such as nucleic acid and proteins. The unique properties of tumor cells and membranes make them widely used in drug loading, membrane fusion and vaccines. In particular, personalized vectors prepared using the editable properties of cells can help in the design of personalized vaccines. This review focuses on recent research on TDMV technology and its application in personalized immunotherapy. We elucidate the strengths and challenges of TDMVs to promote their application from theory to clinical practice.

Keywords: tumor-derived membrane vesicles; cancer therapy; tumor vaccine; personalized immunotherapy

1. Introduction

Cancer is the leading cause of human death globally and a significant disease reducing life expectancy. According to the International Agency for Research on Cancer (IARC), 19.3 million new cases and millions of cancer deaths were estimated worldwide in 2020 [1]. Clinically, the primary treatments for cancers are surgical resection, radiotherapy and chemotherapy, but these methods may cause tumor recurrence, damage to normal tissues, and toxic side effects caused by a lack of precise targeting [2]. In contrast to conventional treatments, tumor immunotherapy, which refers to the regulation of the patient's immune system to fight against tumors, has become the mainstream of research and clinical practice. Immunotherapy by activating immune cells to trigger a systemic anti-tumor immune response can eradicate primary and distant tumors, establishing long-term immune memory to prevent tumor recurrence [3]. Tumor immunotherapy has now yielded exciting results in hematological cancers, lymphoma and myeloma [4]. Monoclonal antibodies, immune checkpoint therapy (ICT) and chimeric antigen receptor (CAR) T cell therapy have achieved significant clinical efficacy [5,6]. However, there remain many challenges to the widespread clinical application of immunotherapy. Monoclonal antibodies can exhibit off-target toxicity and adverse immunological effects. Only 13% of patients showed a significant immune response to ICT [7]. Effective CAR T-cell therapy for hematological cancers has not significantly impacted the treatment of more prevalent solid epithelial cancers [8]. Combined immunotherapy has better therapeutic effects while at the cost of more acute inflammatory side effects [9,10]. Therefore, how to safely and effectively drive the immune response against cancer remains an urgent issue for tumor immunotherapy.

The gap between the tumor microenvironment in the body is the main reason for the significant gap in the efficacy of tumor immunotherapy. In particular, the immunosuppressive microenvironment and high interstitial pressure in solid tumors make it difficult for drugs to penetrate and act inside the tumor, thus contributing to the immune escape of tumor cells and making treatment very difficult. Tumors can be divided into three types [11]: the first is the immune desert type, which lacks tumor-infiltrating lymphocytes (TILs) in the central and peripheral regions. PD-1/PD-L1 therapy is clinically ineffective for this type. The second is the immune-excluded type, which has many TILs at the tumor edge but forms an immune desert in the central area. After treatment with anti-PD-L1/PD-1, stroma-associated T cells can show signs of activation and proliferation without deeper infiltration. The third, the immunoinflammatory type, has TILs in the central and peripheral regions and contains effectors such as monocytes and pro-inflammatory factors around the tumor.

Nevertheless, tumor escape suppresses the immune response. Tumor mutational burden (TMB) due to intratumoral heterogeneity also has implications for treatment. As TMB increases, more neoantigens are released, triggering more robust T cell responses for better therapeutic effects [12,13]. The amount and type of gut microbiota affect the incidence of cancer and the body's susceptibility to treatment. The study showed that ICT had no significant effect on tumor-bearing mice lacking gut microbes [14–16]. The higher the abundance of probiotics and the more $CD8^+$ T and $CD4^+$ T cells in the surrounding blood, the better effect of anti-PD-1 on melanoma.

Fortunately, the development of nanomaterials has opened up more options for tumor immunotherapy. Protein particles, vesicles, liposomes, micelles, inorganic particles and metal-organic frameworks (MOFs) are used to enhance tumor immunogenicity and inhibit tumor growth [17–19]. However, the foreign substances and the carriers involved in drug transport are also easy to be eliminated by the immune system [20]. Polyethylene glycol (PEG) is commonly used to modify the surface of nanoparticles. It can protect the nanoparticles from clearance by the immune system and prolong drug half-life. However, recent studies found that PEG can accelerate the blood clearance effect, reducing the drug's efficacy [21]. The major limitation to the broader success of immunotherapy treatments is not the lack of rational therapeutic targets but rather how to successfully reach these targets at the right time and place. Therefore, it is necessary to develop personalized therapeutic modalities that promote systemic and durable anti-tumor immunity to eradicate malignancies and prevent metastasis and recurrence completely [22].

Cell-derived membrane vesicles carry abundant recognition units that endow them with high biological specificity. Membrane vesicle camouflage can bypass clearance by immune cells, has a longer circulation time and upon reaching the tumor site, its bilayer lipid structure can fuse directly with tumor cells to utilize the treatment [2,23,24]. Membrane vesicles can improve bioavailability, effectively target treatment sites, reduce drug side effects and promote drug retention and sustained release in tissues [25–27]. In addition, several clinical results suggest that membrane vesicles of their own origin are virtually immunogenic and non-toxic, while synthetic materials still have unavoidable safety concerns in terms of immunogenicity and toxicity [28]. A variety of cell-derived membrane vesicle nanoparticles have been studied, including erythrocytes, stem cells, dendritic cells, natural killer cells, fibroblasts and tumor cells [29,30]. In particular, tumor cells can expand indefinitely and can isolate membrane vesicles in large batches of cultures in vitro. Unlike other membrane vesicles, tumor-derived membrane vesicles have properties that are highly similar to those of homologous tumors. TDMVs can be divided into tumor cell membrane vesicles (TCMVs) and tumor extracellular vesicles (TEVs). TCMVs carry a comprehensive and complete set of proteins and surface antigens that can stimulate the body's immune response and have great potential as cancer vaccines [25,31]. TEVs are significant players in intercellular signaling and information exchange, regulating tumor progression by promoting tumor invasion, extracellular matrix remodeling, angiogenesis and immunosuppression [23,32].

Personalized therapies have emerged in response to differences in the efficacy of immunotherapy for different individuals. Delivering personalized drugs to patients based on genomic alterations, specific biomolecules and biomarkers can ensure maximum therapeutic efficacy and minimal side effects, eliminating the time wastage caused by ineffective drugs. Due to their excellent homotargeting capabilities, TDMVs can solve the challenge of precise targeting of personalized therapies and overcome the complex and cumbersome synthesis process of stimulus-responsive nanomedicines [33]. An example of personalized nanomedicine based on cancer cell membranes was obtained using B16F10 and red blood cells (RBC) membrane fusion vesicles and coating hollow copper sulfide nanoparticles loaded with doxorubicin (DOX) [34]. This study showed that the nanoparticle system had significant homotypic targeting with increasing cycle time and could effectively kill tumors.

For tumor therapy, tumor cell-derived membrane vesicles have promising application prospects and unique advantages (Figure 1). This review introduces the use of tumor cell-derived membrane vesicles, including cell membranes (TCMVs), exosomes (TEXs), microvesicles (TMVs) and apoptotic bodies in immunotherapy, discussing their benefits and limitations. Finally, a brief summary of the current challenges and prospects for using cancer cell-derived membrane vesicles to improve immunotherapy is presented.

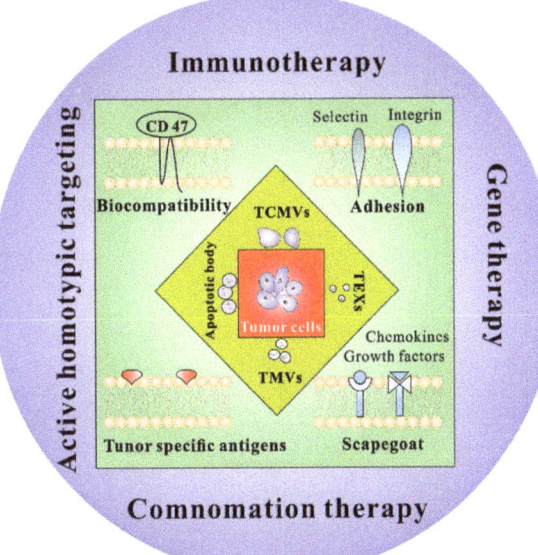

Figure 1. Properties and application prospects of TDMVs. TCMVs, tumor-derived cell membrane vesicles; TEXs, tumor-derived exosomes; TMVs, tumor-derived microvesicles.

2. Tumor Cell-Derived Membrane Vesicles

2.1. Tumor Cell Membrane Vesicles

Immunotherapy not only kills tumors in situ but also inhibits tumor metastasis and recurrence. However, how to precisely target tumor cells across the tumor extracellular matrix has been the main reason limiting the further development of immunotherapy. Due to the presence of large amounts of collagen, the extracellular matrix (ECM) of tumors is denser than normal cells, and the dense ECM makes it difficult for drugs to reach the core of tumors. The ECM can also bind to many drugs, further reducing the therapeutic effect [35,36]. At the same time, the rapid proliferation of the tumor makes the lymphatic reflux function absent, and the hydraulic pressure in the interstitial space of tumor tissue increases, making it difficult for the drugs injected intravenously to penetrate the tumor to achieve the therapeutic effect [37,38].

Tumor cells have the ability to self-target and adhere to homologous tumor tissue, known as "homologous adhesion" of tumor cells [39–41]. Many studies have shown that the abnormal expression of specific antigens on the surface of tumor cells (galactose lectin-3, N-calmucin, immunoglobulin-like cell-adhesion molecule) and cell adhesion molecules (epithelial cell adhesion molecules) contribute to this adhesion effect [41–43]. In particular, the immunoglobulin-like cell-adhesion molecule (Ig-CAM), which is overexpressed on the surface of tumor cells, supports homologous adhesion through homologous interactions with each of the other proteins (e.g., calmodulin, integrins) on the surface of adjacent cells [44–46]. This homologous adhesion confers specific self-recognition and self-targeting capabilities to tumor cells, which will provide a precise self-targeting function for immunotherapy.

TCMVs are tumor cell membranes extracted by squeezing using ultrasound and filter head to form nanoscale bilayer lipid structured vesicles that do not carry tumor cell genetic material. TCMVs have the properties of immune escape, unlimited growth capacity, anti-cell death, prolonged circulation time and homologous targeting. These properties allow TCMVs-based drug delivery systems to be highly aggregated at tumor sites (Table 1). TCMVs encapsulate adriamycin or paclitaxel and target tumor sites by exploiting homologous targeting of tumor cells [47,48]. Wan et al. delivered DOX and sorafenib (Sfn) with TMCVs to modulate the tumor microenvironment to sensitize the immune response against tumor immunogenic cell death (ICD). TMCVs delivery vehicle shows high stability, biocompatibility and excellent anticancer properties [49,50]. Cell membrane vesicle surface proteins provide antigen, recruit and activate antigen-presenting cells (APCs), while the wrapped drug can be released to kill tumor cells. MCF-7 cell membrane-encapsulated indocyanine green (ICG) nanoparticles were used in a diagnostic and therapeutic platform [41]. Thanks to the homologous targeting of cancer cell membranes, the particles aggregated heavily at tumor sites and reduced aggregation in the liver and kidney, showing good photothermal response and excellent imaging properties. Rao et al. designed a nanoprobe of MDA-MB-435 cancer cell membrane-encapsulated upconversion nanoparticles [51]. Lu et al. devised a highly sensitive multicellular miRNA imaging strategy for the first time by simultaneously encapsulating Au nanoparticles and DSN modified with miRNA fluorescent detection probes into tumor cell capsules to achieve ultrasensitive multiplex miRNA imaging in living cells [52]. Zhang et al. overexpressed PD-1 on cancer cell membranes to enhance anti-tumor responses by disrupting the PD-1/PD-L1 immunosuppressive axis [53]. Jiang et al. expressed CD80 on the surface of tumor cell membranes to make them into antigen-presentable particles [54]. The particles could directly stimulate activated tumor antigen-specific T cells by binding to the T cell receptor and CD28, and activated T cells suppress tumor growth by killing tumor cells expressing the same antigen. Zhu et al. designed a viral mimetic ternary nanoengineering constructed from DNA, Gd (III) and tumor cell membranes to enable host-specific gene therapy [54]. Membrane fusion technology expands the application of TCMVs. The particles obtained by fusing erythrocyte membranes with TCMVs have the biocompatibility of erythrocytes and the precise targeting ability of tumor cells and are loaded with photosensitizers to obtain excellent anti-tumor effects [34,55,56]. TCMVs carry all the antigenic proteins of tumor cells, but their immunogenicity is low. Researchers have fused TCMVs with biological membranes such as bacterial membranes, dendritic cell membranes and macrophage membranes to improve the immunogenicity of the particles and enhance antigen delivery, obtaining better immune effects [2,57–59].

Table 1. Representative applications of TCMVS in tumor therapy.

TCMVs Source	Engineering Strategy	Drug	Application	Ref.
Ovarian cancer cell	DC/TCMVs Fusion; PLGA core	CpG ODN	Vaccine	[60]
4T1 cell	DC/TCMVs fusion; MOF core	photosensitizer	PDT and vaccine	[61]
4T1 cell	DC/TCMVs fusion; MOF core	-	vaccine	[62]
Glioblastoma cell	$Cu_{2-x}Se$ NPs core	PD-L1 inhibitor and indoximod	ICT, PDT and ICD	[63]
Osteosarcoma cell	Macrophage cell membrane/TCMVs fusion; PLGA core	PTX	targeted tumor	[64]
solid tumor	Bacterial membrane/ TCMVs fusion	-	vaccine	[64,65]
B16F10 cell	Bacterial membrane/TCMVs fusion; PLGA core	ICG	Vaccine and PTT	[66]
B16F10	RBC/TCMVs fusion; CuS NPs core	DOX	Chemo-immunotherapy	[34]
4T1 cell	PLGA core	R837	vaccine	[67,68]
Ovarian cancer cell	RBC/TCMVs fusion; Fe_3O_4 core	ICG	PTT and Immunotherapy	[69]
4T1 cell	RBC/TCMVs fusion; Fe_3O_4 core	CSF-1R inhibitor:	Immunotherapy	[70]
HepG2 cell	Prussian blue Nps core	-	PTT	[56]
4T1 cell	alginate gel encapsulation	anti-PD-1 antibodies	vaccine	[71]
4T1 cell	PAMAM core	DOX	targeting and anti-metastasis treatment	[72]
HCT116	F127 core	R837	vaccine	[33]
4T1 cell and B16F10 cell	Encoded SIRPα and PD-1	-	ICT and CD47 blockade	[73]
B16F10	-	DMA and Cdk5 inhibitor	ICT	[74]
Hela cell	PLGA core	PTX and siRNA	Chemo-immunotherapy	[48]
B16-OVA cell	OVA assembly core	Ce6	PDT	[75]
lung carcinoma cell	-	Dox and Sorafenib	ICD and ICT	[49]
4T1 cell	Surface-anchored CD80 and IL-12	-	vaccine	[76]
MCF-7	Au NPs core	MicroRNA	cancer diagnosis	[52]
4T1 cell and B16F10 cell	thermosensitive hydrogel encapsulation	black phosphorus	Vaccine, PTT and ICT	[77]
B16F10 cell	cationic polymers core	DOX	Chemo-immunotherapy	[78]
Tumor cell	Surface-anchored anti CD205	-	vaccine	[79]
B16-OVA	Surface-anchored mannose; PLGA core	R837	vaccine	[80]
B16F10	PLGA core	CpG	vaccine	[81]

ICD, Immunogenic cell death; ICT, immune checkpoint therapy; NPs, nanoparticles; PDT, photodynamic therapy; PTT, photothermal therapy.

2.2. Tumor Extracellular Vesicles

Extracellular vesicles (EVs) are nano- or micron-sized particles composed of phospholipid bilayers constitutively or inducibly released by all cells, including exosomes, microvesicles and apoptotic bodies (Table 2). The components of natural extracellular vesicles mainly contain proteins, nucleic acids, lipids and metabolites, which act as message transmitters, regulate recipient cells' physiological and pathological states by delivering signaling molecules to other cells, and participate in the development and progression of many diseases [82–84]. They reflect the metabolic state of the organism and the function of cells under different pathological conditions and have potential clinical diagnostic value. Meanwhile, extracellular vesicles are the organism's components with low immunogenicity and good biocompatibility, exhibiting tissue targeting mediated by surface molecules (integral proteins and glycan) and the ability to transport biomolecules to recipient cells promising for drug delivery applications [85]. Currently, therapeutic drugs are loaded into extracellular vesicles by incubation, extrusion, electroporation, ultrasound and genetic modification for therapeutic research in diseases such as cardiac repair, liver diseases, lung diseases and tumors [86–88].

Table 2. Classification of different types of extracellular vesicles.

	Exosomes	Microvesicles	Apoptotic Bodies
Size	20–100 nm	50–1000 nm	500–2000 nm
Biogenesis	The inner membrane forms multivesicles within the cell that fuses with the plasma membrane to release exosomes into the extracellular compartment	Local changes in plasma membrane stiffness and curvature, cell surface shrinkage and outward blistering	Released by belting of apoptotic cell membrane
Contents	mRNA, microRNA, cytoplasmic and membrane protein, MHC	mRNA, miroRNA, noncoding RNAs, cytoplasmic and membrane protein	nuclear fractions, cytoplasmic protein, cell organelles
Biomakers	Tetraspanins, ESCRT peoteins, flotillin, TSG101	Integrins, seltctins, CD40 ligand	Phosphatidylserine, annexin V
Ref.	[89,90]	[91,92]	[93,94]

TEVs secreted by tumor cells play an essential role in tumor development. TEVs interacting with ECM can induce tumor cell adhesion and targeted migration [95]. On the other hand, TEVs carry a variety of bioactive substances (proteins, RNA, lipids) that enhance vascular permeability and create a microenvironment conducive to tumor cell metastasis [96–98]. For example, lung cancer cell exosome miRNA-9 promotes endothelial cell migration and angiogenesis through the downregulation of the SOCS5-JAK-STAT pathway [99]. Glioma or breast cancer cells secrete glutaminyl transferase-containing microvesicles that can alter the tumor microenvironment and promote tumorigenesis [100]. Tumor cells secrete DNA-containing apoptotic vesicles capable of transferring from source cells to normal cells, triggering the expression of oncogenes in fibroblasts [101]. In addition, EVs from tumor cells such as melanoma, breast and lung cancer have been reported to carry the immunosuppressive molecule PD-L1, which promotes tumor growth by misfiring T cells through the binding of the PD-L1 structural domain to PD-1 [102].

TEVs can be used not only as biomarkers or drug delivery vehicles due to their unique advantages but also for tumor immunotherapy. Many clinical trials evaluate the composition of TEVs as biomarkers for determining cancer staging and the effectiveness of oncology drug therapy (Table 3). Researchers are evaluating the expression profiles of exosomal miRNA and PD-L1 before and after immunotherapy in patients with non-small cell lung cancer and exploring the potential of exosomes as biomarkers for predicting the efficacy of anticancer drugs (NCT04427475). Koh et al. designed an extracellular vesicle-based immune checkpoint inhibitor that achieved tumor regression by blocking CD47 with SIRPα on phagocytes, leading to more extensive CD8$^+$ T cell infiltration in tumors [103]. TEVs carry tumor-associated antigens (TAA) that stimulate in vivo through the Fas/FasL signaling pathway CD8$^+$ T cells to kill tumors. Meanwhile, TEVs enhance antigen uptake by DCs and trigger more robust immune responses by inducing specific CD4$^+$ T cell proliferation. TEVs play an important role in regulating immune cells in the tumor microenvironment as mediators between tumor and immune cells.

Table 3. Representative applications of TEVs in tumor therapy.

TEVs Sourse	Engineering Strategy	Drug	Application	Ref.
MDA-MB-231 cells	alpha-lactalbumin-engineered TEVs	ELANE and Hiltonol	Vaccine and ICD	[104]
Colorectal cancer cell	-	microRNA 424	immunotherapy	[105]
CT26 cell	thermosensitive liposomes/gene-engineered TEVs Fusion	-	PTT and CD47 blockade	[106]
HEPA1–6	-	HMGN1	vaccine	[107]
4T1 cell	AIE luminogen/TEVs fusion	Dexamethasone	PDT	[108]
EL4 cell	gold-silver nanorods core	CpG	PTT and immunotherapy	[109]
HER2 expressing breast cancer	encoded anti-CD3 and anti-HER2 antibodies	-	immunotherapy	[110]
Serum exosomes from tumor-bearing mice	-	black phosphorus	PTT and vaccine	[111]
B16BL6 cells	encoding streptavidin lactadherin protein	CpG	immunotherapy	[112]

2.2.1. Exosomes

Compared to synthetic nanoparticles, exosomes have the natural advantage of less toxicity and less rejection by the immune system. In addition, it allows them to cross some barriers, such as the placental barrier and blood–brain barrier [113–115]. Exosomes are not formed by direct outgrowth or shedding from the plasma membrane; instead, they are formed by inward outgrowth from the inner membrane, resulting in the formation of intracellular multi-vesicular vesicles, which then fuse with the plasma membrane and release exosomes into the extracellular compartment [89,90]. Exosomes are common membrane-bound nanovesicles that contain a variety of biomolecules such as lipids, proteins and nucleic acids. Exosome surface-bound proteins are derived from the cytoplasmic membrane from which they originate, and thus exosomes released from antigen-presenting cells, DCs and tumor cells have promising applications in vaccine development [116]. In addition, exosomes have characteristics such as lipid membranes and particle sizes in the nanoscale size, which can reduce the clearance or damage of their contents by complement or macrophages, thus prolonging the circulating half-life and improving biological activity. Chemical or biological modification of exosomes can enhance the potential therapeutic capacity of exosomes. Thus, exosomes can be used as drug delivery vehicles to treat diseases [117]. Exosomes have advantages such as good biocompatibility, low immunogenicity and the ability to cross the blood–brain barrier, which facilitate the delivery of nucleic acids or drugs. Exosomes carry tumor necrosis factor-related apoptosis-inducing ligands that transduce pro-apoptotic signals to different tumor cells, thereby inducing apoptosis in cancer cells and ultimately inhibiting tumor progression [118]. In addition, exosomes can transport small molecule compound drugs, such as paclitaxel and adriamycin, across the blood–brain barrier for targeted delivery [114,119]. Exosomes can eliminate the drug resistance properties of tumor cells, such as wrapping chemotherapeutic drugs into tumor cell-derived exosomes. They are preferentially internalized by tumor cells and subsequently release anti-tumor drugs, thereby reversing tumor cell resistance in vitro. There are differences in the surface protein composition of exosomes of different cellular origins, and their ability to transport RNA-like drugs varies. Mesenchymal cell-derived exosomes expressing the CD47 protein that protects cells from phagocytosis enhanced the ability to deliver miRNAs to pancreatic tumors, significantly improving overall survival in a mouse model [120].

The secretion of tumor-derived exosomes (TEXs) is mainly attributed to the overexpression of Rab3D and the acidic tumor microenvironment [121], which carries information characteristic of malignant tumors, such as NKG2-D-ligand on the surface of melanoma-derived exosomes [122]. It shows that TEXs play a crucial role in cancer metastasis and proliferation [123]. However, TEXs mode of communication with cells is still not fully understood. Current scholarship suggests that TEXs rely mainly on lipid rafts in the cytoplasmic membrane of target cells [124], cholesterol homeostasis [125] or membrane fusion [121] to enter the recipient cells. Uptake of TEXs by ordinary endothelial cells activates angiogenic signaling pathways in the cells to stimulate new blood vessel formation and promote tumor growth [126]. At the same time, TEXs can be secreted into the tumor microenvironment via autocrine and paracrine signaling to initiate epithelial-mesenchymal transition (EMT), which has a high potential to form tumor metastases once it spreads to the systemic circulation [127]. In addition, TEXs can evade immune surveillance and promote irrepressible metastatic progression [128]. TEVs can influence tumor progression by affecting the role of immune cells. It found that TEVs carry NKG2D ligands that bind directly to natural killer (NK) cells, downregulate NKG2D expression, inhibit NK cell activation and significantly reduce the recognition and killing effect of NK cells on tumors [129].TEVs can regulate macrophage polarization, organize phagocytosis of tumor cells by macrophages and enhance tumor cell drug resistance [130,131]. TEVs act on $CD8^+$ T and $CD4^+$ T cells through PD-L1 on the membrane surface, resulting in suppression of T cell function, a significant reduction in secreted effector cytokines (TNF-α, IL-2, TNF-α), and a significant reduction in the expression of CD69 and CD25, markers of $CD8^+$ T cell and $CD4^+$ T cell activation [132–134].

Engineered exosomes enhance anti-tumor capacity through precise targeting, high bioavailability and enhanced efficiency. Surface modification of TEXs through cellular transgene expression, chemical modification and electrostatic interactions can further enhance the targeting efficiency of exosomes to cancer cells. TEVs have been used as delivery systems for small molecule drugs, proteins and nucleic acids [135,136]. In addition, TEXs promote resistance to various chemotherapeutic agents and antibodies, which provides a multi-component diagnostic window for tumor detection [137,138]. Currently, more than 40 clinical trials of TEXs biomarkers are in progress, according to the Clinical Trials Registry website (clinicaltrials.gov).

2.2.2. Microvesicles

Unlike exosomes, microvesicles are a type of Evs formed directly by the cytoplasmic membrane through outward outgrowth form [139]. The biogenesis of microvesicles involves local stiffness and curvature changes caused by the rearrangement of lipids and proteins on the cytoplasmic membrane, followed by the vertical transport of molecular material to the plasma membrane to form specific contents, and finally, the use of surface contraction mechanisms to squeeze leading to the outward blistering of the plasma membrane to produce vesicles [91,92]. Microvesicles not only randomly wrap the cell contents but also selectively incorporate proteins and nucleic acids, etc., into the vesicles. It has been shown that ARF6 is one of the microvesicle regulatory selective proteins [140], which binds to Ras-related small GTP and is involved in the activation and regulation of intracellular somatic recycling and extracellular peripheral actin remodeling [141]. EGFR, Akt, MT1-MMP and other complex kinase receptors, $\beta 1$ integrin receptor, MHC-I, VAMP3 and others enter microvesicles via ARF6-regulated intracellular somatic recycling [142–144]. Meanwhile, AFR6 can translocate the ARF6-Exportin5 axis of miRNA into microvesicles [145].

Tumor-derived microvesicles (TMVs) can deliver biologically active components, including oncoproteins, oncogenes, soluble factors, chemokine receptors, specific enzymes and microRNAs [146–148]. TMVs help tumor cells evade by exposing FasL proteins, tumor necrosis factor (TNF)-associated regulatory ligands, etc., to induce apoptosis in $CD8^+$ T cells' immune response [149,150]. Breast cancer cells or glioma cells secrete glutamyltransferase microvesicles to promote tumorigenesis and improve the tumor microenvironment [100]. In breast cancer cells cultured in a hypoxic environment, Rab22a is co-localized with microvesicles by a situation that regulates microvesicle formation and material sorting [151]. VEGF released from tumor cells is an influential factor in promoting tumor angiogenesis [152]. TMVs were reported to carry CD147 to promote VEGF secretion and thus induce angiogenesis in ovarian cancer [153].

Nevertheless, Zhang et al. observed that miRNA-29a/c carried by TMV inhibited the growth of vascular cells by suppressing VEGF expression in gastric cancer cells [154]. Thus, miRNA-loaded microvesicles could be designed to suppress tumor growth by blocking blood vessel generation. Multidrug resistance mediated by the plasma membrane multidrug efflux transporter, P-glycoprotein (P-gp), often leads to tumor treatment failure [155]. In breast cancer, the transient receptor potential channel 5 (TRPC5) protein carried by TMV was demonstrated to regulate the expression of P-gp and promote tumor drug resistance [156]. Dong et al. found that the TRPC5 blocking antibody T5E3 reduced P-gp expression in human breast P-gp production in human epithelial cells and converted drug-resistant cells to non-drug-resistant cells [157]. MVs can also merge with other biological membranes to transport anti-tumor drugs into cells as a type of EVs. Therefore, TMVs with homologous targeting might be suitable vehicles for anti-tumor therapy [76]. Meanwhile, TMVs can serve as vehicles carrying biological signals or molecules that facilitate tumor cell invasion and metastasis and serve as biomarkers to predict cancer patient prognosis [158].

2.2.3. Apoptotic Bodies

Apoptotic vesicles refer to the condensation of chromatin during apoptosis leading to blistering of the plasma membrane enclosing the cell contents into distinct membrane-enveloped vesicles, which prevent toxic components of dying cells from damaging the cells [159,160]. Apoptotic vesicles are the largest extracellular vesicles, approximately 500–2000 nm in size, and typically contain DNA fragments, histones and cytoplasmic organelle fragments [93]. The markers of apoptotic vesicles are usually considered to be Annexin V, thrombospondin and C3b [94,161,162]. In the normal state, apoptotic vesicles are cleared by phagocytosis through specific interactions between recognition receptors on and specific changes in the membrane composition of apoptotic cells [162–164]. Recent studies have indicated that apoptotic vesicles are implicated in tumor progression, metastasis and microenvironment formation. Apoptotic vesicles carry DNA fragments capable of transferring at the level of adjacent but different cell types. Apoptotic vesicles can transport tumor DNA from human C-MYC and H-RASV12-transfected rat fibroblasts to wild-type mouse fibroblasts, activating the full tumorigenic potential of wild-type cells [165]. DNA packaged into lymphoma-derived apoptotic vesicles is phagocytosed by surrounding fibroblasts, leading to the fusion of lymphoma-derived DNA into the genome of fibroblasts [166]. In addition, apoptotic vesicles can transfer proteins to phagocytic cells such as macrophages and DCs for immunomodulation [167–169]. For example, macrophages can phagocytose apoptotic vesicles containing auto-antigens, suggesting that auto-antigens can be transferred to specialized phagocytes, providing new ideas for tumor vaccine research [170].

3. Engineering Tumor Cell-Derived Membrane Vesicles in Cancer Treatment
3.1. Encapsulation

In 2011, Zhang took the lead in proposing a camouflage strategy, using erythrocyte membrane wrapping material to obtain camouflage to evade the clearance of nanocarriers by immune cells, thus deriving a biomimetic delivery platform for nanocarriers modified with cell membranes [171]. At the same time, the encapsulated nanocarriers also help provide physical support for membrane vesicles, ensuring that the functional components are embedded in the membrane function. A variety of materials, including mesoporous silicon, polymers, magnetic nanoparticles, MOFs, gold nanoparticles and upconversion nanoparticles, are encapsulated to function in membrane vesicles [72,171–175]. Kroll et al. used TCMVs to encapsulate PLGA nanoparticles loaded with immune adjuvant CpG and achieved significant therapeutic and preventive effects (Figure 2) [81]. The use of PLGA nanoparticles with small particle sizes is beneficial to lymph node drainage, and CpG can efficiently induce the maturation of APCs cells to break the immunosuppression of the tumor microenvironment. TCMVs that retain cell surface antigenic proteins are wrapped on the surface of nanoparticles to more realistically mimic the surface structure of tumor cells and induce anti-tumor immune responses more efficiently. Li et al. developed a novel cancer vaccine with Fe_3O_4 magnetic nanoclusters as the core and anti-CD205-modified TCMVs as the coat [79]. Vaccine homing in lymph nodes was achieved using Fe_3O_4 magnetism. Meanwhile, camouflaged TCMVs act as reservoirs for various antigens, enabling subsequent multi-antigen responses. In addition, the modified anti-CD205 directed more nanoparticles to $CD8^+$ DCs, promoting antigen cross-presentation. These specific benefits lead to the considerable proliferation of T cells with clonal diversity and cytotoxic activity.

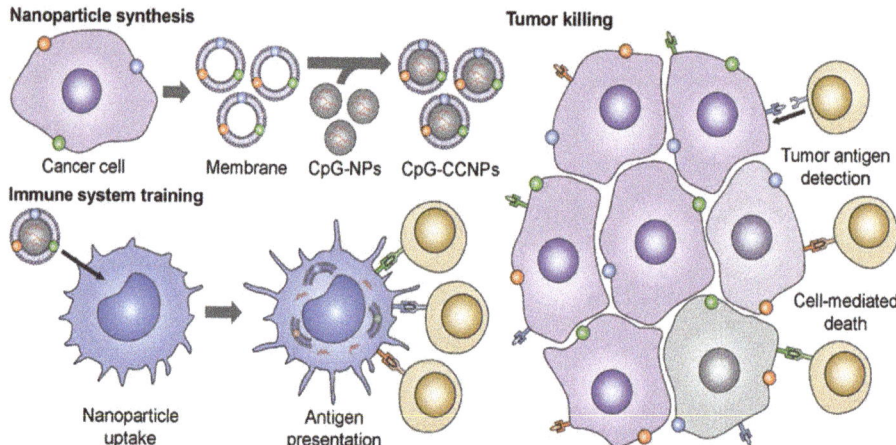

Figure 2. Schematic diagram of TCMVs-based CpG-anti-tumor vaccines. Use of cancer cell membranes carrying tumor-specific antigens to wrap CpG-loaded nanoparticles to generate nanoparticle tumor vaccines. The tumor-specific antigens on the surface of TCMVs promote uptake and presentation by antigen-presenting cells, activating multiple specific T cells that act to monitor and kill tumor cells. Reproduced with permission [81]. Copyright 2017, Wiley-VCH.

3.2. Surface Modification

The surface of cell-derived membrane vesicles is composed of polysaccharides, proteins, lipids, etc. They provide various surface properties that allow modification by foreign materials. For example, thiol and amine groups on the membrane surface can interact with maleimide-modified nanoparticles on the membrane surface via thiol and carboxylation reactions [80,176,177]. Jia et al. engineered an integrated glioma exosome-based diagnostic and therapeutic platform that carried curcumin (Cur) and superparamagnetic iron oxide nanoparticles (SPIONs) [178]. These TEXs were conjugated to peptides targeting neuropilin-1 by click chemistry for glioma-targeted exosome imaging and therapeutic function. Experiments with glioma cells and in-suit glioma models demonstrate that such engineered TEXs can smoothly cross the blood–brain barrier, providing favorable conditions for targeted imaging and treatment of gliomas. Chemical coupling does not destroy the integrity of membrane vesicles and has the advantages of high selectivity and fast reaction speed. However, conditions such as osmotic pressure and temperature must be strictly controlled during the reaction. Additionally, the residual solvents should be removed to avoid rupture or denaturation of membrane vesicles after the reaction [179]. The surface modification of membrane vesicles by physical means such as hydrophobic interaction, receptor–ligand binding and electrostatic interaction is also a commonly used method [103,180]. Membrane vesicles have lipid bilayers and negative charges, enabling hydrophobic and positively charged materials to adsorb on membrane vesicles stably. Physical strategies are readily achieved by direct co-incubation with cells or EVs within a specific temperature range. DSPE-PEG is a commonly used auxiliary phospholipid, which can bind to RBD, maleimide, folic acid and other ligands to enhance the targeting of materials [181–183]. Yang et al. used mannose-modified DSPE-PEG to insert into TCMVs to enhance antigen presentation by utilizing mannose receptors carried on the surface of APCs [175]. Nakase binds cationic lipids to the surface of exosomes via electrostatic interactions, facilitating the uptake of exosomes [184]. Although the physical strategy is easy to operate and has high safety, it still suffers from the difficulty in controlling the adhesion strength, and the resulting vesicles may dissociate due to in vivo shear forces.

3.3. Membrane Fusion

To enhance the effect of tumor cell-derived membrane vesicles, the researchers used different kinds of materials to fuse them. In addition to excellent biocompatibility, senescent or damaged red blood cells are eliminated by cells such as macrophages and DCs in the spleen, providing spleen targeting capabilities [69,185]. Wang et al. designed a pH-responsive copolymer micelle camouflaged by the erythrocyte and TCMVs hybrid membranes. In the acidic tumor microenvironment, the micelle exhibited a membrane escape effect, which could promote recognition and interaction with tumor-associated macrophages [70]. Han et al. obtained a personalized vaccine by fusing red blood cells with TCMVs by ultrasound and extrusion. The vaccine particles can be effectively delivered to the spleen and activate the T cell immune response [186]. The fusion vesicles of DCs-derived cell membranes and TCMVs retain the antigens of tumor cells and carry costimulatory substances such as MHC-I, MHC-II, CD80 and CD86, and retain the antigen presentation and T cell activation functions of DCs [60–62,187]. The macrophages are highly infiltrating and can induce better tumor treatment and recurrence prevention after fusion with TCMVs [64,188]. The vesicles obtained by fusion of multiple TCMVs carry multiple tumor-specific antigens, which can treat multiple tumors and prevent recurrence [73,189]. Years of research have found a large number of pathogen-associated molecular patterns (PAMPs) on the surface of bacterial membranes, such as lipopolysaccharides, mannose, lifters and lectins. These PAMPs can induce the recognition and binding of highly expressed pattern recognition receptors (PRRs) on the surface of innate immune cells, thereby activating innate and adaptive immunity and clearing tumors [2,190]. Chen et al. designed hybrid vesicles of attenuated Salmonella fused to TCMVs [66]. This hybrid vesicle inherits the immune functions of both parents and exhibits a robust immune response to tumor cells. In addition, loading indocyanine green (ICG) inside the hybrid vesicles can induce local photothermal effects, effectively destroying solid tumors and inhibiting tumor recurrence. Zuo et al. constructed hybrid vesicles fused with E. coli membranes and TCMVs to inhibit tumor metastasis (Figure 3) [191]. Due to the immunogenicity of bacterial membranes, hybrid vesicles are more likely to be accumulated in the draining lymph nodes than single TCMVs. The activated innate immune system further activates the adaptive immune response involving T lymphocytes, effectively inhibiting tumor growth, recurrence and metastasis to the lung. Furthermore, hybrid vesicles induced adaptive immune responses in a syngeneic bilateral tumor model, reversibly demonstrating the effect of individualized immunotherapy.

3.4. Genetic Engineering

Genetic engineering has higher controllability, safety and flexibility than membrane fusion technology. Genetic engineering transfers the genetic information of living cells into membrane vesicles through physical methods such as viral vectors, cationic polymers, electroporation and microinjection [53,54,192,193]. Rao et al. fused TCMVs containing SiRPα variant, M1 macrophage membrane and platelet membrane to obtain hybrid fusion vesicles. By blocking the CD47/SIRP innate immune pathway and promoting M2 to M1 repolarization in the tumor microenvironment, local recurrence and metastasis of malignant melanoma were significantly prevented [194]. Meng et al. constructed a fusion cell vesicle of a high-affinity SIRPα variant and PD-1 (Figure 4) [73]. First, 4T1 cells and B16F10 cells could express SIRPα and PD-1, respectively, by gene editing, and the cell membranes of the two were fused to obtain fused TCMVs. Simultaneously blocking the CD47/SIRP and PD-1/PD-L1 immunosuppressive axis via SIPRα and PD-1 promotes antigen presentation by macrophages and DCs and enhances anti-tumor T cell immunity.

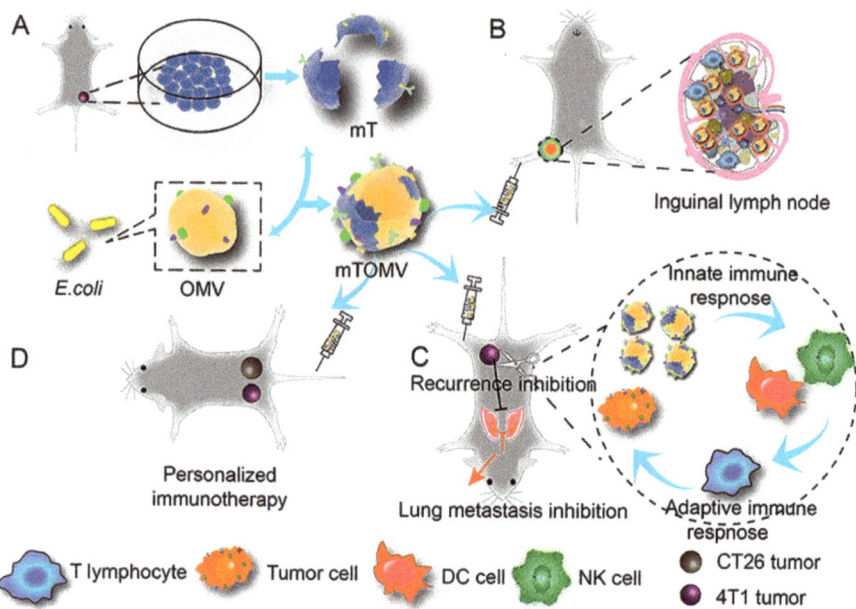

Figure 3. Schematic illustration of fusion vesicles of bacterial outer membrane and TCMVs for personalized immunotherapy. (**A**) The fabrication of fusion vesicles. (**B**) Accumulation and retention behavior of inguinal lymph nodes following right posterior intraplantar injection. (**C**) Fusion vesicles inhibit tumor lung metastasis. (**D**) Bilateral tumor model to validate the effect of fusion vesicle personalized immunotherapy. Reproduced with permission [191]. Copyright 2021, American Chemical Society.

Similarly, taking advantage of the targeting properties of TEVs, introducing genetic information such as small interfering RNA (siRNA) and miRNA from other cells into TEVs can induce the expression of transgenic proteins in target cells and prevent RNA from being degraded by RNases [194–197]. Ohno targeted miRNA delivery to EGFR-expressing cancer tissues using modified exosomes with GE11 peptide or EGF on the surface [198]. Morishita et al. genetically engineered melanoma cells by transfection with a plasmid encoding a streptavidin-lacadherin fusion protein to generate genetically engineered exosomes. A vaccine combining these engineered exosomes with a biotinylated CpG adjuvant in vitro induced strong anti-tumor effects in a mouse model of melanoma [112]. High mobility group nucleosome-binding protein 1 (HMGN1) is a protein adjuvant that can enhance the response of DCs to exogenous antigens and continuously induce Th1 immune responses [199]. Zuo et al. directly anchored the functional N-terminal domain of HMGN1 (N1ND) to TEXs through CP05, an exosome anchoring peptide, which enhanced the maturation and activation of DCs and accelerated the generation of memory T cells. The approach generated strong and durable anti-tumor immunity [107]. Shi et al. found that genetically engineered exosomes with anti-CD3 and anti-HER2 antibodies led SMART-Exos to efficiently and selectively induce HER2-expressing tumor-specific immunity, thereby providing a new tumor immunotherapy idea for HER2-positive breast cancer [200,201].

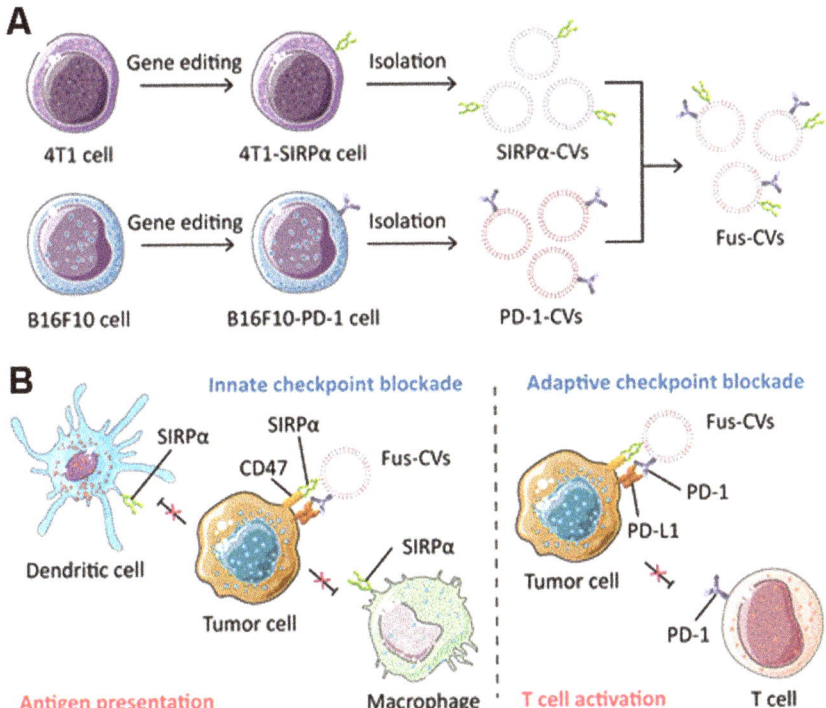

Figure 4. Gene-edited fusion vesicles for multi-targeted immune checkpoint therapy. (**A**) SIRPα variants CV1 and PD-1 were overexpressed on 4T1 and B16F10 cancer cells, respectively, and fusion vesicles were then prepared. (**B**) Fusion vesicles promote antigen uptake and presentation by antigen-presenting cells and enhance anti-tumor T-cell immunity by blocking CD47/SIRPα and PD-1/PD-L1immunosuppressive axis. Reproduced with permission [73]. Copyright 2021, Wiley-VCH.

4. The Application of Tumor Cell-Derived Membrane Vesicles to Personalized Immunotherapy

Personalized therapy is the most suitable therapy for the patient, taking into account the individual circumstances of the patient's genetic information, epigenetic and environmental factors. It also ensures the effectiveness of prescriptions, reduces the adverse reactions caused by traditional treatments and costs more time for treatment [202]. The development of tumor cell-derived membrane vesicles technology provides precise targeting of tumor tissue for personalized immunotherapy. In addition, tumor cell-derived membrane vesicles can combine with stimuli-responsive treatments such as light, sound, magnetism, pH and reactive oxygen species to improve tumor personalized treatment effects, promote tumor regression and inhibit metastasis and recurrence [74,203,204].

4.1. Cancer Vaccines

As emerging tumor immunotherapy, tumor vaccines utilize the administration of tumor cell-associated antigens and other immune stimulatory signals to train the body's immune system to recognize and fight tumors [65,205,206]. It possesses the advantages of high specificity, low cost and few adverse reactions. Corresponding tumor vaccines such as breast and bladder cancer have also entered the clinical trial stage. Considerable inherited heterogeneity exists between patients with the same type of cancer [71,207]. The complexity and diversity of antigens result in significant differences in antigen presentation between individuals with the same tumor type, leading to various efficacy between different populations. Vaccines from lysates of tumor tissues or tumor cell lines contain intact tumor cell-specific antigens.

Tumor cell-derived membrane vesicles-coated drugs are a potent anticancer weapon. In addition to inducing a highly specific immune response, they also can target homologous tumor cells [81,110]. Ye et al. used melanoma tumor cell lysate as antigen combined with photothermal therapy to enhance antigen uptake by DCs, promote T cell migration and local pro-inflammatory cytokine production and effectively target primary and distal secondary primary tumors [208]. Yang et al. proposed to coat imiquimod adjuvant nanoparticles with mannose-modified TCMVs, so that the vaccine can be taken up and presented by antigen-presenting cells in large quantities, triggering an anti-tumor immune response [175]. Ma et al. prepared a tumor cell lysate-based nanovaccine, which induced tumor-specific T cell responses, and both adaptive and innate immune responses against cancer cells were activated by the nanovaccine [209]. DCs are important immune cells linking innate and adaptive immunity and serve as vaccine targets. Lu et al. reported a hydrogel personalized vaccine loaded with granulocyte-macrophage colony-stimulating factor (GM-CSF) using surgically resected tumor cell lysates as antigens. DCs are recruited by releasing GM-CSF from the hydrogel, thereby providing a fully personalized tumor antigen repertoire, exhibiting excellent tumor-suppressive effects in postoperative tumor models [210].

However, the complex intracellular proteins and organelle components in whole-cell lysates can disrupt the recognition and presentation of antigens [211]. In contrast to whole cell lysates, TCMVs have complete cell membrane protein antigens (including neoantigens) and do not contain complex cytoplasmic proteins and components, making them the best tumor vaccine candidates. TCMVs vaccine triggers individualized immune responses against corresponding tumors and induces more effective and durable anti-tumor immune responses while avoiding tumor cytoplasmic protein interference and immune escape caused by downregulation of partial antigen expression [67,212]. Kroll et al. designed a nanovaccine with TCMVs encapsulating CpG, using the antigenic proteins on TCMVs to activate the body-specific immune response, leading to an anti-tumor effect [81]. Xiong et al. reported a calmodulin-expressing TCMVs wrapper-loaded R837 nanovaccine that used calmodulin exposed on the surface of TCMVs to induce active uptake of the vaccine by DCs, enabling simultaneous delivery of adjuvant and antigen and departure of a personalized immune response against 4T1 tumors [67]. Xu et al. constructed a fluorinated polymer-based personalized tumor vaccine that showed a robust immune memory effect in several postoperative models and effectively protected against tumor recurrence [213]. Zhang et al. fused the Toll-like receptor agonist monophosphoryl lipid A (MPLA) into the phospholipid bilayer of TCMVs to increase the activity of APCs, thereby activating $CD8^+$ T cells to kill tumors [86]. Liu et al. prepared a DCs and TCMVs fusion vesicle tumor vaccine (Figure 5) [62]. The fusion of the two immune-associated cells resulted in high expression of tumor antigen complexes and immune costimulatory molecules on the fusion vesicles, allowing the vaccine particles to exert APCs to stimulate T cell immune activation and induce a favorable immune response. In addition, eukaryotic-prokaryotic nanovaccines constructed using TCMVs with bacterial extracellular vesicles showed powerful therapeutic and therapeutic effects, providing new perspectives on the design of tumor immunogenicity, adjuvant and scalable vaccine platforms [66].

The immunogenicity of TEXs could be improved by gene editing [214]. TEXs loaded with IL-2 and IL-18 cytokine genes could induce potent specific killing responses [215,216]. Yin et al. anchored the TLR4 agonist HMGN1 short functional peptide to TEXs from different sources through the exosome anchoring peptide CP05 and obtained a more immunogenic DC vaccine, especially in the middle and late stages with low immune response rate. In the mouse model of hepatocellular carcinoma, the tumor microenvironment was significantly improved, and long-term immune response and tumor inhibition were obtained [107]. ICD can enhance tumor antigen exposure, promote the release of immune-stimulating tumor cell content, and facilitate the uptake of dying tumor cells by DCs. Huang et al. constructed a combination of TLR3 agonist Hiltonol and ICD inducer

ELANE to engineer TEXs that can activate DCs in situ in a mouse xenograft model of poorly immunogenic triple-negative breast cancer and tumor organs derived from patients with hot tears; both produced effective tumor suppression [104]. In conclusion, engineered tumor-cell-derived membrane vesicles have a promising application in developing anti-tumor vaccines due to their great advantage of carrying tumor-specific antigens.

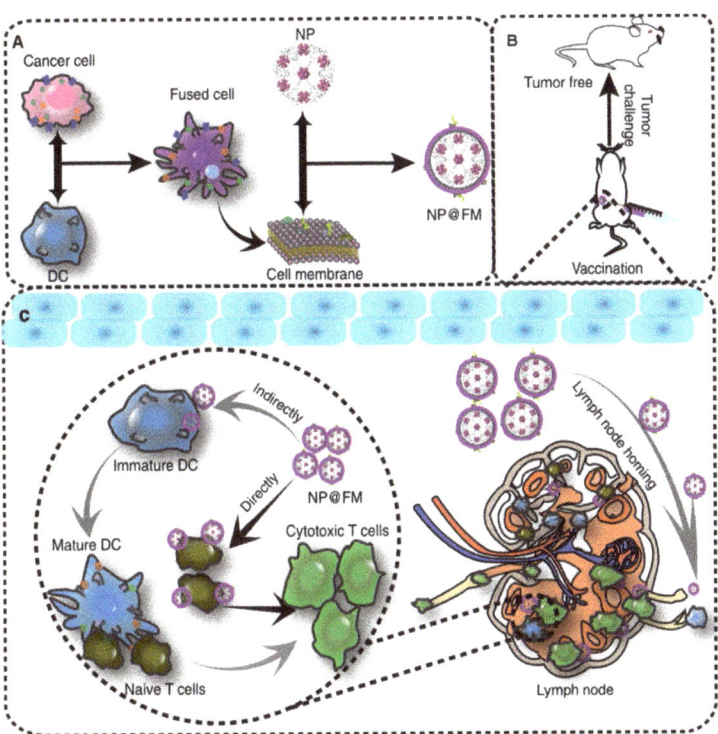

Figure 5. Fusion vesicles encapsulating MOFs for tumor prevention. (**A**) Preparation of fused vesicles encapsulating MOFs. (**B**) Fusion vesicle vaccination for tumor prophylaxis. (**C**) Mechanisms by which fusion vesicles induce immune response. Reprinted/adapted with permission from Ref. [62]. 2019, Springer Nature.

4.2. Immune Checkpoint Therapy

Immune checkpoint therapy (ICT) has achieved therapeutic effects in a variety of tumor models, but in clinical trials, the response rates of different patients to ICT vary widely, and most patients cannot benefit from ICT therapy. The development of tumor cell-derived membrane vesicles technology provides a new idea for ICT. Li et al. designed an injectable hydrogel based on TCMVs with the powerful ability to simultaneously reprogram local tumors and circulating exosomal PD-L1 to facilitate PD-L1-based immune checkpoint therapy (Figure 6) [74]. Using sodium oxidized alginate-modified TCMVs as a gelling agent, hydrogels were formed in vivo with Ca^{2+} channel inhibitors (DMA) and cell cycle protein-dependent kinase 5 (Cdk5) inhibitors to create an immune ecology as an antigen pool. Reducing the amount of circulating exosomal PD-L1, decreasing genetic PD-L1 expression in tumor cells, attenuating IFN-γ-induced PD-L1 adaptive immune tolerance and achieving downregulation of PD-L1 expression in tumor cells and exosomes.

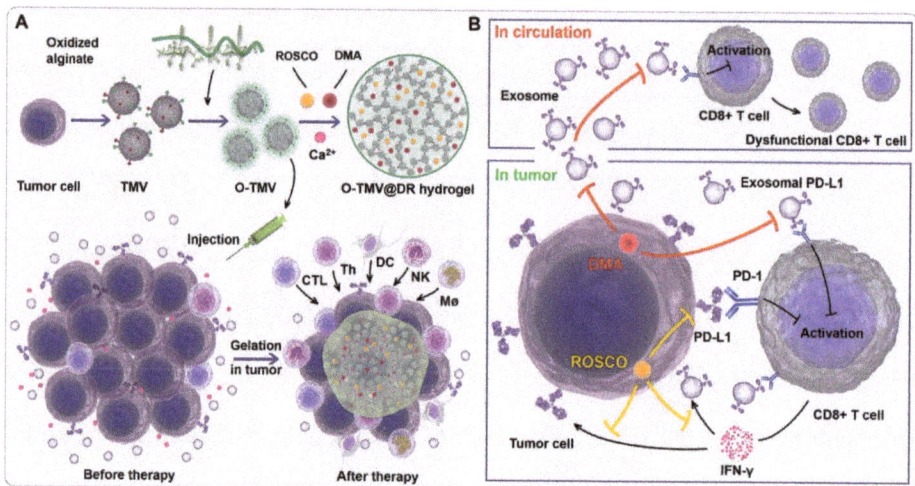

Figure 6. Schematic diagram of TCMVs-based injectable hydrogels for ICT. (**A**) Oxidized sodium alginate is adsorbed on the surface of TCMVs to form a gel, and after injection into the tumor, Ca^{2+} in the microenvironment would chelate with the particles to form a gel, causing an antigen reservoir effect and continuous recruitment to activate antigen-presenting cells and lymphocytes. (**B**) Adding DMA and ROSCO to the gel blocks Ca^{2+} entry into tumor cells and inhibits the secretion of circulating PD-L1 and tumor PD-L1 exosomes. Reproduced with permission [74]. Copyright 2021, Wiley-VCH.

miRNA-424 in TEVs inhibits the CD80/86-CD28 costimulatory pathway in DCs and T cells, resulting in resistance to ICT. TEVs with knockdown of miRNA-424 increase the efficacy of immune checkpoint blockade therapy and stimulate anti-tumor immunity [105]. CD47 is overexpressed on a variety of tumor cells and activates "don't eat me" signaling by binding to SIRPα, causing immune escape of tumor cells from the mononuclear phagocyte system. Researchers designed exosomes containing SIRPα variants as immune checkpoint blockers, thereby antagonizing the interaction between CD47 and SIRPα, inducing enhanced tumor phagocytosis, and triggering an effective anti-tumor T-cell response [53,103,106].

4.3. Combination Therapy

In order to achieve complementary advantages and functional amplification of various therapeutic methods, researchers have conducted many studies on the combination of immunotherapy with other methods such as chemotherapy, photothermal and photodynamic therapy [217–220]. Wu et al. developed a chemoimmunotherapy-based TCMVs nanoparticle, using the homotypic targeting ability of TCMVs to deliver DOX to the tumor site, causing tumor cell death to form a tumor in situ vaccine [78]. TEVS-loaded chemotherapy drugs can promote drug uptake and reverse drug resistance in tumor-regenerative or stem-like cancer cells [221–223]. Remarkable achievements have been made in photodynamic and photothermal tumor therapy by exploiting the homologous targeting properties of TEVs [77,108,111,224]. Wang used TCMVs to encapsulate ovalbumin-assembled nanoparticles encapsulating the photosensitizer Ce6 [75]. The ROS generated after illumination significantly enhances the cross-presentation efficiency of antigens, which can effectively initiate immune cascade reactions and improve the effectiveness of traditional photodynamic therapy. Zheng et al. fed cells with attached CpG gold nanorods and then produced apoptotic bodies loaded with gold nanorods by UV light irradiation of cells [109]. Upon near-infrared light irradiation, the photothermal effect triggered by the gold nanorods effectively eliminated the tumor.

At the same time, the strategy relied on co-stimulation with immune agonist, CpG, and tumor-associated antigens released by photothermal therapy in situ, promising to elicit a practical, durable tumor-specific immune response advantageous for alleviating immunosuppression. Zhen et al. constructed a biomimetic nanoparticle (CS-I/J@CM NPs) combining light, sound and immune checkpoint therapy for the treatment of glioblastoma (Figure 7) [63]. The encapsulation of TCMVs can improve the targeting ability and enrichment of particles at tumor sites. Cu2-xSe particles possess the properties of light-responsive Fenton-like catalytic induction of immunogenic cell death and alleviation of tumor hypoxia, repolarizing M2 macrophages to M1 type, thereby alleviating the immunosuppressive microenvironment of glioblastoma. The release of indoximod effectively blocked IDO-induced Treg cell infiltration in tumor sites. JQ1 can reduce the expression of PD-L1 on cancer cells. Under NIR II light irradiation, nanoparticles transformed glioblastoma from cold tumor to hot tumor, and the CD8$^+$ T cells in the tumor increased significantly, showing a good therapeutic effect.

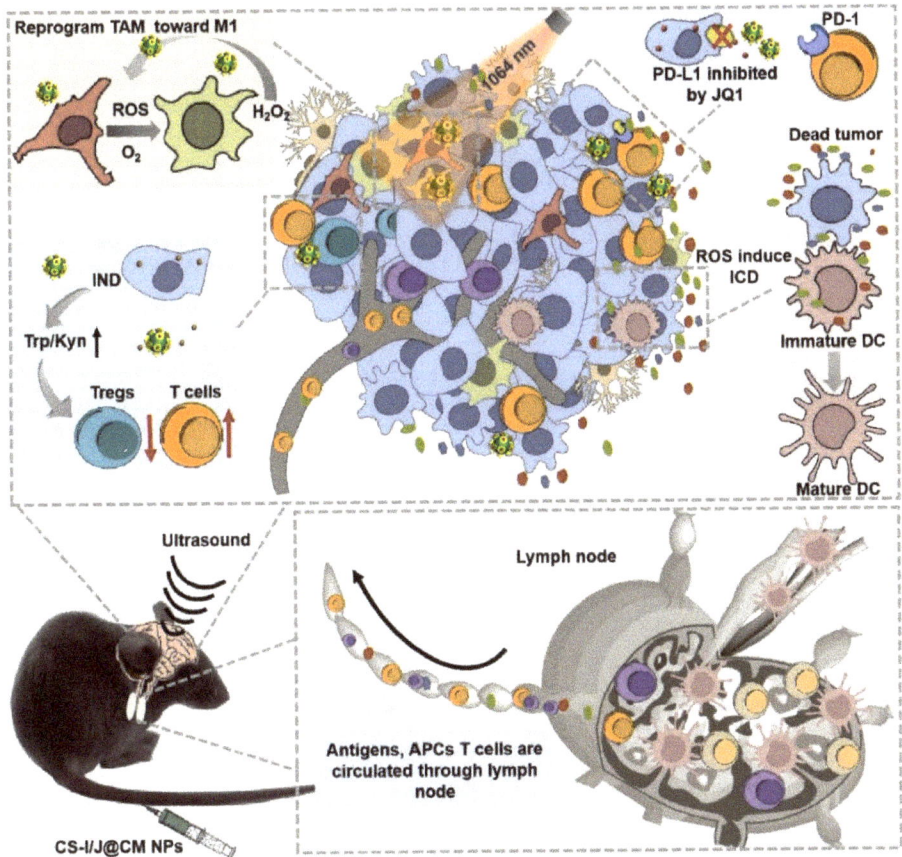

Figure 7. Integrated CS-I/J@CM NPs remodel the tumor immunosuppressive microenvironment to improve glioblastoma immunotherapy [63].

5. Concluding Remarks and Future Perspectives

From synthetic materials such as functionalized liposomes and micelles inspired by biomembranes to tumor cell-derived membrane vesicle-coated nanoparticles that bind to cell membranes, researchers have pursued suitable carrier materials for tumor immunotherapy. This review focuses on TDMV technology and its application in personalized immunotherapy. Tumor immunotherapy has yielded exciting results in several clinical trials. At the same time, achieving precise targeting and universal efficacy is also a problem for tumor immunotherapies in clinical trials. The choice of any TDMVs can target homologous tumors, overcoming the disadvantages of synthetic particles. TDMVs exploit the biological properties of cells, such as the ability to cross biological barriers, circulate in the body for long periods, interact with other cells and the capability to pass through biological barriers. In particular, the ability to pass through biological barriers and modify tissue toxicity effectively protects the drug from its effects. Unique approaches are utilized by introducing integrated biological components and functions that have synergistic effects and enhance the performance of TDMVs. For example, ligands composed of antibodies, peptides and proteins can be integrated into cell membranes to improve the function of cancer immunotherapy. TDMVs carry tumor cell proteins or genetic material, and their modification enables personalized therapy for all patients, especially for the development of tumor vaccines.

Cancer immunotherapy based on TDMVs technology is an attractive option due to the excellent biocompatibility and versatility, but in practice, there are many challenges to overcome to achieve widespread clinical application. First, the mechanism of action of TDMVs with tumor cells has not yet been fully explained. For example, the biological information carried by TEVs is stochastic in nature, and the mechanism of carrying is still unclear to achieve effective and precise regulation. Its mode of communication with the cell remains unclear. Second, whether the batch reproducibility, homogeneity and storage stability of TDMVs meet the quality manufacturing specification (GMP) standards also limit their further clinical translation. Third, biosafety issues are owing to unknown biological mechanisms. The current system for evaluating biosafety in the clinical setting is not robust, making the safety assessment of TDMVs unconvincing. In addition, personalized immunotherapies based on TDMVs currently have long lead times and high costs, and further exploration of optimization options is needed. However, with greater understanding and creative ideas, the field of TDMV -based nanotechnology can certainly circumvent these issues and drive cell membrane nanotechnology closer to accurate clinical applications.

Funding: This research was funded by China Postdoctoral Science Foundation, grant number 2020M683194.

Data Availability Statement: Data sharing not applicable.

Conflicts of Interest: The authors declare no conflict of interest.

References

1. Sung, H.; Ferlay, J.; Siegel, R.L.; Laversanne, M.; Soerjomataram, I.; Jemal, A.; Bray, F. Global Cancer Statistics 2020: GLOBOCAN Estimates of Incidence and Mortality Worldwide for 36 Cancers in 185 Countries. *CA Cancer J. Clin.* **2021**, *71*, 209–249. [CrossRef] [PubMed]
2. Luo, G.-F.; Chen, W.-H.; Zeng, X.; Zhang, X.-Z. Cell primitive-based biomimetic functional materials for enhanced cancer therapy. *Chem. Soc. Rev.* **2020**, *50*, 945–985. [CrossRef] [PubMed]
3. Tan, S.; Li, D.; Zhu, X. Cancer immunotherapy: Pros, cons and beyond. *Biomed. Pharmacother.* **2020**, *124*, 109821. [CrossRef] [PubMed]
4. Melenhorst, J.J.; Chen, G.M.; Wang, M.; Porter, D.L.; Chen, C.; Collins, M.A.; Gao, P.; Bandyopadhyay, S.; Sun, H.; Zhao, Z.; et al. Decade-long leukaemia remissions with persistence of CD4+ CAR T cells. *Nature* **2022**, *602*, 503–509. [CrossRef] [PubMed]
5. Maude, S.L.; Frey, N.; Shaw, P.A.; Aplenc, R.; Barrett, D.M.; Bunin, N.J.; Chew, A.; Gonzalez, V.E.; Zheng, Z.; Lacey, S.F.; et al. Chimeric antigen receptor T cells for sustained remissions in leukemia. *N. Engl. J. Med.* **2014**, *371*, 1507–1517. [CrossRef]
6. Yarchoan, M.; Hopkins, A.; Jaffee, E.M. Tumor Mutational Burden and Response Rate to PD-1 Inhibition. *N. Engl. J. Med.* **2017**, *377*, 2500–2501. [CrossRef]

7. Haslam, A.; Prasad, V. Estimation of the Percentage of US Patients with Cancer Who Are Eligible for and Respond to Checkpoint Inhibitor Immunotherapy Drugs. *JAMA Netw. Open* **2019**, *2*, e192535. [CrossRef]
8. Rafiq, S.; Hackett, C.S.; Brentjens, R.J. Engineering strategies to overcome the current roadblocks in CAR T cell therapy. *Nat. Rev. Clin. Oncol.* **2019**, *17*, 147–167. [CrossRef]
9. Larkin, J.; Hodi, F.S.; Wolchok, J.D. Combined Nivolumab and Ipilimumab or Monotherapy in Untreated Melanoma. *N. Engl. J. Med.* **2015**, *373*, 1270–1271. [CrossRef]
10. Postow, M.A.; Sidlow, R.; Hellmann, M.D. Immune-Related Adverse Events Associated with Immune Checkpoint Blockade. *N. Engl. J. Med.* **2018**, *378*, 158–168. [CrossRef]
11. Chen, D.S.; Mellman, I. Elements of cancer immunity and the cancer-immune set point. *Nature* **2017**, *541*, 321–330. [CrossRef]
12. Jensen, C.; Madsen, D.H.; Hansen, M.; Schmidt, H.; Svane, I.M.; Karsdal, M.A.; Willumsen, N. Non-invasive biomarkers derived from the extracellular matrix associate with response to immune checkpoint blockade (anti-CTLA-4) in metastatic melanoma patients. *J. Immunother. Cancer* **2018**, *6*, 152. [CrossRef] [PubMed]
13. Linette, G.P.; Becker-Hapak, M.; Skidmore, Z.L.; Baroja, M.L.; Xu, C.; Hundal, J.; Spencer, D.H.; Fu, W.; Cummins, C.; Robnett, M.; et al. Immunological ignorance is an enabling feature of the oligo-clonal T cell response to melanoma neoantigens. *Proc. Natl. Acad. Sci. USA* **2019**, *116*, 23662–23670. [CrossRef] [PubMed]
14. Matson, V.; Fessler, J.; Bao, R.; Chongsuwat, T.; Zha, Y.; Alegre, M.-L.; Luke, J.J.; Gajewski, T.F. The commensal microbiome is associated with anti-PD-1 efficacy in metastatic melanoma patients. *Science* **2018**, *359*, 104–108. [CrossRef] [PubMed]
15. Sivan, A.; Corrales, L.; Hubert, N.; Williams, J.B.; Aquino-Michaels, K.; Earley, Z.M.; Benyamin, F.W.; Lei, Y.M.; Jabri, B.; Alegre, M.-L.; et al. Commensal Bifidobacterium promotes antitumor immunity and facilitates anti-PD-L1 efficacy. *Science* **2015**, *350*, 1084–1089. [CrossRef]
16. Han, S.; Huang, K.; Gu, Z.; Wu, J. Tumor immune microenvironment modulation-based drug delivery strategies for cancer immunotherapy. *Nanoscale* **2019**, *12*, 413–436. [CrossRef]
17. Delfi, M.; Sartorius, R.; Ashrafizadeh, M.; Sharifi, E.; Zhang, Y.; De Berardinis, P.; Zarrabi, A.; Varma, R.S.; Tay, F.R.; Smith, B.R.; et al. Self-assembled peptide and protein nanostructures for anti-cancer therapy: Targeted delivery, stimuli-responsive devices and immunotherapy. *Nano Today* **2021**, *38*, 101119. [CrossRef]
18. Ghosh, B.; Biswas, S. Polymeric micelles in cancer therapy: State of the art. *J. Control. Release* **2021**, *332*, 127–147. [CrossRef]
19. Liang, C.; Zhang, X.; Wang, Z.; Wang, W.; Yang, M.; Dong, X.-C. Organic/inorganic nanohybrids rejuvenate photodynamic cancer therapy. *J. Mater. Chem. B* **2020**, *8*, 4748–4763. [CrossRef]
20. Karmali, P.P.; Simberg, D. Interactions of nanoparticles with plasma proteins: Implication on clearance and toxicity of drug delivery systems. *Expert Opin. Drug Deliv.* **2011**, *8*, 343–357. [CrossRef]
21. Emam, S.E.; Elsadek, N.E.; Abu Lila, A.S.; Takata, H.; Kawaguchi, Y.; Shimizu, T.; Ando, H.; Ishima, Y.; Ishida, T. Anti-PEG IgM production and accelerated blood clearance phenomenon after the administration of PEGylated exosomes in mice. *J. Control. Release* **2021**, *334*, 327–334. [CrossRef] [PubMed]
22. Xue, Y.; Che, J.; Ji, X.; Li, Y.; Xie, J.; Chen, X. Recent advances in biomaterial-boosted adoptive cell therapy. *Chem. Soc. Rev.* **2022**, *51*, 1766–1794. [CrossRef] [PubMed]
23. Théry, C.; Ostrowski, M.; Segura, E. Membrane vesicles as conveyors of immune responses. *Nat. Rev. Immunol.* **2009**, *9*, 581–593. [CrossRef] [PubMed]
24. Chen, Z.; Wang, Z.; Gu, Z. Bioinspired and Biomimetic Nanomedicines. *Accounts Chem. Res.* **2019**, *52*, 1255–1264. [CrossRef] [PubMed]
25. Fang, R.H.; Kroll, A.V.; Gao, W.W.; Zhang, L.F. Cell Membrane Coating Nanotechnology. *Adv. Mater.* **2018**, *30*, e1706759. [CrossRef] [PubMed]
26. Thanuja, M.Y.; Anupama, C.; Ranganath, S.H. Bioengineered cellular and cell membrane-derived vehicles for actively targeted drug delivery: So near and yet so far. *Adv. Drug Deliv. Rev.* **2018**, *132*, 57–80. [CrossRef]
27. Zhang, P.; Liu, G.; Chen, X. Nanobiotechnology: Cell membrane-based delivery systems. *Nano Today* **2016**, *13*, 7–9. [CrossRef]
28. Tominaga, N.; Yoshioka, Y.; Ochiya, T. A novel platform for cancer therapy using extracellular vesicles. *Adv. Drug Deliv. Rev.* **2015**, *95*, 50–55. [CrossRef]
29. Srivatsav, A.T.; Kapoor, S. The Emerging World of Membrane Vesicles: Functional Relevance, Theranostic Avenues and Tools for Investigating Membrane Function. *Front. Mol. Biosci.* **2021**, *8*, 640355. [CrossRef]
30. Liu, X.; Liu, C.; Zheng, Z.; Chen, S.; Pang, X.; Xiang, X.; Tang, J.; Ren, E.; Chen, Y.; You, M.; et al. Vesicular Antibodies: A Bioactive Multifunctional Combination Platform for Targeted Therapeutic Delivery and Cancer Immunotherapy. *Adv. Mater.* **2019**, *31*, e1808294. [CrossRef]
31. Noh, Y.-W.; Kim, S.-Y.; Kim, J.-E.; Kim, S.; Ryu, J.; Kim, I.; Lee, E.; Um, S.H.; Lim, Y.T. Multifaceted Immunomodulatory Nanoliposomes: Reshaping Tumors into Vaccines for Enhanced Cancer Immunotherapy. *Adv. Funct. Mater.* **2017**, *27*, 1605398. [CrossRef]
32. Möller, A.; Lobb, R.J. The evolving translational potential of small extracellular vesicles in cancer. *Nat. Cancer* **2020**, *20*, 697–709. [CrossRef]
33. Park, W.; Seong, K.Y.; Han, H.H.; Yang, S.Y.; Hahn, S.K. Dissolving microneedles delivering cancer cell membrane coated nanoparticles for cancer immunotherapy. *RSC Adv.* **2021**, *11*, 10393–10399. [CrossRef]

34. Wang, D.; Dong, H.; Li, M.; Cao, Y.; Yang, F.; Zhang, K.; Dai, W.; Wang, C.; Zhang, X. Erythrocyte–Cancer Hybrid Membrane Camouflaged Hollow Copper Sulfide Nanoparticles for Prolonged Circulation Life and Homotypic-Targeting Photothermal/Chemotherapy of Melanoma. *ACS Nano* **2018**, *12*, 5241–5252. [CrossRef]
35. Durymanov, M.; Rosenkranz, A.; Sobolev, A.S. Current Approaches for Improving Intratumoral Accumulation and Distribution of Nanomedicines. *Theranostics* **2015**, *5*, 1007–1020. [CrossRef] [PubMed]
36. Sun, Q.; Zhou, Z.; Qiu, N.; Shen, Y. Rational Design of Cancer Nanomedicine: Nanoproperty Integration and Synchronization. *Adv. Mater.* **2017**, *29*, 1606628. [CrossRef]
37. Kalluri, R.; Zeisberg, M. Fibroblasts in cancer. *Nat. Rev. Cancer* **2006**, *6*, 392–401. [CrossRef]
38. Wilhelm, S.; Tavares, A.J.; Dai, Q.; Ohta, S.; Audet, J.; Dvorak, H.F.; Chan, W.C.W. Analysis of nanoparticle delivery to tumours. *Nat. Rev. Mater.* **2016**, *1*, 16014. [CrossRef]
39. Zhang, M.; Ye, J.; Li, C.; Xia, Y.; Wang, Z.; Feng, J.; Zhang, X. Cytomembrane-Mediated Transport of Metal Ions with Biological Specificity. *Adv. Sci.* **2019**, *6*, 1900835. [CrossRef]
40. Xia, J.; Cheng, Y.; Zhang, H.; Li, R.; Hu, Y.; Liu, B. The role of adhesions between homologous cancer cells in tumor progression and targeted therapy. *Expert Rev. Anticancer Ther.* **2017**, *17*, 517–526. [CrossRef]
41. Chen, Z.; Zhao, P.; Luo, Z.; Zheng, M.; Tian, H.; Gong, P.; Gao, G.; Pan, H.; Liu, L.; Ma, A.; et al. Cancer Cell Membrane–Biomimetic Nanoparticles for Homologous-Targeting Dual-Modal Imaging and Photothermal Therapy. *ACS Nano* **2016**, *10*, 10049–10057. [CrossRef] [PubMed]
42. Khaldoyanidi, S.K.; Glinsky, V.; Sikora, L.; Glinskii, A.B.; Mossine, V.V.; Quinn, T.P.; Glinsky, G.V.; Sriramarao, P. MDA-MB-435 Human Breast Carcinoma Cell Homo- and Heterotypic Adhesion under Flow Conditions Is Mediated in Part by Thomsen-Friedenreich Antigen-Galectin-3 Interactions. *J. Biol. Chem.* **2003**, *278*, 4127–4134. [CrossRef] [PubMed]
43. Qiu, W.-X.; Zhang, M.-K.; Liu, L.-H.; Gao, F.; Zhang, L.; Li, S.; Xie, B.-R.; Zhang, C.; Feng, J.; Zhang, X.-Z. A self-delivery membrane system for enhanced anti-tumor therapy. *Biomaterials* **2018**, *161*, 81–94. [CrossRef] [PubMed]
44. Aggarwal, S.; Sharma, S.C.; Das, S.N. Galectin-1 and galectin-3: Plausible tumour markers for oral squamous cell carcinoma and suitable targets for screening high-risk population. *Clin. Chim. Acta* **2015**, *442*, 13–21. [CrossRef] [PubMed]
45. Bombardelli, L.; Cavallaro, U. Immunoglobulin-like cell adhesion molecules: Novel signaling players in epithelial ovarian cancer. *Int. J. Biochem. Cell Biol.* **2010**, *42*, 590–594. [CrossRef]
46. Gao, J.; Zheng, Q.; Xin, N.; Wang, W.; Zhao, C. CD 155, an onco-immunologic molecule in human tumors. *Cancer Sci.* **2017**, *108*, 1934–1938. [CrossRef]
47. Sun, H.; Su, J.; Meng, Q.; Yin, Q.; Chen, L.; Gu, W.; Zhang, P.; Zhang, Z.; Yu, H.; Wang, S.; et al. Cancer-Cell-Biomimetic Nanoparticles for Targeted Therapy of Homotypic Tumors. *Adv. Mater.* **2016**, *28*, 9581–9588. [CrossRef]
48. Xu, C.; Liu, W.; Hu, Y.; Li, W.; Di, W. Bioinspired tumor-homing nanoplatform for co-delivery of paclitaxel and siRNA-E7 to HPV-related cervical malignancies for synergistic therapy. *Theranostics* **2020**, *10*, 3325–3339. [CrossRef]
49. Wan, J.; Wang, J.; Zhou, M.; Rao, Z.; Ling, X. A cell membrane vehicle co-delivering sorafenib and doxorubicin remodel the tumor microenvironment and enhance immunotherapy by inducing immunogenic cell death in lung cancer cells. *J. Mater. Chem. B* **2020**, *8*, 7755–7765. [CrossRef]
50. Wang, H.; Liu, Y.; He, R.; Xu, D.; Zang, J.; Weeranoppanant, N.; Dong, H.; Li, Y. Cell membrane biomimetic nanoparticles for inflammation and cancer targeting in drug delivery. *Biomater. Sci.* **2019**, *8*, 552–568. [CrossRef]
51. Rao, L.; Bu, L.-L.; Cai, B.; Xu, J.-H.; Li, A.; Zhang, W.-F.; Sun, Z.-J.; Guo, S.-S.; Liu, W.; Wang, T.-H.; et al. Cancer Cell Membrane-Coated Upconversion Nanoprobes for Highly Specific Tumor Imaging. *Adv. Mater.* **2016**, *28*, 3460–3466. [CrossRef] [PubMed]
52. Lu, H.; Guo, K.; Cao, Y.; Yang, F.; Wang, D.; Dou, L.; Liu, Y.; Dong, H. Cancer Cell Membrane Vesicle for Multiplex MicroRNA Imaging in Living Cells. *Anal. Chem.* **2019**, *92*, 1850–1855. [CrossRef] [PubMed]
53. Zhang, X.; Wang, C.; Wang, J.; Hu, Q.; Langworthy, B.; Ye, Y.; Sun, W.; Lin, J.; Wang, T.; Fine, J.; et al. PD-1 Blockade Cellular Vesicles for Cancer Immunotherapy. *Adv. Mater.* **2018**, *30*, e1707112. [CrossRef]
54. Jiang, Y.; Krishnan, N.; Zhou, J.; Chekuri, S.; Wei, X.; Kroll, A.V.; Yu, C.L.; Duan, Y.; Gao, W.; Fang, R.H.; et al. Engineered Cell-Membrane-Coated Nanoparticles Directly Present Tumor Antigens to Promote Anticancer Immunity. *Adv. Mater.* **2020**, *32*, e2001808. [CrossRef] [PubMed]
55. Zhu, J.-Y.; Zhang, M.-K.; Ding, X.-G.; Qiu, W.-X.; Yu, W.-Y.; Feng, J.; Zhang, X.-Z. Virus-Inspired Nanogenes Free from Man-Made Materials for Host-Specific Transfection and Bio-Aided MR Imaging. *Adv. Mater.* **2018**, *30*, e1707459. [CrossRef]
56. Wang, P.; Kankala, R.K.; Chen, B.; Zhang, Y.; Zhu, M.; Li, X.; Long, R.; Yang, D.; Krastev, R.; Wang, S.; et al. Cancer Cytomembrane-Cloaked Prussian Blue Nanoparticles Enhance the Efficacy of Mild-Temperature Photothermal Therapy by Disrupting Mitochondrial Functions of Cancer Cells. *ACS Appl. Mater. Interfaces* **2021**, *13*, 37563–37577. [CrossRef]
57. Browning, M.J. Antigen presenting cell/tumor cell fusion vaccines for cancer immunotherapy. *Hum. Vaccines Immunother.* **2013**, *9*, 1545–1548. [CrossRef]
58. Han, L.; Peng, K.; Qiu, L.-Y.; Li, M.; Ruan, J.-H.; He, L.-L.; Yuan, Z.-X. Hitchhiking on Controlled-Release Drug Delivery Systems: Opportunities and Challenges for Cancer Vaccines. *Front. Pharmacol.* **2021**, *12*, 679602. [CrossRef]
59. Zhang, L.; Yin, T.; Zhang, B.; Yan, C.; Lu, C.; Liu, L.; Chen, Z.; Ran, H.; Shi, Q.; Pan, H.; et al. Cancer-macrophage hybrid membrane-camouflaged photochlor for enhanced sonodynamic therapy against triple-negative breast cancer. *Nano Res.* **2022**, *15*, 4224–4232. [CrossRef]

60. Zhang, L.; Zhao, W.; Huang, J.; Li, F.; Sheng, J.; Song, H.; Chen, Y. Development of a Dendritic Cell/Tumor Cell Fusion Cell Membrane Nano-Vaccine for the Treatment of Ovarian Cancer. *Front. Immunol.* **2022**, *13*, 828263. [CrossRef]
61. Liu, W.; Zou, M.; Liu, T.; Zeng, J.; Li, X.; Yu, W.; Li, C.; Ye, J.; Song, W.; Feng, J.; et al. Expandable Immunotherapeutic Nano-platforms Engineered from Cytomembranes of Hybrid Cells Derived from Cancer and Dendritic Cells. *Adv. Mater.* **2019**, *31*, e1900499. [CrossRef] [PubMed]
62. Liu, W.-L.; Zou, M.-Z.; Liu, T.; Zeng, J.-Y.; Li, X.; Yu, W.-Y.; Li, C.-X.; Ye, J.-J.; Song, W.; Feng, J.; et al. Cytomembrane nano-vaccines show therapeutic effects by mimicking tumor cells and antigen presenting cells. *Nat. Commun.* **2019**, *10*, 3199. [CrossRef] [PubMed]
63. Wang, T.; Zhang, H.; Qiu, W.; Han, Y.; Liu, H.; Li, Z. Biomimetic nanoparticles directly remodel immunosuppressive microenvironment for boosting glioblastoma immunotherapy. *Bioact. Mater.* **2022**, *16*, 418–432. [CrossRef] [PubMed]
64. Cai, J.-X.; Liu, J.-H.; Wu, J.-Y.; Li, Y.-J.; Qiu, X.-H.; Xu, W.-J.; Xu, P.; Xiang, D.-X. Hybrid Cell Membrane-Functionalized Bio-mimetic Nanoparticles for Targeted Therapy of Osteosarcoma. *Int. J. Nanomed.* **2022**, *17*, 837–854. [CrossRef] [PubMed]
65. Saxena, M.; van der Burg, S.H.; Melief, C.J.M.; Bhardwaj, N. Therapeutic cancer vaccines. *Nat. Rev. Cancer* **2021**, *21*, 360–378. [CrossRef]
66. Chen, Q.; Huang, G.; Wu, W.; Wang, J.; Hu, J.; Mao, J.; Chu, P.; Bai, H.; Tang, G. A Hybrid Eukaryotic-Prokaryotic Nano-platform with Photothermal Modality for Enhanced Antitumor Vaccination. *Adv. Mater.* **2020**, *32*, e1908185. [CrossRef]
67. Xiao, L.; Huang, Y.; Yang, Y.; Miao, Z.; Zhu, J.; Zhong, M.; Feng, C.; Tang, W.; Zhou, J.; Wang, L.; et al. Biomimetic cy-tomembrane nanovaccines prevent breast cancer development in the long term. *Nanoscale* **2021**, *13*, 3594–3601. [CrossRef]
68. Xiong, X.; Zhao, J.; Pan, J.; Liu, C.; Guo, X.; Zhou, S. Personalized Nanovaccine Coated with Calcinetin-Expressed Cancer Cell Membrane Antigen for Cancer Immunotherapy. *Nano Lett.* **2021**, *21*, 8418–8425. [CrossRef]
69. Xiong, J.; Wu, M.; Chen, J.; Liu, Y.; Chen, Y.; Fan, G.; Liu, Y.; Cheng, J.; Wang, Z.; Wang, S.; et al. Cancer-Erythrocyte Hybrid Membrane-Camouflaged Magnetic Nanoparticles with Enhanced Photothermal-Immunotherapy for Ovarian Cancer. *ACS Nano* **2021**, *15*, 19756–19770. [CrossRef]
70. Wang, Y.; Luan, Z.; Zhao, C.; Bai, C.; Yang, K. Target delivery selective CSF-1R inhibitor to tumor-associated macrophages via erythrocyte-cancer cell hybrid membrane camouflaged pH-responsive copolymer micelle for cancer immunotherapy. *Eur. J. Pharm. Sci.* **2019**, *142*, 105136. [CrossRef]
71. Tian, Y.; Xu, C.; Feng, J.; Huangfu, Y.; Wang, K.; Zhang, Z.-L. Personalized gel-droplet monocyte vaccines for cancer immunotherapy. *Lab Chip* **2021**, *21*, 4414–4426. [CrossRef] [PubMed]
72. Sancho-Albero, M.; Encinas-Giménez, M.; Sebastián, V.; Pérez, E.; Luján, L.; Santamaría, J.; Martin-Duque, P. Transfer of photothermal nanoparticles using stem cell derived small extracellular vesicles for in vivo treatment of primary and multinodular tumours. *J. Extracell. Vesicles* **2022**, *11*, e12193. [CrossRef] [PubMed]
73. Meng, Q.; Zhao, Y.; Dong, C.; Liu, L.; Pan, Y.; Lai, J.; Liu, Z.; Yu, G.; Chen, X.; Rao, L. Genetically Programmable Fusion Cel-lular Vesicles for Cancer Immunotherapy. *Angew. Chem. Int. Ed.* **2021**, *60*, 26320–26326. [CrossRef] [PubMed]
74. Li, Q.; Zhao, Z.; Qin, X.; Zhang, M.; Du, Q.; Li, Z.; Luan, Y. A Checkpoint-Regulatable Immune Niche Created by Injectable Hydrogel for Tumor Therapy. *Adv. Funct. Mater.* **2021**, *31*, 2104630. [CrossRef]
75. Wang, H.; Wang, K.; He, L.; Liu, Y.; Dong, H.; Li, Y. Engineering antigen as photosensitiser nanocarrier to facilitate ROS triggered immune cascade for photodynamic immunotherapy. *Biomaterials* **2020**, *244*, 119964. [CrossRef]
76. Pack, C.D.; Bommireddy, R.; Munoz, L.E.; Patel, J.M.; Bozeman, E.N.; Dey, P.; Radhakrishnan, V.; Vartabedian, V.F.; Venkat, K.; Ramachandiran, S.; et al. Tumor membrane-based vaccine immunotherapy in combination with anti-CTLA-4 antibody confers protection against immune checkpoint resistant murine triple-negative breast cancer. *Hum. Vaccines Immunother.* **2020**, *16*, 3184–3193. [CrossRef]
77. Ye, X.; Liang, X.; Chen, Q.; Miao, Q.; Chen, X.; Zhang, X.; Mei, L. Surgical Tumor-Derived Personalized Photothermal Vac-cine Formulation for Cancer Immunotherapy. *ACS Nano* **2019**, *13*, 2956–2968. [CrossRef]
78. Wu, M.; Liu, X.; Bai, H.; Lai, L.; Chen, Q.; Huang, G.; Liu, B.; Tang, G. Surface-Layer Protein-Enhanced Immunotherapy Based on Cell Membrane-Coated Nanoparticles for the Effective Inhibition of Tumor Growth and Metastasis. *ACS Appl. Mater. In-terfaces* **2019**, *11*, 9850–9859. [CrossRef]
79. Li, F.; Nie, W.; Zhang, F.; Lu, G.; Lv, C.; Lv, Y.; Bao, W.; Zhang, L.; Wang, S.; Gao, X.; et al. Engineering Magnetosomes for High-Performance Cancer Vaccination. *ACS Central Sci.* **2019**, *5*, 796–807. [CrossRef]
80. Kooijmans, S.A.A.; Gitz-Francois, J.J.J.M.; Schiffelers, R.M.; Vader, P. Recombinant phosphatidylserine-binding nanobodies for targeting of extracellular vesicles to tumor cells: A plug-and-play approach. *Nanoscale* **2018**, *10*, 2413–2426. [CrossRef]
81. Kroll, A.V.; Fang, R.H.; Jiang, Y.; Zhou, J.; Wei, X.; Gao, J.; Luk, B.T.; Dehaini, D.; Gao, W.; et al. Nanoparticulate Delivery of Cancer Cell Membrane Elicits Multiantigenic Antitumor Immunity. *Adv. Mater.* **2017**, *29*, 1703969. [CrossRef] [PubMed]
82. Elsharkasy, O.M.; Nordin, J.Z.; Hagey, D.W.; De Jong, O.G.; Schiffelers, R.M.; Andaloussi, S.E.; Vader, P. Extracellular vesi-cles as drug delivery systems: Why and how? *Adv. Drug Deliv. Rev.* **2020**, *159*, 332–343. [CrossRef] [PubMed]
83. Veerman, R.E.; Akpinar, G.G.; Eldh, M.; Gabrielsson, S. Immune Cell-Derived Extracellular Vesicles-Functions and Thera-peutic Applications. *Trends Mol. Med.* **2019**, *25*, 382–394. [CrossRef]
84. Skotland, T.; Sagini, K.; Sandvig, K.; Llorente, A. An emerging focus on lipids in extracellular vesicles. *Adv. Drug Deliv. Rev.* **2020**, *159*, 308–321. [CrossRef]

85. Wu, P.; Zhang, B.; Ocansey, D.K.W.; Xu, W.; Qian, H. Extracellular vesicles: A bright star of nanomedicine. *Biomaterials* **2020**, *269*, 120467. [CrossRef]
86. Zhao, Y.; Li, Y.; Jiang, L.; Gu, Y.; Liu, J. Cell-derived biomimetic nanocarriers for targeted cancer therapy: Cell membranes and extracellular vesicles. *Drug Deliv.* **2021**, *28*, 1237–1255. [CrossRef]
87. Lima Correa, B.; El Harane, N.; Gomez, I.; Rachid Hocine, H.; Vilar, J.; Desgres, M.; Bellamy, V.; Keirththana, K.; Guillas, C.; Perotto, M.; et al. Extracellular vesicles from human cardiovascular progenitors trigger a reparative immune response in infarcted hearts. *Cardiovasc. Res.* **2020**, *117*, 292–307. [CrossRef]
88. Barenholz-Cohen, T.; Merkher, Y.; Haj, J.; Shechter, D.; Kirchmeier, D.; Shaked, Y.; Weihs, D. Lung mechanics modifications facilitating metastasis are mediated in part by breast cancer-derived extracellular vesicles. *Int. J. Cancer* **2020**, *147*, 2924–2933. [CrossRef]
89. Sun, Y.; Liu, J. Potential of Cancer Cell-Derived Exosomes in Clinical Application: A Review of Recent Research Advances. *Clin. Ther.* **2014**, *36*, 863–872. [CrossRef]
90. Kowal, J.; Arras, G.; Colombo, M.; Jouve, M.; Morath, J.P.; Primdal-Bengtson, B.; Dingli, F.; Loew, D.; Tkach, M.; Théry, C. Proteomic comparison defines novel markers to characterize heterogeneous populations of extracellular vesicle subtypes. *Proc. Natl. Acad. Sci. USA* **2016**, *113*, E968–E977. [CrossRef]
91. D'Souza-Schorey, C.; Clancy, J.W. Tumor-derived microvesicles: Shedding light on novel microenvironment modulators and prospective cancer biomarkers. *Genes Dev.* **2012**, *26*, 1287–1299. [CrossRef] [PubMed]
92. Revenfeld, A.L.S.; Bæk, R.; Nielsen, M.H.; Stensballe, A.; Varming, K.; Jørgensen, M. Diagnostic and Prognostic Potential of Extracellular Vesicles in Peripheral Blood. *Clin. Ther.* **2014**, *36*, 830–846. [CrossRef] [PubMed]
93. Chen, B.; Li, Q.; Zhao, B.; Wang, Y. Stem Cell-Derived Extracellular Vesicles as a Novel Potential Therapeutic Tool for Tis-sue Repair. *STEM CELLS Transl. Med.* **2017**, *6*, 1753–1758. [CrossRef]
94. Wlodkowic, D.; Telford, W.; Skommer, J.; Darzynkiewicz, Z. Apoptosis and Beyond: Cytometry in Studies of Programmed Cell Death. *Methods Cell Biol.* **2011**, *103*, 55–98. [CrossRef] [PubMed]
95. Sung, B.H.; Ketova, T.; Hoshino, D.; Zijlstra, A.; Weaver, A.M. Directional cell movement through tissues is controlled by exosome secretion. *Nat. Commun.* **2015**, *6*, 7164. [CrossRef]
96. Tkach, M.; Théry, C. Communication by Extracellular Vesicles: Where We Are and Where We Need to Go. *Cell* **2016**, *164*, 1226–1232. [CrossRef]
97. Raposo, G.; Stoorvogel, W. Extracellular vesicles: Exosomes, microvesicles, and friends. *J. Cell Biol.* **2013**, *200*, 373–383. [CrossRef] [PubMed]
98. van Dommelen, S.M.; Vader, P.; Lakhal, S.; Kooijmans, S.; van Solinge, W.W.; Wood, M.J.; Schiffelers, R.M. Microvesicles and exosomes: Opportunities for cell-derived membrane vesicles in drug delivery. *J. Control. Release* **2012**, *161*, 635–644. [CrossRef] [PubMed]
99. Zhuang, G.; Wu, X.; Jiang, Z.; Kasman, I.; Yao, J.; Guan, Y.; Oeh, J.; Modrusan, Z.; Bais, C.; Sampath, D.; et al. Tu-mour-secreted miR-9 promotes endothelial cell migration and angiogenesis by activating the JAK-STAT pathway. *EMBO J.* **2012**, *31*, 3513–3523. [CrossRef]
100. Antonyak, M.A.; Li, B.; Boroughs, L.K.; Johnson, J.L.; Druso, J.E.; Bryant, K.L.; Holowka, D.A.; Cerione, R.A. Cancer cell-derived microvesicles induce transformation by transferring tissue transglutaminase and fibronectin to recipient cells. *Proc. Natl. Acad. Sci. USA* **2011**, *108*, 4852–4857. [CrossRef]
101. Reich, C.F.; Pisetsky, D.S. The content of DNA and RNA in microparticles released by Jurkat and HL-60 cells undergoing in vitro apoptosis. *Exp. Cell Res.* **2009**, *315*, 760–768. [CrossRef]
102. Chen, G.; Huang, A.C.; Zhang, W.; Zhang, G.; Wu, M.; Xu, W.; Yu, Z.; Yang, J.; Wang, B.; Sun, H.; et al. Exosomal PD-L1 con-tributes to immunosuppression and is associated with anti-PD-1 response. *Nature* **2018**, *560*, 382–386. [CrossRef] [PubMed]
103. Koh, E.; Lee, E.J.; Nam, G.-H.; Hong, Y.; Cho, E.; Yang, Y.; Kim, I.-S. Exosome-SIRPα, a CD47 blockade increases cancer cell phagocytosis. *Biomaterials* **2017**, *121*, 121–129. [CrossRef] [PubMed]
104. Huang, L.; Rong, Y.; Tang, X.; Yi, K.; Qi, P.; Hou, J.; Liu, W.; He, Y.; Gao, X.; Yuan, C.; et al. Engineered exosomes as an in situ DC-primed vaccine to boost antitumor immunity in breast cancer. *Mol. Cancer* **2022**, *21*, 45. [CrossRef]
105. Zhao, X.; Yuan, C.; Wangmo, D.; Subramanian, S. Tumor-Secreted Extracellular Vesicles Regulate T-Cell Costimulation and Can Be Manipulated To Induce Tumor-Specific T-Cell Responses. *Gastroenterology* **2021**, *161*, 560–574.e11. [CrossRef]
106. Cheng, L.; Zhang, X.; Tang, J.; Lv, Q.; Liu, J. Gene-engineered exosomes-thermosensitive liposomes hybrid nanovesicles by the blockade of CD47 signal for combined photothermal therapy and cancer immunotherapy. *Biomaterials* **2021**, *275*, 120964. [CrossRef]
107. Zuo, B.; Qi, H.; Lu, Z.; Chen, L.; Sun, B.; Yang, R.; Zhang, Y.; Liu, Z.; Gao, X.; You, A.; et al. Alarmin-painted exosomes elicit persistent antitumor immunity in large established tumors in mice. *Nat. Commun.* **2020**, *11*, 1790. [CrossRef]
108. Zhu, D.-M.; Duo, Y.; Suo, M.; Zhao, Y.; Xia, L.; Zheng, Z.; Li, Y.; Tang, B.Z. Tumor-Exocytosed Exosome/Aggregation-Induced Emission Luminogen Hybrid Nanovesicles Facilitate Efficient Tumor Penetration and Photodynamic Therapy. *Angew. Chem. Int. Ed.* **2020**, *59*, 13836–13843. [CrossRef]
109. Zheng, L.; Hu, X.; Wu, H.; Mo, L.; Xie, S.; Li, J.; Peng, C.; Xu, S.; Qiu, L.; Tan, W. In Vivo Monocyte/Macrophage-Hitchhiked Intratumoral Accumulation of Nanomedicines for Enhanced Tumor Therapy. *J. Am. Chem. Soc.* **2019**, *142*, 382–391. [CrossRef]

110. He, L.; Nie, T.; Xia, X.; Liu, T.; Huang, Y.; Wang, X.; Chen, T. Designing Bioinspired 2D MoSe 2 Nanosheet for Efficient Photothermal-Triggered Cancer Immunotherapy with Reprogramming Tumor-Associated Macrophages. *Adv. Funct. Mater.* **2019**, *29*, 1901240. [CrossRef]
111. Liu, Q.; Fan, T.; Zheng, Y.; Yang, S.-L.; Yu, Z.; Duo, Y.; Zhang, Y.; Adah, D.; Shi, L.; Sun, Z.; et al. Immunogenic exo-some-encapsulated black phosphorus nanoparticles as an effective anticancer photo-nanovaccine. *Nanoscale* **2020**, *12*, 19939–19952. [CrossRef]
112. Morishita, M.; Takahashi, Y.; Matsumoto, A.; Nishikawa, M.; Takakura, Y. Exosome-based tumor antigens-adjuvant co-delivery utilizing genetically engineered tumor cell-derived exosomes with immunostimulatory CpG DNA. *Biomaterials* **2016**, *111*, 55–65. [CrossRef]
113. Davidson, S.M. Benefit of Extracellular Vesicles at the Blood-Brain Barrier. *Arter. Thromb. Vasc. Biol.* **2021**, *41*, 1146–1148. [CrossRef]
114. Saint-Pol, J.; Gosselet, F.; Duban-Deweer, S.; Pottiez, G.; Karamanos, Y. Targeting and Crossing the Blood-Brain Barrier with Extracellular Vesicles. *Cells* **2020**, *9*, 851. [CrossRef]
115. Terstappen, G.C.; Meyer, A.H.; Bell, R.D.; Zhang, W. Strategies for delivering therapeutics across the blood-brain barrier. *Nat. Rev. Drug Discov.* **2021**, *20*, 362–383. [CrossRef]
116. Gurung, S.; Perocheau, D.; Touramanidou, L.; Baruteau, J. The exosome journey: From biogenesis to uptake and intracellular signalling. *Cell Commun. Signal.* **2021**, *19*, 47. [CrossRef]
117. Batrakova, E.V.; Kim, M.S. Using exosomes, naturally-equipped nanocarriers, for drug delivery. *J. Control. Release* **2015**, *219*, 396–405. [CrossRef]
118. Luan, X.; Sansanaphongpricha, K.; Myers, I.; Chen, H.; Yuan, H.; Sun, D. Engineering exosomes as refined biological nanoplatforms for drug delivery. *Acta Pharmacol. Sin.* **2017**, *38*, 754–763. [CrossRef]
119. Das, C.K.; Jena, B.C.; Banerjee, I.; Das, S.; Parekh, A.; Bhutia, S.K.; Mandal, M. Exosome as a Novel Shuttle for Delivery of Therapeutics across Biological Barriers. *Mol. Pharm.* **2018**, *16*, 24–40. [CrossRef]
120. Chopra, N.; Arya, B.D.; Jain, N.; Yadav, P.; Wajid, S.; Singh, S.P.; Choudhury, S. Biophysical Characterization and Drug Delivery Potential of Exosomes from Human Wharton's Jelly-Derived Mesenchymal Stem Cells. *ACS Omega* **2019**, *4*, 13143–13152. [CrossRef]
121. Yang, J.; Liu, W.; Lu, X.; Fu, Y.; Li, L.; Luo, Y. High expression of small GTPase Rab3D promotes cancer progression and me-tastasis. *Oncotarget* **2015**, *6*, 11125–11138. [CrossRef]
122. López-Cobo, S.; Campos-Silva, C.; Moyano, A.; Oliveira-Rodríguez, M.; Paschen, A.; Yáñez-Mó, M.; Blanco-López, M.C.; Valés-Gómez, M. Immunoassays for scarce tumour-antigens in exosomes: Detection of the human NKG2D-Ligand, MICA, in tetraspanin-containing nanovesicles from melanoma. *J. Nanobiotechnol.* **2018**, *16*, 47. [CrossRef]
123. Subramanian, A.; Gupta, V.; Sarkar, S.; Maity, G.; Banerjee, S.; Ghosh, A.; Harris, L.; Christenson, L.K.; Hung, W.; Bansal, A.; et al. Exosomes in carcinogenesis: Molecular palkis carry signals for the regulation of cancer progression and metastasis. *J. Cell Commun. Signal.* **2016**, *10*, 241–249. [CrossRef]
124. Svensson, K.J.; Christianson, H.C.; Wittrup, A.; Bourseau-Guilmain, E.; Lindqvist, E.; Svensson, L.M.; Mörgelin, M.; Belting, M. Exosome Uptake Depends on ERK1/2-Heat Shock Protein 27 Signaling and Lipid Raft-mediated Endocytosis Negatively Regulated by Caveolin-1. *J. Biol. Chem.* **2013**, *288*, 17713–17724. [CrossRef]
125. Plebanek, M.P.; Mutharasan, R.K.; Volpert, O.; Matov, A.; Gatlin, J.C.; Thaxton, C.S. Nanoparticle Targeting and Cholesterol Flux Through Scavenger Receptor Type B-1 Inhibits Cellular Exosome Uptake. *Sci. Rep.* **2015**, *5*, 15724. [CrossRef]
126. Whiteside, T.L. Tumor-Derived Exosomes and Their Role in Cancer Progression. *Adv. Clin. Chem.* **2016**, *74*, 103–141. [CrossRef]
127. Syn, N.; Wang, L.; Sethi, G.; Thiery, J.-P.; Goh, B.-C. Exosome-Mediated Metastasis: From Epithelial-Mesenchymal Transi-tion to Escape from Immunosurveillance. *Trends Pharmacol. Sci.* **2016**, *37*, 606–617. [CrossRef]
128. Zhang, L.; Zhang, S.; Yao, J.; Lowery, F.J.; Zhang, Q.; Huang, W.-C.; Li, P.; Li, M.; Wang, X.; Zhang, C.; et al. Microenviron-ment-induced PTEN loss by exosomal microRNA primes brain metastasis outgrowth. *Nature* **2015**, *527*, 100–104. [CrossRef]
129. Clayton, A.; Mitchell, J.P.; Court, J.; Linnane, S.; Mason, M.D.; Tabi, Z. Human Tumor-Derived Exosomes Down-Modulate NKG2D Expression. *J. Immunol.* **2008**, *180*, 7249–7258. [CrossRef]
130. Zhang, X.; Chen, Y.; Hao, L.; Hou, A.; Chen, X.; Li, Y.; Wang, R.; Luo, P.; Ruan, Z.; Ou, J.; et al. Macrophages induce resistance to 5-fluorouracil chemotherapy in colorectal cancer through the release of putrescine. *Cancer Lett.* **2016**, *381*, 305–313. [CrossRef]
131. Dong, N.; Shi, X.; Wang, S.; Gao, Y.; Kuang, Z.; Xie, Q.; Li, Y.; Deng, H.; Wu, Y.; Li, M.; et al. M2 macrophages mediate soraf-enib resistance by secreting HGF in a feed-forward manner in hepatocellular carcinoma. *Br. J. Cancer* **2019**, *121*, 22–33. [CrossRef]
132. Wen, S.W.; Sceneay, J.; Lima, L.G.; Wong, C.S.; Becker, M.; Krumeich, S.; Lobb, R.J.; Castillo, V.; Ni Wong, K.; Ellis, S.; et al. The Biodistribution and Immune Suppressive Effects of Breast Cancer-Derived Exosomes. *Cancer Res.* **2016**, *76*, 6816–6827. [CrossRef]
133. Zhou, K.; Guo, S.; Li, F.; Sun, Q.; Liang, G. Exosomal PD-L1: New Insights Into Tumor Immune Escape Mechanisms and Therapeutic Strategies. *Front. Cell Dev. Biol.* **2020**, *8*, 569219. [CrossRef]
134. Ricklefs, F.L.; Alayo, Q.; Krenzlin, H.; Mahmoud, A.B.; Speranza, M.C.; Nakashima, H.; Hayes, J.L.; Lee, K.; Balaj, L.; Passaro, C.; et al. Immune evasion mediated by PD-L1 on glioblastoma-derived extracellular vesicles. *Sci. Adv.* **2018**, *4*, eaar2766. [CrossRef]
135. Pi, Y.-N.; Xia, B.-R.; Jin, M.-Z.; Jin, W.-L.; Lou, G. Exosomes: Powerful weapon for cancer nano-immunoengineering. *Biochem. Pharmacol.* **2021**, *186*, 114487. [CrossRef]

136. Sun, D.; Zhuang, X.; Xiang, X.; Liu, Y.; Zhang, S.; Liu, C.; Barnes, S.; Grizzle, W.; Miller, D.; Zhang, H.-G. A Novel Nanoparticle Drug Delivery System: The Anti-inflammatory Activity of Curcumin Is Enhanced When Encapsulated in Exosomes. *Mol. Ther.* **2010**, *18*, 1606–1614. [CrossRef]
137. Boelens, M.C.; Wu, T.J.; Nabet, B.Y.; Xu, B.; Qiu, Y.; Yoon, T.; Azzam, D.J.; Victor, C.T.-S.; Wiemann, B.Z.; Ishwaran, H.; et al. Exosome Transfer from Stromal to Breast Cancer Cells Regulates Therapy Resistance Pathways. *Cell* **2014**, *159*, 499–513. [CrossRef]
138. Cesselli, D.; Parisse, P.; Aleksova, A.; Veneziano, C.; Cervellin, C.; Zanello, A.; Beltrami, A.P. Extracellular Vesicles: How Drug and Pathology Interfere with Their Biogenesis and Function. *Front. Physiol.* **2018**, *9*, 1394. [CrossRef]
139. Heijnen, H.F.; Schiel, A.E.; Fijnheer, R.; Geuze, H.J.; Sixma, J.J. Activated Platelets Release Two Types of Membrane Vesicles: Microvesicles by Surface Shedding and Exosomes Derived from Exocytosis of Multivesicular Bodies and -Granules. *Blood* **1999**, *94*, 3791–3799. [CrossRef]
140. Muralidharan-Chari, V.; Clancy, J.; Plou, C.; Romao, M.; Chavrier, P.; Raposo, G.; D'Souza-Schorey, C. ARF6-Regulated Shedding of Tumor Cell-Derived Plasma Membrane Microvesicles. *Curr. Biol.* **2009**, *19*, 1875–1885. [CrossRef]
141. Donaldson, J.G. Multiple Roles for Arf6: Sorting, Structuring, and Signaling at the Plasma Membrane. *J. Biol. Chem.* **2003**, *278*, 41573–41576. [CrossRef] [PubMed]
142. Muralidharan-Chari, V.; Clancy, J.; Sedgwick, A.; D'Souza-Schorey, C. Microvesicles: Mediators of extracellular communication during cancer progression. *J. Cell Sci.* **2010**, *123*, 1603–1611. [CrossRef] [PubMed]
143. Ikonomidis, J.S.; Nadeau, E.K.; Akerman, A.W.; Stroud, R.E.; Mukherjee, R.; Jones, J.A. Regulation of membrane type-1 matrix metalloproteinase activity and intracellular localization in clinical thoracic aortic aneurysms. *J. Thorac. Cardiovasc. Surg.* **2016**, *153*, 537–546. [CrossRef]
144. Al-Nedawi, K.; Meehan, B.; Micallef, J.; Lhotak, V.; May, L.; Guha, A.; Rak, J. Intercellular transfer of the oncogenic receptor EGFRvIII by microvesicles derived from tumour cells. *Nat. Cell Biol.* **2008**, *10*, 619–624. [CrossRef] [PubMed]
145. Clancy, J.; Zhang, Y.; Sheehan, C.; D'Souza-Schorey, C. An ARF6-Exportin-5 axis delivers pre-miRNA cargo to tumour microvesicles. *Nat. Cell Biol.* **2019**, *21*, 856–866. [CrossRef]
146. Bian, X.; Xiao, Y.-T.; Wu, T.; Yao, M.; Du, L.; Ren, S.; Wang, J. Microvesicles and chemokines in tumor microenvironment: Mediators of intercellular communications in tumor progression. *Mol. Cancer* **2019**, *18*, 50. [CrossRef]
147. Willms, E.; Cabañas, C.; Mäger, I.; Wood, M.J.A.; Vader, P. Extracellular Vesicle Heterogeneity: Subpopulations, Isolation Techniques, and Diverse Functions in Cancer Progression. *Front. Immunol.* **2018**, *9*, 738. [CrossRef]
148. Baj-Krzyworzeka, M.; Szatanek, R.; Weglarczyk, K.; Baran, J.; Urbanowicz, B.; Brański, P.; Ratajczak, M.Z.; Zembala, M. Tumour-derived microvesicles carry several surface determinants and mRNA of tumour cells and transfer some of these determinants to monocytes. *Cancer Immunol. Immunother.* **2005**, *55*, 808–818. [CrossRef]
149. Wieckowski, E.; Whiteside, T.L. Human Tumor-Derived vs. Dendritic Cell-Derived Exosomes Have Distinct Biologic Roles and Molecular Profiles. *Immunol. Res.* **2006**, *36*, 247–254. [CrossRef]
150. Yi, M.; Xu, L.; Jiao, Y.; Luo, S.; Li, A.; Wu, K. The role of cancer-derived microRNAs in cancer immune escape. *J. Hematol. Oncol.* **2020**, *13*, 25. [CrossRef]
151. Wang, T.; Gilkes, D.M.; Takano, N.; Xiang, L.; Luo, W.; Bishop, C.J.; Chaturvedi, P.; Green, J.J.; Semenza, G.L. Hypoxia-inducible factors and RAB22A mediate formation of microvesicles that stimulate breast cancer invasion and metastasis. *Proc. Natl. Acad. Sci. USA* **2014**, *111*, E3234–E3242. [CrossRef] [PubMed]
152. Finley, S.D.; Popel, A.S. Effect of Tumor Microenvironment on Tumor VEGF during Anti-VEGF Treatment: Systems Biology Predictions. *JNCI J. Natl. Cancer Inst.* **2013**, *105*, 802–811. [CrossRef] [PubMed]
153. Szubert, S.; Szpurek, D.; Moszynski, R.; Nowicki, M.; Frankowski, A.; Sajdak, S.; Michalak, S. Extracellular matrix metalloproteinase inducer (EMMPRIN) expression correlates positively with active angiogenesis and negatively with basic fibroblast growth factor expression in epithelial ovarian cancer. *J. Cancer Res. Clin. Oncol.* **2013**, *140*, 361–369. [CrossRef]
154. Zhang, H.; Bai, M.; Deng, T.; Liu, R.; Wang, X.; Qu, Y.; Duan, J.; Zhang, L.; Ning, T.; Ge, S.; et al. Cell-derived microvesicles mediate the delivery of miR-29a/c to suppress angiogenesis in gastric carcinoma. *Cancer Lett.* **2016**, *375*, 331–339. [CrossRef] [PubMed]
155. Jorfi, S.; Inal, J.M. The role of microvesicles in cancer progression and drug resistance. *Biochem. Soc. Trans.* **2013**, *41*, 293–298. [CrossRef]
156. Ma, X.; Cai, Y.; He, D.; Zou, C.; Zhang, P.; Lo, C.Y.; Xu, Z.; Chan, F.L.; Yu, S.; Chen, Y.; et al. Transient receptor potential channel TRPC5 is essential for P-glycoprotein induction in drug-resistant cancer cells. *Proc. Natl. Acad. Sci. USA* **2012**, *109*, 16282–16287. [CrossRef] [PubMed]
157. Dong, Y.; Pan, Q.; Jiang, L.; Chen, Z.; Zhang, F.; Liu, Y.; Xing, H.; Shi, M.; Li, J.; Li, X.; et al. Tumor endothelial expression of P-glycoprotein upon microvesicular transfer of TrpC5 derived from adriamycin-resistant breast cancer cells. *Biochem. Biophys. Res. Commun.* **2014**, *446*, 85–90. [CrossRef]
158. Balaj, L.; Lessard, R.; Dai, L.; Cho, Y.-J.; Pomeroy, S.L.; Breakefield, X.O.; Skog, J. Tumour microvesicles contain retrotransposon elements and amplified oncogene sequences. *Nat. Commun.* **2011**, *2*, 180. [CrossRef]
159. Wickman, G.; Julian, L.; Olson, M.F. How apoptotic cells aid in the removal of their own cold dead bodies. *Cell Death Differ.* **2012**, *19*, 735–742. [CrossRef]
160. Xu, X.; Lai, Y.; Hua, Z.-C. Apoptosis and apoptotic body: Disease message and therapeutic target potentials. *Biosci. Rep.* **2019**, *39*, BSR20180992. [CrossRef]

161. Takizawa, F.; Tsuji, S.; Nagasawa, S. Enhancement of macrophage phagocytosis upon iC3b deposition on apoptotic cells. *FEBS Lett.* **1996**, *397*, 269–272. [CrossRef]
162. Erwig, L.-P.; Henson, P.M. Clearance of apoptotic cells by phagocytes. *Cell Death Differ.* **2007**, *15*, 243–250. [CrossRef] [PubMed]
163. Taylor, R.C.; Cullen, S.P.; Martin, S.J. Apoptosis: Controlled demolition at the cellular level. *Nat. Rev. Mol. Cell Biol.* **2008**, *9*, 231–241. [CrossRef] [PubMed]
164. Vandivier, R.W.; Ogden, C.A.; Fadok, V.A.; Hoffmann, P.R.; Brown, K.K.; Botto, M.; Walport, M.; Fisher, J.H.; Henson, P.M.; Greene, K.E. Role of Surfactant Proteins A, D, and C1q in the Clearance of Apoptotic Cells In Vivo and In Vitro: Calreticulin and CD91 as a Common Collectin Receptor Complex. *J. Immunol.* **2002**, *169*, 3978–3986. [CrossRef] [PubMed]
165. Bergsmedh, A.; Szeles, A.; Henriksson, M.; Bratt, A.; Folkman, M.J.; Spetz, A.-L.; Holmgren, L. Horizontal transfer of onco-genes by uptake of apoptotic bodies. *Proc. Natl. Acad. Sci. USA* **2001**, *98*, 6407–6411. [CrossRef] [PubMed]
166. Holmgren, L.; Szeles, A.; Rajnavölgyi, E.; Folkman, J.; Klein, G.; Ernberg, I.; Falk, K.I. Horizontal Transfer of DNA by the Uptake of Apoptotic Bodies. *Blood* **1999**, *93*, 3956–3963. [CrossRef] [PubMed]
167. Turnier, J.L.; Kahlenberg, J.M. Using autoantibody signatures to define cancer risk in dermatomyositis. *J. Clin. Investig.* **2022**, *132*, e156025. [CrossRef]
168. Gregory, C.D.; Dransfield, I. Apoptotic Tumor Cell-Derived Extracellular Vesicles as Important Regulators of the On-co-Regenerative Niche. *Front. Immunol.* **2018**, *9*, 1111. [CrossRef]
169. McGaha, T.L.; Karlsson, M.C.I. Apoptotic cell responses in the splenic marginal zone: A paradigm for immunologic reac-tions to apoptotic antigens with implications for autoimmunity. *Immunol. Rev.* **2015**, *269*, 26–43. [CrossRef]
170. Tran, H.B.; Ohlsson, M.; Beroukas, D.; Hiscock, J.; Bradley, J.; Buyon, J.P.; Gordon, T.P. Subcelluar Redistribution of La/SSB Autoantigen During Rhysiologic Apoptosis in the Fetal Mouse Heart and Conduction System. *Arthr. Rheum.* **2002**, *46*, 202–208. [CrossRef]
171. Hu, C.-M.J.; Zhang, L.; Aryal, S.; Cheung, C.; Fang, R.H.; Zhang, L. Erythrocyte membrane-camouflaged polymeric nano-particles as a biomimetic delivery platform. *Proc. Natl. Acad. Sci. USA* **2011**, *108*, 10980–10985. [CrossRef] [PubMed]
172. Huang, J.; Yang, B.; Peng, Y.; Huang, J.; Wong, S.H.D.; Bian, L.; Zhu, K.; Shuai, X.; Han, S. Nanomedicine-Boosting Tumor Immunogenicity for Enhanced Immunotherapy. *Adv. Funct. Mater.* **2021**, *31*, 2011171. [CrossRef]
173. Silva, A.K.A.; Kolosnjaj-Tabi, J.; Bonneau, S.; Marangon, I.; Boggetto, N.; Aubertin, K.; Clément, O.; Bureau, M.F.; Luciani, N.; Gazeau, F.; et al. Magnetic and Photoresponsive Theranosomes: Translating Cell-Released Vesicles into Smart Nanovectors for Cancer Therapy. *ACS Nano* **2013**, *7*, 4954–4966. [CrossRef] [PubMed]
174. Tan, Y.; Huang, J.; Li, Y.; Li, S.; Luo, M.; Luo, J.; Lee, A.W.; Fu, L.; Hu, F.; Guan, X. Near-Infrared Responsive Membrane Nanovesicles Amplify Homologous Targeting Delivery of Anti-PD Immunotherapy against Metastatic Tumors. *Adv. Health Mater.* **2021**, *11*, 2101496. [CrossRef]
175. Yang, R.; Xu, J.; Xu, L.; Sun, X.; Chen, Q.; Zhao, Y.; Peng, R.; Liu, Z. Cancer Cell Membrane-Coated Adjuvant Nanoparticles with Mannose Modification for Effective Anticancer Vaccination. *ACS Nano* **2018**, *12*, 5121–5129. [CrossRef]
176. Taherkhani, S.; Mohammadi, M.; Daoud, J.; Martel, S.; Tabrizian, M. Covalent Binding of Nanoliposomes to the Surface of Magnetotactic Bacteria for the Synthesis of Self-Propelled Therapeutic Agents. *ACS Nano* **2014**, *8*, 5049–5060. [CrossRef]
177. Liu, L.; He, H.; Luo, Z.; Zhou, H.; Liang, R.; Pan, H.; Ma, Y.; Cai, L. In Situ Photocatalyzed Oxygen Generation with Photo-synthetic Bacteria to Enable Robust Immunogenic Photodynamic Therapy in Triple-Negative Breast Cancer. *Adv. Funct. Mater.* **2020**, *30*, 1910176. [CrossRef]
178. Jia, G.; Han, Y.; An, Y.; Ding, Y.; He, C.; Wang, X.; Tang, Q. NRP-1 targeted and cargo-loaded exosomes facilitate simultane-ous imaging and therapy of glioma in vitro and in vivo. *Biomaterials* **2018**, *178*, 302–316. [CrossRef]
179. Pham, T.C.; Jayasinghe, M.K.; Pham, T.T.; Yang, Y.; Wei, L.; Usman, W.M.; Chen, H.; Pirisinu, M.; Gong, J.; Kim, S.; et al. Covalent conjugation of extracellular vesicles with peptides and nanobodies for targeted therapeutic delivery. *J. Extracell. Vesicles* **2021**, *10*, e12057. [CrossRef]
180. Nie, W.; Wu, G.; Zhang, J.; Huang, L.; Ding, J.; Jiang, A.; Zhang, Y.; Liu, Y.; Li, J.; Pu, K.; et al. Responsive Exosome Nano-bioconjugates for Synergistic Cancer Therapy. *Angew. Chem. Int. Ed.* **2019**, *59*, 2018–2022. [CrossRef]
181. Higashi, K.; Mibu, F.; Saito, K.; Limwikrant, W.; Yamamoto, K.; Moribe, K. Composition-dependent structural changes and antitumor activity of ASC-DP/DSPE-PEG nanoparticles. *Eur. J. Pharm. Sci.* **2017**, *99*, 24–31. [CrossRef] [PubMed]
182. Hadidi, N.; Moghadam, N.S.; Pazuki, G.; Parvin, P.; Shahi, F. In Vitro Evaluation of DSPE-PEG (5000) Amine SWCNT Tox-icity and Efficacy as a Novel Nanovector Candidate in Photothermal Therapy by Response Surface Methodology (RSM). *Cells* **2021**, *10*, 2874. [CrossRef] [PubMed]
183. Maeda, N.; Takeuchi, Y.; Takada, M.; Namba, Y.; Oku, N. Synthesis of angiogenesis-targeted peptide and hydrophobized polyethylene glycol conjugate. *Bioorganic Med. Chem. Lett.* **2004**, *14*, 1015–1017. [CrossRef] [PubMed]
184. Nakase, I.; Futaki, S. Combined treatment with a pH-sensitive fusogenic peptide and cationic lipids achieves enhanced cy-tosolic delivery of exosomes. *Sci. Rep.* **2015**, *5*, 10112. [CrossRef] [PubMed]
185. Banz, A.; Cremel, M.; Rembert, A.; Godfrin, Y. In situ targeting of dendritic cells by antigen-loaded red blood cells: A novel approach to cancer immunotherapy. *Vaccine* **2010**, *28*, 2965–2972. [CrossRef]
186. Han, X.; Shen, S.; Fan, Q.; Chen, G.; Archibong, E.; Dotti, G.; Liu, Z.; Gu, Z.; Wang, C. Red blood cell-derived nanoerythro-some for antigen delivery with enhanced cancer immunotherapy. *Sci. Adv.* **2019**, *5*, eaaw6870. [CrossRef] [PubMed]

187. Gong, J.; Chen, D.; Kashiwaba, M.; Kufe, D. Induction of antitumor activity by immunization with fusions of dendritic and carcinoma cells. *Nat. Med.* **1997**, *3*, 558–561. [CrossRef]
188. He, H.; Guo, C.; Wang, J.; Korzun, W.J.; Wang, X.-Y.; Ghosh, S.; Yang, H. Leutusome: A Biomimetic Nanoplatform Integrat-ing Plasma Membrane Components of Leukocytes and Tumor Cells for Remarkably Enhanced Solid Tumor Homing. *Nano Lett.* **2018**, *18*, 6164–6174. [CrossRef]
189. Rao, L.; Wu, L.; Liu, Z.; Tian, R.; Yu, G.; Zhou, Z.; Yang, K.; Xiong, H.-G.; Zhang, A.; Yu, G.-T.; et al. Hybrid cellular mem-brane nanovesicles amplify macrophage immune responses against cancer recurrence and metastasis. *Nat. Commun.* **2020**, *11*, 4909. [CrossRef]
190. Li, Z.; Wang, Y.; Liu, J.; Rawding, P.; Bu, J.; Hong, S.; Hu, Q. Chemically and Biologically Engineered Bacteria-Based Deliv-ery Systems for Emerging Diagnosis and Advanced Therapy. *Adv. Mater.* **2021**, *33*, 2102580. [CrossRef]
191. Zou, M.-Z.; Li, Z.-H.; Bai, X.-F.; Liu, C.-J.; Zhang, X.-Z. Hybrid Vesicles Based on Autologous Tumor Cell Membrane and Bacterial Outer Membrane to Enhance Innate Immune Response and Personalized Tumor Immunotherapy. *Nano Lett.* **2021**, *21*, 8609–8618. [CrossRef] [PubMed]
192. Li, L.; Miao, Q.; Meng, F.; Li, B.; Xue, T.; Fang, T.; Zhang, Z.; Zhang, J.; Ye, X.; Kang, Y.; et al. Genetic engineering cellular vesicles expressing CD64 as checkpoint antibody carrier for cancer immunotherapy. *Theranostics* **2021**, *11*, 6033–6043. [CrossRef] [PubMed]
193. Chen, Z.; Hu, Q.; Gu, Z. Leveraging Engineering of Cells for Drug Delivery. *Acc. Chem. Res.* **2018**, *51*, 668–677. [CrossRef] [PubMed]
194. Mizrak, A.; Bolukbasi, M.F.; Ozdener, G.B.; Brenner, G.J.; Madlener, S.; Erkan, E.P.; Ströbel, T.; Breakefield, X.O.; Saydam, O. Genetically Engineered Microvesicles Carrying Suicide mRNA/Protein Inhibit Schwannoma Tumor Growth. *Mol. Ther.* **2013**, *21*, 101–108. [CrossRef]
195. Ridder, K.; Sevko, A.; Heide, J.; Dams, M.; Rupp, A.-K.; Macas, J.; Starmann, J.; Tjwa, M.; Plate, K.H.; Sultmann, H.; et al. Extracellular vesicle-mediated transfer of functional RNA in the tumor microenvironment. *Oncoimmunology* **2015**, *4*, e1008371. [CrossRef] [PubMed]
196. Yang, M.; Chen, J.; Su, F.; Yu, B.; Su, F.; Lin, L.; Liu, Y.; Huang, J.-D.; Song, E. Microvesicles secreted by macrophages shuttle invasion-potentiating microRNAs into breast cancer cells. *Mol. Cancer* **2011**, *10*, 117. [CrossRef]
197. Kooijmans, S.A.A.; Aleza, C.G.; Roffler, S.R.; Van Solinge, W.; Vader, P.; Schiffelers, R.M. Display of GPI-anchored an-ti-EGFR nanobodies on extracellular vesicles promotes tumour cell targeting. *J. Extracell. Vesicles* **2016**, *5*, 31053. [CrossRef]
198. Ohno, S.-I.; Takanashi, M.; Sudo, K.; Ueda, S.; Ishikawa, A.; Matsuyama, N.; Fujita, K.; Mizutani, T.; Ohgi, T.; Ochiya, T.; et al. Systemically Injected Exosomes Targeted to EGFR Deliver Antitumor MicroRNA to Breast Cancer Cells. *Mol. Ther.* **2013**, *21*, 185–191. [CrossRef]
199. Yang, D.; Postnikov, Y.V.; Li, Y.; Tewary, P.; De La Rosa, G.; Wei, F.; Klinman, D.; Gioannini, T.; Weiss, J.; Furusawa, T.; et al. High-mobility group nucleosome-binding protein 1 acts as an alarmin and is critical for lipopolysaccharide-induced im-mune responses. *J. Exp. Med.* **2011**, *209*, 157–171. [CrossRef]
200. Cheng, Q.; Shi, X.; Han, M.; Smbatyan, G.; Lenz, H.-J.; Zhang, Y. Reprogramming Exosomes as Nanoscale Controllers of Cellular Immunity. *J. Am. Chem. Soc.* **2018**, *140*, 16413–16417. [CrossRef]
201. Shi, X.; Cheng, Q.; Hou, T.; Han, M.; Smbatyan, G.; Lang, J.E.; Epstein, A.L.; Lenz, H.-J.; Zhang, Y. Genetically Engineered Cell-Derived Nanoparticles for Targeted Breast Cancer Immunotherapy. *Mol. Ther.* **2019**, *28*, 536–547. [CrossRef] [PubMed]
202. Mathur, S.; Sutton, J. Personalized medicine could transform healthcare. *Biomed. Rep.* **2017**, *7*, 3–5. [CrossRef] [PubMed]
203. Ding, B.; Zheng, P.; Li, D.; Wang, M.; Jiang, F.; Wang, Z.; Ma, P.; Lin, J. Tumor microenvironment-triggered in situ cancer vaccines inducing dual immunogenic cell death for elevated antitumor and antimetastatic therapy. *Nanoscale* **2021**, *13*, 10906–10915. [CrossRef] [PubMed]
204. Ochyl, L.J.; Bazzill, J.D.; Park, C.; Xu, Y.; Kuai, R.; Moon, J.J. PEGylated tumor cell membrane vesicles as a new vaccine plat-form for cancer immunotherapy. *Biomaterials* **2018**, *182*, 157–166. [CrossRef] [PubMed]
205. Badrinath, S.; Dellacherie, M.O.; Li, A.; Zheng, S.; Zhang, X.; Sobral, M.; Pyrdol, J.W.; Smith, K.L.; Lu, Y.; Haag, S.; et al. A vaccine targeting resistant tumours by dual T cell plus NK cell attack. *Nature* **2022**, *606*, 992–998. [CrossRef]
206. Islam, M.A.; Rice, J.; Reesor, E.; Zope, H.; Tao, W.; Lim, M.; Ding, J.; Chen, Y.; Aduluso, D.; Zetter, B.R.; et al. Adjuvant-pulsed mRNA vaccine nanoparticle for immunoprophylactic and therapeutic tumor suppression in mice. *Biomaterials* **2020**, *266*, 120431. [CrossRef]
207. Burrell, R.A.; McGranahan, N.; Bartek, J.; Swanton, C. The causes and consequences of genetic heterogeneity in cancer evo-lution. *Nature* **2013**, *501*, 338–345. [CrossRef]
208. Ye, Y.; Wang, C.; Zhang, X.; Hu, Q.; Zhang, Y.; Liu, Q.; Wen, D.; Milligan, J.; Bellotti, A.; Huang, L.; et al. A mela-nin-mediated cancer immunotherapy patch. *Sci. Immunol.* **2017**, *2*, eaan5692. [CrossRef]
209. Ma, L.; Diao, L.; Peng, Z.; Jia, Y.; Xie, H.; Li, B.; Ma, J.; Zhang, M.; Cheng, L.; Ding, D.; et al. Immunotherapy and Prevention of Cancer by Nanovaccines Loaded with Whole-Cell Components of Tumor Tissues or Cells. *Adv. Mater.* **2021**, *33*, 2104849. [CrossRef]
210. Lu, Y.; Wu, C.; Yang, Y.; Chen, X.; Ge, F.; Wang, J.; Deng, J. Inhibition of tumor recurrence and metastasis via a surgical tumor-derived personalized hydrogel vaccine. *Biomater. Sci.* **2022**, *10*, 1352–1363. [CrossRef]

211. Fang, R.H.; Hu, C.-M.J.; Luk, B.T.; Gao, W.; Copp, J.A.; Tai, Y.; O'Connor, D.E.; Zhang, L. Cancer Cell Membrane-Coated Nanoparticles for Anticancer Vaccination and Drug Delivery. *Nano Lett.* **2014**, *14*, 2181–2188. [CrossRef] [PubMed]
212. Fang, R.H.; Jiang, Y.; Fang, J.C.; Zhang, L. Cell membrane-derived nanomaterials for biomedical applications. *Biomaterials* **2017**, *128*, 69–83. [CrossRef] [PubMed]
213. Xu, J.; Lv, J.; Zhuang, Q.; Yang, Z.; Cao, Z.; Xu, L.; Pei, P.; Wang, C.; Wu, H.; Dong, Z.; et al. A general strategy towards per-sonalized nanovaccines based on fluoropolymers for post-surgical cancer immunotherapy. *Nat. Nanotechnol.* **2020**, *15*, 1043–1052. [CrossRef]
214. Liu, Y.; Gu, Y.; Cao, X. The exosomes in tumor immunity. *OncoImmunology* **2015**, *4*, e1027472. [CrossRef]
215. Yang, Y.; Xiu, F.; Cai, Z.; Wang, J.; Wang, Q.; Fu, Y.; Cao, X. Increased induction of antitumor response by exosomes derived from interleukin-2 gene-modified tumor cells. *J. Cancer Res. Clin. Oncol.* **2007**, *133*, 389–399. [CrossRef] [PubMed]
216. Dai, S.; Zhou, X.; Wang, B.; Wang, Q.; Fu, Y.-X.; Chen, T.; Wan, T.; Yu, Y.; Cao, X. Enhanced induction of dendritic cell matu-ration and HLA-A*0201-restricted CEA-specific CD8+ CTL response by exosomes derived from IL-18 gene-modified CEA-positive tumor cells. *Klin. Wochenschr.* **2006**, *84*, 1067–1076. [CrossRef]
217. Yang, Y.; Wang, L.; Cao, H.; Li, Q.; Li, Y.; Han, M.; Wang, H.; Li, J. Photodynamic Therapy with Liposomes Encapsulating Photosensitizers with Aggregation-Induced Emission. *Nano Lett.* **2019**, *19*, 1821–1826. [CrossRef]
218. Han, X.; Chen, J.; Chu, J.; Liang, C.; Ma, Q.; Fan, Q.; Liu, Z.; Wang, C. Platelets as platforms for inhibition of tumor recur-rence post-physical therapy by delivery of anti-PD-L1 checkpoint antibody. *J. Control. Release* **2019**, *304*, 233–241. [CrossRef]
219. Cazares-Cortes, E.; Cabana, S.; Boitard, C.; Nehlig, E.; Griffete, N.; Fresnais, J.; Wilhelm, C.; Abou-Hassan, A.; Ménager, C. Recent insights in magnetic hyperthermia: From the "hot-spot" effect for local delivery to combined magne-to-photo-thermia using magneto-plasmonic hybrids. *Adv. Drug Deliv. Rev.* **2018**, *138*, 233–246. [CrossRef]
220. Marangoni, V.S.; Bernardi, J.C.; Reis, I.B.; Fávaro, W.J.; Zucolotto, V. Photothermia and Activated Drug Release of Natural Cell Membrane Coated Plasmonic Gold Nanorods and β-Lapachone. *ACS Appl. Bio Mater.* **2019**, *2*, 728–736. [CrossRef]
221. Ma, J.; Zhang, Y.; Tang, K.; Zhang, H.; Yin, X.; Li, Y.; Xu, P.; Sun, Y.; Ma, R.; Ji, T.; et al. Reversing drug resistance of soft tu-mor-repopulating cells by tumor cell-derived chemotherapeutic microparticles. *Cell Res.* **2016**, *26*, 713–727. [CrossRef] [PubMed]
222. Kim, M.S.; Haney, M.J.; Zhao, Y.; Mahajan, V.; Deygen, I.; Klyachko, N.L.; Inskoe, E.; Piroyan, A.; Sokolsky, M.; Okolie, O.; et al. Development of exosome-encapsulated paclitaxel to overcome mdr in cancer cells. *Nanomed. Nanotechnol. Biol. Med.* **2016**, *12*, 655–664. [CrossRef] [PubMed]
223. Liu, J.; Ye, Z.; Xiang, M.; Chang, B.; Cui, J.; Ji, T.; Zhao, L.; Li, Q.; Deng, Y.; Xu, L.; et al. Functional extracellular vesicles en-gineered with lipid-grafted hyaluronic acid effectively reverse cancer drug resistance. *Biomaterials* **2019**, *223*, 119475. [CrossRef] [PubMed]
224. Bose, R.J.; Kumar, S.U.; Zeng, Y.; Afjei, R.; Robinson, E.; Lau, K.; Bermudez, A.; Habte, F.; Pitteri, S.J.; Sinclair, R.; et al. Tumor Cell-Derived Extracellular Vesicle-Coated Nanocarriers: An Efficient Theranostic Platform for the Cancer-Specific Delivery of Anti-miR-21 and Imaging Agents. *ACS Nano* **2018**, *12*, 10817–10832. [CrossRef]

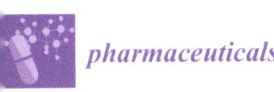

Article

Sesamol Loaded Albumin Nanoparticles: A Boosted Protective Property in Animal Models of Oxidative Stress

Sara Zaher [1], Mahmoud E. Soliman [2,3], Mahmoud Elsabahy [4] and Rania M. Hathout [2,*]

1. Assiut International Center of Nanomedicine, Al-Rajhy Liver Hospital, Assiut University, Assiut 71515, Egypt; sarazaher914@gmail.com
2. Department of Pharmaceutics and Industrial Pharmacy, Faculty of Pharmacy, Ain Shams University, Cairo 11566, Egypt; mahmoud.e.soliman@pharma.asu.edu.eg
3. Pharm D Program, Egypt-Japan University of Science and Technology (EJUST), New Borg El Arab, Alexandria 21934, Egypt
4. School of Biotechnology and Science Academy, Badr University in Cairo, Badr City, Cairo 11829, Egypt; mahmoud.elsabahy@buc.edu.eg
* Correspondence: rania.hathout@pharma.asu.edu.eg

Abstract: The current study evaluated the ability of sesamol-loaded albumin nanoparticles to impart protection against oxidative stress induced by anthracyclines in comparison to the free drug. Albumin nanoparticles were prepared via the desolvation technique and then freeze-dried with the cryoprotectant, trehalose. Albumin concentration, pH, and type of desolvating agent were assessed as determining factors for successful albumin nanoparticle fabrication. The optimal nanoparticles were spherical in shape, and they had an average particle diameter of 127.24 ± 2.12 nm with a sesamol payload of 96.89 ± 2.4 µg/mg. The drug cellular protection was tested on rat hepatocytes pretreated with 1 µM doxorubicin, which showed a 1.2-fold higher protective activity than the free sesamol. In a pharmacokinetic study, the loading of a drug onto nanoparticles resulted in a longer half-life and mean residence time, as compared to the free drug. Furthermore, in vivo efficacy and biochemical assessment of lipid peroxidation, cardiac biomarkers, and liver enzymes were significantly ameliorated after administration of the sesamol-loaded albumin nanoparticles. The biochemical assessments were also corroborated with the histopathological examination data. Sesamol-loaded albumin nanoparticles, prepared under controlled conditions, may provide an enhanced protective effect against off-target doxorubicin toxicity.

Keywords: sesamol; albumin nanoparticles; doxorubicin; oxidative stress; antioxidants

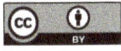

1. Introduction

Excessive free radical generation and cellular oxidative stress are implicated as a causative or as an adjuvant of various pathologies, such as hepatic fibrosis, pulmonary inflammation, cardiomyopathy, diabetic complications, renal disease, brain aging, and neurodegenerative conditions [1–3]. Several chemotherapeutic agents are a potential source of free radicals and reactive species, which impede their therapeutic use [4]. Free radicals are involved in cellular respiration, cell growth regulation, intracellular signaling, and biomolecule synthesis [5].

Doxorubicin (DOX), a secondary metabolite of *Streptomyces peucetius* that belongs to the family of anthracycline drugs, is a potent antineoplastic agent that is widely used to treat different adult and pediatric tumors, including solid tumors, leukemias, breast cancer, and Hodgkin's and non-Hodgkin's lymphoma. It works by multiple cytotoxic pathways and the most potent is targeting topoisomerase II α, which is highly expressed in cancer cells, to inhibit DNA replication [6]. Unfortunately, DOX is metabolized by cytochrome P450 and flavin-monooxygenase enzymes to its semiquinone form, which interacts with oxygen molecules to generate reactive oxygen species (ROS) [4,7]. Additionally, DOX molecules interact with iron (Fe^{2+}) forming a free radical complex, which is usually involved in the production of hydroxyl radical (HO•). Excessive ROS generation triggers the lipid peroxidation and the depletion of endogenous antioxidant enzymes, resulting in mitochondrial dysfunction, cellular injury, and multi-organ toxicity [8]. Hence, searching for a protective agent remains a challenge [9].

Currently, there is great interest toward the combination of natural antioxidants such as, curcumin, silibinin, or sesamol (SML), and conventional antineoplastic agents such as, cisplatin, and doxorubicin as prospects for chemotherapy to avoid harmful [10] effects, which can be toxic to healthy cells [11–14]. Sesamol (3,4-methylenedioxy phenol, SML), a phenolic antioxidant agent, is a major component of sesame seed oil. SML has a potent antioxidant, anti-inflammatory, and free radical scavenging activity [10,15].

Several researchers have demonstrated the protective effect of SML on oxidative stress caused by DOX. It has been reported to possess various physiological activities as a hepatoprotective, cardioprotective, antiatherogenic, and anti-aging agent by attenuating oxidative stress and systemic inflammation [16]. However, SML has poor intracellular bioavailability (F_{ic}) due to its hydrophilic nature [17]. SML also suffers from rapid clearance that is associated with the appearance of its metabolites such as sesamol sulphate/glucuronide within four hours [18,19]. Hence, a sustained release formulation can provide a controlled and a steady release manner to maintain SML plasma concentration that is stable for a prolonged time. Albumin nanoparticles that can be internalized and engulfed by cells may provide sustained drug release and prolonged efficacy.

Human serum albumin (HSA) is an endogenous, non-toxic, biodegradable, nonimmunogenic, water-soluble polymer (Generally Regarded As Safe (GRAS)) that possesses serum stability and a long half-life [20]. In addition, HSA provides sites for the binding of various polar and nonpolar drugs. Further, albumin-based nanoparticles (ANPs) play a vital role in passive targeting, and they accumulate in solid tumors and inflamed tissues due to the enhanced permeability and retention effect [21]. The aforementioned preferable properties of albumin form the rationale for developing albumin-based drug delivery systems [20]. Clinically, several drugs have been loaded onto ANPs and approved for use as DOX, methotrexate, and paclitaxel.

It is worth noting that HSA possesses direct and indirect antioxidant effects. It works directly as a free radical scavenger as the free thiol groups in the Cys-34 residue are able to trap different types of ROS and six methionine groups, which are easily oxidized. Moreover, HSA can act indirectly by binding bilirubin that inhibit lipid peroxidation and free metals such as iron and copper, which catalyze aggressive ROS formation [22].

The work in this study comprised the fabrication of a series of SML-loaded ANPs (SML-ANPs) formulations adopting the desolvation technique. A systematic optimization concerning the influence of albumin concentration, pH of the medium, and the type of desolvation reagent on the physicochemical characteristics of nanoparticles was carried out to allow preparation of a colloidal system with well-defined physicochemical characteristics. In vitro and in vivo assessments were carried out in animal models of oxidative stress induced by DOX.

2. Results

2.1. Characterization of SML-ANPs and Statistical Modeling

The desolvation technique allowed fabrication of homogenous SML-ANPs with a drug loading capacity ranging from 14.8 to 116.7 µg/mg HSA. All the prepared formulations showed particle diameters ranging from 111.5 to 367.1 nm, with an acceptable PDI < 0.3 and zeta potential. The morphological appearance using SEM imaging revealed that the particles have almost a regular spherical shape with a smooth surface, as shown in Figure 1.

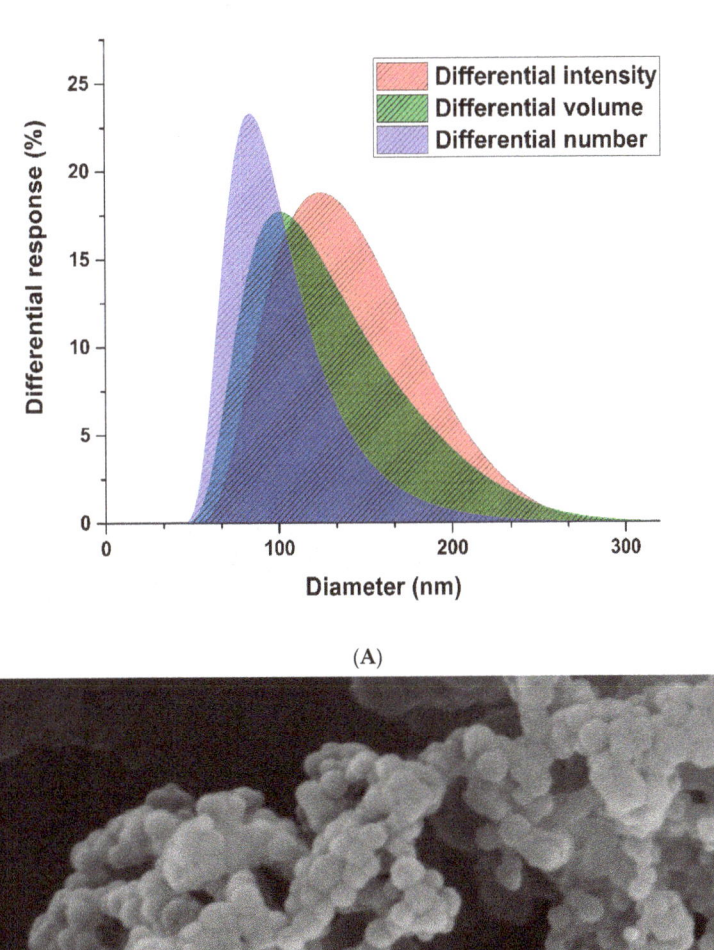

Figure 1. Size distribution histograms, the intensity-, volume-, and number-averaged hydrodynamic diameter histograms of a selected SML-ANPs (**A**), scanning electron micrograph (**B**).

Figure 2 summarizes the effect of the three tested variables on the fabrication of SML-ANPS. Although the increase in pH had a fluctuating effect on the particle size and the loading capacity, it was observed to cause a marked increase in the negative charge of the produced ANPS. However, optimizing HSA mass to get small monodisperse ANPS with a high loading capacity was more significant (Supplementary material, Table S1). The

D-optimal design reveals the importance of each of the variables, and it jointly tests their interactions (Supplementary material, Table S2). Each response was fitted to the suggested model generated by the optimal design. The generated equations according to the DOD (Equations (S9)–(S14)) are mentioned in the supplementary file [23,24].

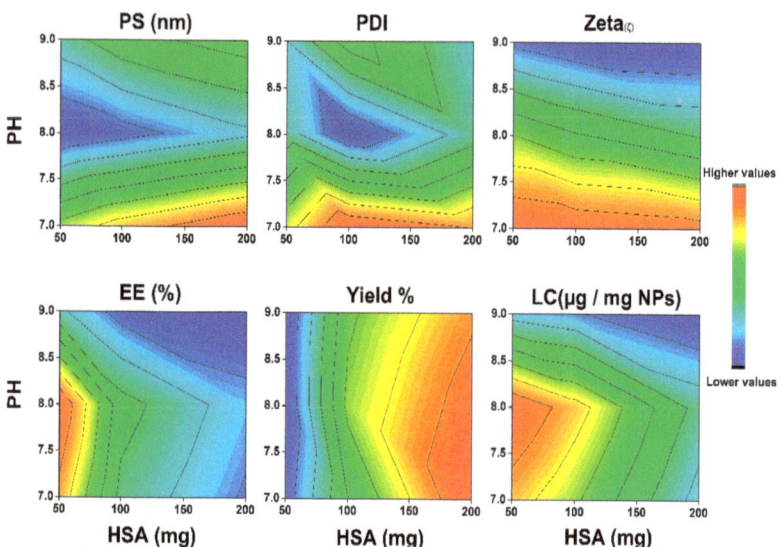

Figure 2. Contour plots generated by the D-optimal design demonstrating the effect of albumin concentration and aqueous medium pH using ethanol acetone as a desolvating agent on the albumin nanoparticles diameter (PS), polydispersity index (PDI), Zeta potential, sesamol encapsulation efficiency (EE%), albumin nanoparticles percent yield, and sesamol loading in albumin nanoparticles (LC).

Multiple regression analysis of the results of the measured responses was performed, as shown in Table 1. The R2 values represent the amount of variation around the mean explained by the model. Most of the presented models were significant (p value < 0.001), with a good predictability ($R^2 > 0.94$), demonstrating fittingness of the models except the PDI model which was insignificant. An ANOVA test was used to verify the adequacy of these models. The term "adequate precision" is a measure of the range of a predicted response relative to its associated error, which measures the signal-to-noise ratio [25]. Most of the models showed a ratio higher than 4.0, which implies an adequate signal that can navigate the design space using that model [26]. The results showed that changing the three tested factors (HSA concentration, pH, and changing type of desolvating agent) had a statistically significant impact on the physicochemical properties of the prepared SML-ANPs. The Predicted R^2 was in reasonable agreement with the Adjusted R^2; i.e., the difference was less than 0.2, which showed a strong correlation between the independent parameters and the responses.

Table 1. Characteristics of the generated response surface models.

Responses	PS	PDI	Zeta	%EE	%Yield	LC [1]
Order	Quadratic	Quadratic	Linear	Quadratic	Quadratic	Quadratic
Significance	extremely significant ($p < 0.001$)	ns	extremely significant ($p < 0.001$)	extremely significant ($p < 0.001$)	extremely significant ($p < 0.001$)	extremely significant ($p < 0.001$)
R^2	0.994	0.649	0.969	0.972	0.983	0.942
Adjusted R^2	0.989	0.338	0.963	0.947	0.968	0.890
Predicted R^2	0.969	−0.468	0.953	0.871	0.923	0.736
Adequate precision	45.801	3.998	34.93	18.01	23.926	12.855 [2]

[1] Abbreviations: DL: Drug loading; EE%: Percent of entrapment efficiency; SML-ANPS: Sesamol-loaded albumin nanoparticles; PDI: Polydispersity index; PS: Particle size; Y%: Percent of yield; and ZP: Zeta potential. [2] "ns" presents that no significant differences.

Using Design-Expert software® and by applying the D-optimal design desirability function, the optimum conditions for SML-ANPs fabrications were 131 mg/mL concentrations of HSA, pH 8.12, and ethanol acetone mixture as a desolvating agent with a desirability rate of 0.734. Moreover, the optimum formulation according to the predetermined parameters in the design and data analysis scored 127 nm, 0.07, −26.2 δ, 87.9%, 81.92%, and 96.9 µg/mg in particles size, PDI, zeta potential, percentage encapsulated, yield percentage, and sesamol payload, respectively, which were found to be in considerable agreement with their corresponding predicted values that were obtained by the design expert software. The mean particle size measurements using DSL were in agreement with the SEM imaging observed particle size.

2.2. In Vitro Cumulative Release Study

The in vitro release profiles of SML from the selected SML-ANPs formulations and the free drug solution are shown in Figure 3. SML was released in a biphasic manner with a sustained release subsequent to an initial burst in the first hour. The cumulative percentage of SML released over 72 h was approximately 62.3%. Table S3, summarizes the data derived from the kinetic study, where Higuchi and the Korsmeyer–Peppas model fit the SML release from SML-ANPs rather than the other modules with maximum R2 values of 0.971 and 0.985, respectively, elucidating that SML release followed the diffusion mechanism in the general manner. Besides, the value of the diffusion exponents (n) was 0.336, which corresponds to the Fickian diffusion mechanism of release [27,28].

2.3. Freeze Drying and Stability Studies of SML-ANPs

The freeze-drying of the selected formulation in the absence of cryoprotectants led to a large increase in particle size reaching 386 nm and a lack of homogeneity (PDI, 0.52), as shown in Figure 4. Therefore, freeze-drying without cryoprotectants was determined as not an appropriate technique for stabilizing the suspension of SML-ANPs and enhancing its long-term stability. In the current study, the propensity of three distinct cryoprotectants (sucrose, trehalose, and mannitol) was evaluated at three concentrations of 1%, 2%, and 3% each, while retaining their original state. After reconstitution of the freeze-dried ANPs, 1% sucrose and 1% trehalose were able to maintain the original properties of SML-ANPs suspension with a low non-significant difference at the lowest tested concentration. On the other hand, mannitol showed a significant increase in particle size: 264.7 nm and a PDI of 0.3.

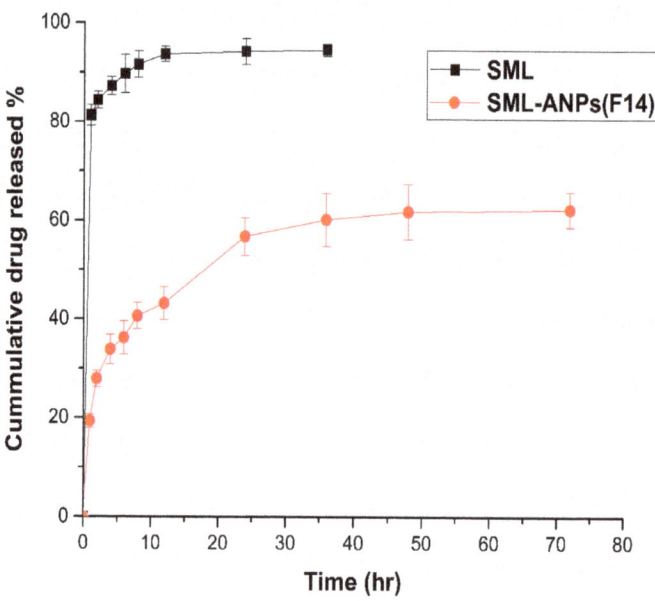

Figure 3. In vitro release profiles of free SML and SML-ANPs (F14). The values are presented as mean ± SD (n in each group = 3).

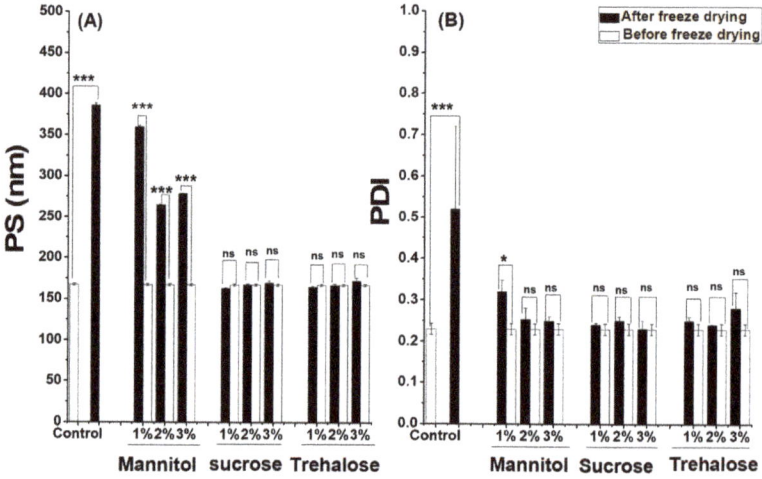

Figure 4. Influence of the freeze-drying process of SML-ANPs (10 mg/mL) in the presence of different excipients on (**A**) particle diameter and (**B**) polydispersity before freeze drying and after reconstitution of the samples in water (mean ± S.D.; n in each group = 3). For all results, ns presents that no significant differences were found and the differences were considered significant when $p < 0.05$, and extremely significant when $p < 0.0001$ presented by *, and ***, respectively.

After reconstitution of the freeze dried SML-ANPs with different types of cryoprotectants, trehalose was able to maintain the properties of SML-ANPs, and it showed a long-term stability of up to six months with a non-significant difference ($p \geq 0.05$). Besides, the data of the short-term stability study showed that SML-ANPs remained stable in water and biologically-relevant media, with no statistically significant changes over the 2-h incubation period in all conditions (results not shown). Regarding the shelf-life testing, three samples of freeze-dried SML-ANPs were tested weekly for 12 weeks. There was no significant change in nanoparticle diameter and PDI over the 12 weeks, except for frozen batches that became micrometric and heterogeneous (PI > 0.3) after 3 weeks of the experiment. Both types of cryoprotectants maintained their physicochemical properties at 4 °C for more than 6 months. There was no significant change in the diameter and PDI ($p < 0.05$) of the formula during the tested period for sucrose and trehalose. All of these results confirmed that sucrose and trehalose would be suitable cryoprotectants for ANPs. On the other hand, when HSA nanoparticles were not stabilized with lyophilization, the resulting carriers were found to be stable for a few weeks, then nanoparticles rapidly aggregated.

2.4. Pharmacokinetic Study Results

Figure 5 depicts the SML plasma concentrations following intravenous administration of SML and SML-ANP at predetermined intervals. Although the clearance patterns of both groups were almost similar, a significant difference of 151.9 and 67.3 µg/mL between SML-treated and SML-ANP-treated groups, respectively, was observed early after 15 min. SML plasma concentration was 10.5 µg/mL after 24 h of an SML-ANPs injection, while SML was barely detected after 8 h in an SML-treated group. Additionally, the SML-treated group displayed a short half-life and a rapid elimination rate of 1.25 h and 0.53 L/h, respectively. As illustrated in Table 2, ANPs can act as an SML reservoir in the bloodstream, with an extended half-life and slower elimination rates of 8.9 h and 0.11 L/h, respectively. When SML-ANPs are gradually degraded, SML is slowly released into the blood stream resulting in a prolonged drug residence time in blood circulation and a higher AUC value of 8.5 h and 88.7 µg·h/L, respectively. Nevertheless, the free SML solution showed a shorter residence time and a lower AUC of 2.6 h and 19.5 µg·h/L, respectively.

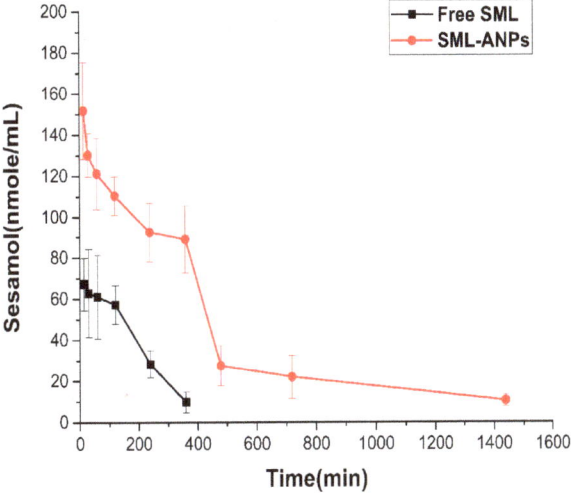

Figure 5. Plasma concentration–time profiles of SML after IV single dose (15 mg/kg) of SML and SML-ANPs. Values are presented as means ± SD (n in each group = 4).

Table 2. Pharmacokinetic parameters of SML concentration after intravenous administration of free SML and SML-ANPs to rats.

Parameters	t1/2(h) *	AUC (µg/mL h) *	MRT(h) *	CL (mL/h) *
Free SML	1.3 ± 0.13	19.5 ± 4.2	2.6 ± 0.03	528.2 ± 115.5
SML-ANPs	6.1 ± 0.44	88.7 ± 12.2	8.5 ± 0.63	114.2 ± 15.9

Abbreviations: t½, half-life; AUC, area under the curve; MRT, mean residence time; CL, clearance, SML: free sesamol and SML-ANPS: Sesamol-loaded albumin nanoparticles. Notes: For all results, the differences between SML-ANPs vs. free SML were considered significant when $p < 0.05$ presented by *. All results expressed mean ± SD, n in each group = 4.

The pharmacokinetic study showed that the average half-life, mean retention time, and AUC were significantly higher ($p < 0.05$) than that of the SML-treated group (Table 2), whereas the clearance rate was lower ($p < 0.05$). The above results indicate that SML-ANPs increased the systemic circulation time leading to a higher amount of SML available for cellular uptake. Moreover, maintaining the plasma SML concentration for a long time with continuous release properties was demonstrated.

2.5. Evaluation of SML-ANPs Hepatoprotection

Figure 6 shows the relative cell protection of SML-ANPs at different concentrations. The results from cultivated rat hepatocytes demonstrated that cell viability was dropped to 25.2 ± 1.3% by incubation with 1 µM DOX for 24 h. Viability percentage, SML hepatoprotection, and enhanced SML-ANP protection capability were counted, as illustrated in Table S4. Treatment with SML showed a percentage of hepatoprotection at concentrations of 100 and 500 µg/mL up to 16.7 ± 4.4 and 30.1 ± 4.6, respectively. However, SML-ANPs showed an enhanced protective activity in comparison to a free SML solution at concentrations of 100 and 500 µg/mL up to 23.2 ± 6.1 and 41.7 ± 4.9 µg/mL, respectively.

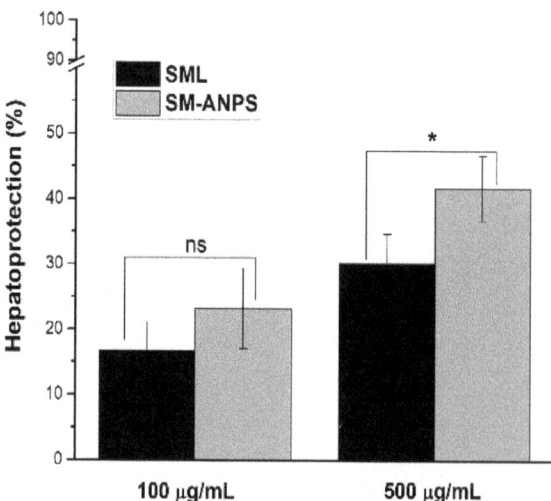

Figure 6. Hepatoprotective effect of SML-ANPs on rat hepatocytes in comparison to free SML solution, measured by the MTS assay. * $p < 0.05$ and ns when no significant difference was found between the SML group and the SML-ANPs group. Results presented as %hepatoprotection and expressed as the mean ± SD (n in each group = 4).

2.6. Biochemical Assessment

By cumulative i.p. injection of DOX, serum levels of CK, LDH, AST, and ALT were significantly elevated to 2.7, 4, 3.3, and 3-fold above the corresponding control values, respectively. However, the co-treatment with SML-ANPs significantly reduced the elevated serum CK and LDH by 59.3 and 64.5%, respectively, while AST and ALT were reduced by 60.5 and 59% in comparison to the corresponding values of the free SML treated group, which were 35.6, 47.2, 49.9, and 41.2%, respectively (Figure 7). These results were accompanied by a significant increase in the MDA levels above the control values by 21.6, 9.4, 114, 7.5, and 8.8-folds in serum, cardiac, liver, kidney, and testis samples, respectively, as illustrated in Figure 7. The protection of doxorubicin-treated rats with SML-ANPs succeeded in normalizing MDA levels, as shown in Figure 7, where MDA activity was significantly reduced in serum, cardiac, liver, kidney, and testis by 88.2, 77.3, 80, 72.3, and 81.2%, respectively, in comparison to the corresponding values of the free SML-treated group: 61.9, 55.9, 59, 41.7, and 86.5%, respectively.

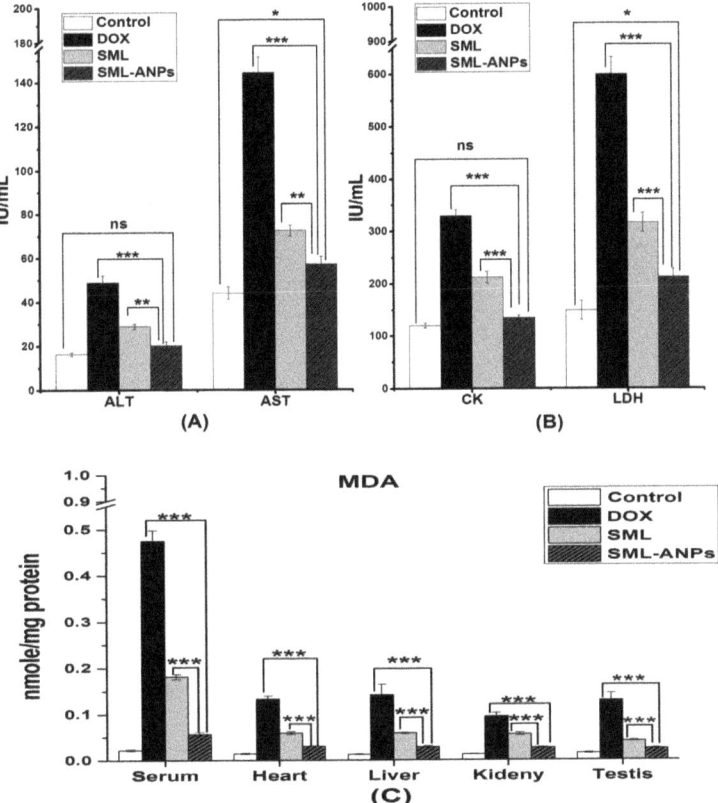

Figure 7. Cardiac (**A**), liver (**B**) and lipid peroxidation (**C**) biomarkers' assessment. * $p < 0.05$, ** $p < 0.001$ and *** $p < 0.0001$ when compared to SML-ANPs group. Data are presented as means ± SE (n in each group = 8).

2.7. Changes in Animal Body Weight and Mortality Rates

As illustrated in Table 3, the body weights (BW) of the experimental animals decreased significantly starting from the first dose in the DOX-treated group compared to the control group ($p < 0.05$). The administration of SML and SML-A NPs controlled this issue. Although there was no significant difference in the animals' body weight between SML-treated or

SML-ANPs-treated animals during the first two weeks, the difference after the third week was highly significant (p value < 0.001). Consequently, these findings pointed to the enhanced protective effect of SML-ANPs at the tested dose. Furthermore, during the study period, there was no mortality in both control GP and SML-ANPs GP. However, throughout the experiment, three animals died; two animals in DOX GP and only one animal in SML GP.

Table 3. Body weights of the experimental animals after the administration of the investigated formulations as compared to the control.

Wt.(g)/Survival Rate	Control GP	DOX GP *	SML GP [ns]	SML-ANPs GP [ns,1,2]
Body weight	151.7 ± 11.02	101.26 ± 5.61	146.5 ± 14.12	162.44 ± 15.49
Survival rate	10/10	8/10	9/10	10/10

[1] Abbreviations: DOX GP: Doxorubicin treated group; SML GP: Sesamol treated group; SML-ANPs GP: Sesamol loaded albumin nanoparticles treated group. [2] For all results, compared to the control group [ns] presents that no significant difference was found and the differences were considered significant when $p < 0.05$ presented by *. Body weight results expressed mean ± SD (n in each group = 10).

Moreover, the DOX treated group showed remarkable degenerative changes at different grades in the cardiac, liver, kidney, and testis tissues in the form of cellular atrophy, cytoplasmic vacuolization, lymphoid cell aggregation, coagulative necrosis, edema, and hemorrhages. Sesamol counteracted the damaging effects of oxidation in SML GP. However, Sesamol-loaded albumin nanoparticles treatment in SML-ANPs GP markedly ameliorated the DOX-induced pathological changes, and they maintained the normal histological picture, as shown in Figure 8. Moreover, the histopathological lesions in the four groups were scored according to the following: 0 = no damage, 1 = (<25% damage) focal, slight changes, 2 = (25–50% damage) multifocal, significant changes, and 3 = (>50% damage) common widespread changes, as illustrated in the Supplementary material, Table S5.

As shown in Figure 8A,B, the liver from the control group showed normal hepatic cells structure organized in cords (Figure 8A) separated by hepatic sinusoids and radiating from the central vein to the portal area (containing branches of heptaic artery, portal vein, and bile duct) (Figure 8B). Kidney sections from the control group (Figure 8C) showed a normal renal cortex with glomeruli and renal tubules. The heart from the control group (Figure 8D) showed normal cardiac muscle histology with its characteristic striated appearance. Th testicular sections from the control group (Figure 8E) showed normal seminiferous tubule with its normal lining epithelium. The liver sections from the DOX group (Figure 8F,G) showed hepatic cell atrophy: particularly, in the centrilobular area, widening of the hepatic sinusoids (arrows), cytoplasmic vacuolization (arrowheads) (Figure 8F), and focal lymphoid cell aggregations in the portal area (arrows) (Figure 8G). The kidney sections from the DOX group (Figure 8H) showed glomerular necrosis (arrow), accumulation of hyaline casts in the Bowman's space and the tubular lumen (arrowheads), and severe renal tubular necrosis. DOX group heart sections (Figure 8I) showed severe myocardial necrosis (arrows) and lymphoid cell infiltration (arrowheads). The testicular sections from the DOX group (Figure 8J) showed severe necrosis of the seminiferous tubule with loss of the spermatogenic cells, intratubular multinucleated spermatids (arrows), and cytoplasmic vacuolization (arrowheads). Liver sections from the SML group (Figure 8K,L) showed moderate atrophy of the hepatocytes in the centrilobular zone, moderate widening of the hepatic sinusoids (arrows) (Figure 8K), mild vacuolated cytoplasm (arrowheads) (Figure 8K), and mild lymphoid cell infiltration in the portal area (arrowheads) (Figure 8L). (M) Kidneys from the SML group showed moderate hyaline cast deposition in the Bowman's space and the tubular lumen (arrowheads) and individual cell necrosis (arrows). The heart sections from the SML group showed mild individual necrosis of the cardiomyocytes (arrow) and moderate cytoplasmic vacuolization (arrowheads) (Figure 8N). The testicular sections from the SML group (Figure 8O) showed almost normal seminiferous tubules and few with depleted spermatogenesis and germ cell detachment from the basal lamina (arrows). The liver sections from the SML-ANPs group (Figure 8P,Q) showed very few hepatocytes with vacuolated cytoplasm (arrowhead) (P) and mild lymphoid cell infiltration in the portal area (arrow) (Q). The SML-ANPs group kidney sections (Figure 8R) showed mild hyaline cast deposition in the tubular lumen (arrowheads). The heart sections from the SML-ANPs group (Figure 8S) showed lymphoid cell infiltration (arrowheads). Finally, the testicular sections from the SML-ANPs group (Figure 8T) showed almost normal seminiferous tubules and spermatogenic cells.

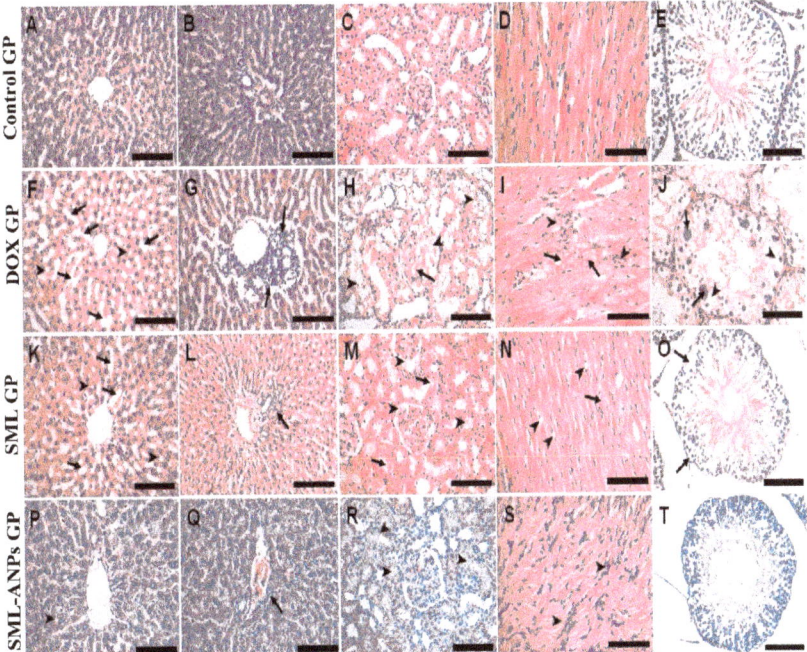

Figure 8. Histopathological changes of heart, liver, kidney, and testes in the control group, doxorubicin treated group (DOX GP), sesamol treated group (SML GP), and sesamol-loaded albumin nanoparticles group (SML-ANPs GP). (**A–E**) represent photomicrographs of the liver, kidney, heart and testis sections, respectively, stained by H & E from the control group. (**F–J**) represent photomicrographs of the liver, kidney, heart and testis sections, respectively, stained by H & E from DOX GP. (**K–O**) represent photomicrographs of the liver, kidney, heart and testis sections, respectively, stained by H & E from SML GP while (**P–T**) represent photomicrographs of the liver, kidney, heart and testis sections, respectively, stained by H & E from SML-ANPs GP.

3. Discussion

ANPS were prepared by a desolvation technique that did not involve the use of heat and high shear strength, which impair drug stability [29]. The operating conditions such as initial pH of the solution, amount of HSA, and type of desolvating agent have been identified as critical factors that influence characteristics of the formed particles. It was previously reported that the isoelectric point (IP) of HSA is 4.9 [30]. At pH < IP, the absence of electrostatic repulsion forces and hydrophobic interactions led to the aggregation of protein molecules and a larger particle size. Decreasing the overall charges by approaching the IP limits the physical stability of the colloidal dispersion and increases the probability of aggregation. On the other hand, in a basic environment, the electrostatic interactions increased the repulsive forces between HSA molecules and, concomitantly, the enhanced protein–solvent interactions decreased the coagulation. As a result, fine HSA particles could be formed accompanied with a higher loading capacity at pH 8. However, at pH 9, enhanced ionization of the albumin molecules occurred and the high negative charges enhanced the repulsion among the HSA molecules due to steric effects that slowed down the aggregation during particle formation and led to an increase in particle size. Moreover, the molecular repulsion caused by a large magnitude of a negative charge can hinder molecules from getting closer thus preventing the production of aggregates with high polydispersity. Furthermore, the accelerated cross-linking process in alkaline conditions (Schiff's base formation) could explain the lower loading capacity and the larger particle size. As amino groups are deprotonated at high pH, free amino groups are available for interaction with the aldehydic groups [31].

Figure 2 demonstrates the contour plots of the D-optimal models. Noticeably, from the plots, a lower concentration of the HSA solution during desolvation significantly decreased ($p < 0.0001$) the particle diameter and increased the loading capacity. Furthermore, increasing the amount of HSA affected the coagulation of the albumin molecules and the formation rate of ANPS. The free albumin molecules start to condense around the protein nuclei, forming albumin particles that start to aggregate with a larger particle size and a high percentage of yield. Upon increasing HSA concentration, the viscosity of the solution increases. As a result, the movements of HSA molecules become slower between the aqueous phase and the desolvating agent. This contributed to a slower nucleation rate and hence larger particles. Changing the desolvation agent from a polar ethanol to an ethanol acetone mixture significantly affected the ANPs zeta potential. Albumin molecules are insoluble in both ethanol and the mixtures of ethanol and acetone [32]. Consequently, this promotes albumin molecules nucleation and then aggregation. The aggregation process results spontaneously in ANPs formation. Notably, the higher hydrophobicity of acetone resulted in particles that possess a lower charge, compared to particles formed with using pure ethanol. The high negative charge of NPs could improve their stability. Efficacy of nanoparticles after injection is mainly dependent on particle size and surface charge. The D-Optimal design allowed analysis of the factors that influence characteristics of the formed nanoparticles.

The experimental results confirmed the ability of using sucrose and trehalose as cryoprotectants to prevent the aggregation of ANPs during the freeze-drying process and to protect them from the deterioration effect of dehydration and the subsequent re-hydration step [33]. Mannitol failed to prevent the particles' aggregation. This could be ascribed to its partial crystallization, mostly during the freeze-drying process. The ability of sucrose and trehalose to form amorphous glasses that are capable of interacting with amorphous proteins, forming a glass matrix around nanoparticles during freeze-drying, could interpret their effectiveness over mannitol [34].

In the in vitro release profile of SML-ANPS, the initial fast release can be attributed to the desorption and the diffusion of SML from the outer surface of ANPS. The initial drug release is necessary for a satisfactory therapeutic effect. The slow release is mainly because of the slow diffusion of SML through the albumin matrix, and this was inconsistent with similar data documented by other authors [35]. On the other side, glutaraldehyde would disperse inside the nanoparticle network throughout the cross-linking process and associate covalently with adjacent amine groups of lysine in albumin residues, leading to a strong stabilization of the matrix of ANPS, resulting in a slow release of SML. During circulation in the blood, slower drug release from the nanoparticles is beneficial as this minimizes the systemic adverse side effects, and it increases ANPs' targeting ability.

SML has been previously tested on different cell lines as an antioxidant to protect them against the damaging effect of cancer therapy. [36]. Sesamol could reduce the oxidative damage and the toxicity to H9c2 cardiomyoblasts caused by doxorubicin [37]. The cellular ability to reduce MTT dye is an indicator of mitochondrial activity, a measure of cellular viability [38]. DOX triggers cellular apoptosis by increasing the levels of intracellular ROS, thus a reduction in cell viability and increasing apoptosis were observed to >70% [39].

However, co-treatment with an antioxidant agent counteracts ROS production and improves the endogenous enzyme levels. Sesamol, being a phenolic compound possessing a methylenedioxy group, is considered a potent inhibitor of cytokine production. Moreover, it is a powerful antioxidant [40]. Furthermore, sesamol was previously reported to elevate mRNA levels and the protein expression of the antioxidant enzymes HO-1 and NQO1 as well as to decrease the inflammatory cytokines TNF-α and IL-1β in D-galactose-treated mice serum. Moreover, the activity of CAT and the GSH level were found to increase in sesamol-treated mice serum. Additionally, sesamol treatment was also found to balance the cellular redox status, protect against mitochondrial dysfunction, and upregulate the antioxidant enzymes by activating the Nrf2 transcriptional pathway [41].

Therefore, treatment with both free and encapsulated sesamol had a protecting effect. However, higher hepato-protectivity of the used antioxidant drug was observed when it was encapsulated in albumin nanoparticles compared to the free drugs. This can be explained by the efficient internalization, localization, and endocytic uptake of albumin nanoparticles via different pathways [42]. Particles with diameters < 200 nm could be phagocytized by cancer cells due to the enhanced permeability and a retention effect [43]. A synergistic antioxidant effect may be also ascribed to the presence of albumin. HSA was reported to possess direct and indirect antioxidant effects. It exerts its direct effect being a free radical scavenger where the free thiol groups in the Cys-34 residue are usually able to trap different types of ROS and due to the presence of six methionine groups that are easily oxidized. HSA can also act indirectly by binding bilirubin that inhibit lipid peroxidation and free metals such as iron and copper, which catalyze aggressive ROS formation [22].

Furthermore, anionic HSA NPs bind to the albumin receptors on the cell surface e.g., Gp60, SPARC. Additionally, binding of albumin to the neonatal Fc receptor (FcRn), a cell membrane bound receptor found on endothelial cells and various organs, such as the kidneys, liver, and intestine, was elucidated by Anderson and co-workers [42]. As SML water solubility impaired its cellular uptake and such molecules need a specific receptor or transporter to transfer it into the cells, it could therefore be hypothesized that ANP improved the availability of SML by prolonging drug residence time and increasing tissue uptake. Antioxidative agents inhibit oxidative damage and death in normal cells by the induction of endogenous antioxidants and/or reactive oxygen species scavenging. Moreover, they prevent the activation of chemical resistance pathways in cancer cells through oxidative stress [44].

SML-ANPs and SML solution pharmacokinetic profiles were studied. SML solution was directly injected, and thus blood exposure resulted in faster elimination. However, the ANPs acted as reservoirs for SML in the blood, where SML-ANP was gradually degraded over time and SML was slowly released into the bloodstream, resulting in an extended residence time, a slower clearance, and higher AUC.

Anticancer agents such as DOX have been demonstrated to exert serious dose impacts on the other non-targeted tissues. Previous reviews corelated DOX's toxic side effects with several factors, such as ROS and RNS generation [25,26]. The semiquinone formed by DOX reacts with molecular oxygen, providing a radical superoxide ($O2^-$) and returns to its quinone form. This cycling process produces several active oxidant species, H_2O_2, OH^-, and $ONOO^-$. The elevated levels of free radicals have a significant potential to initiate lipid peroxidation upon rapid interaction with lipids. Furthermore, it triggers an oxidative stress that affects different biomolecules such as the membrane-bound proteins, enzymes, lipids, mitochondrial genomes, and others. Several studies have shown that oxidative stress and development of iron anthracycline free radicals may be highly responsible for the pathogenesis of DOX-induced cardiotoxicity, hepatotoxicity, nephrotoxicity, and testicular toxicity [45]. DOX-induced cardiotoxicity in rat models is manifested as an escalating level of serum lactate dehydrogenase (LDH), creatine kinase, and cardiac malondialdehyde (MDA), which are associated with the histopathological changes. Coincidentally, DOX has a high affinity for cardiolipin, a phospholipid inserted in the cell membrane of mitochondrial where the DOX-cardiolipin complex act as a substrate and start the lipid peroxidation process. When the hepatocytes are damaged, certain changes occur in cell membrane permeability, which is further correlated with the release of enzymes from the cells, reducing the levels of ALT and AST and increasing their serum levels. A previous study reported an enhanced lipid peroxidation in the kidneys of DOX-treated rats. A recent study provided both biochemical and histological evidence for marked reproductive toxicity caused by DOX through oxidative stress. It was reported that DOX-treated rats showed considerably higher levels of MDA suggesting the strong pro-oxidative activity of DOX. The formation of free radicals is considered to be the rate limiting step in lipid peroxidation. Compared to the DOX-treated group, the administration of SML-ANPS 30 min before DOX showed substantial improvement in the cardiac markers (CK and LDH serum levels) and the biochemical variables. Normally, during DOX therapy, extensive free radical production results in increased membrane permeability of MDA in tissue homogenates as MDA molecules are normally located in the cellular cytoplasm and leak into the serum after tissue damage during inflammation, which can explain histological injuries. Similarly, other studies showed an increase in the levels of biochemical markers with an elevation of LPO in different organs after doxorubicin treatment [11]. It was reported that the therapeutic indices in traditional chemotherapy were enhanced upon co-treatment with antioxidants [44].

4. Materials and Methods

4.1. Materials

The Bradford reagent (Cairo, Egypt), Doxorubicin, was purchased from Thermo Fisher Scientific (Fair Lawn, NJ, USA); Glutaraldehyde, 25 wt.% solution was purchased from Acros Organics (Merelbeke, Belgium); Fetal Bovine serum, gentamycin, HEPES buffer, L-glutamine and RPMI-1640 medium were purchased from Lonza (Verviers, Belgium); HPLC grade acetone, tetrazolium salt (MTT), sesamol and trypan blue dye were purchased Sigma-Aldrich (St. Louis, MO, USA); HPLC grade acetonitrile was purchased from Carl Roth (Karlsruhe, Germany); HPLC grade ethanol was purchased from Thermo Fisher Scientific (Schwerte, Germany); lyophilized HSA were purchased from Alfa Aesar (Kandel, Germany); and the Milli-Q® Integral Water Purification System for Ultrapure Water was purchased from Merck Millipore (Darmstadt, Germany).

4.2. Methods

4.2.1. Fabrication of SML-ANPs

ANPs were prepared using the desolvation process. Briefly, different concentrations of HSA solution were prepared (25, 50 and 100 mg/mL). Then, the pH of drug-polymer solution was adjusted at different pH values (7, 8, and 9) using a phosphate buffered saline solution (PBS). SML was dissolved in the HSA solution and incubated for 4 h under constant stirring. Using a burette, a desolvating agent (ethanol or ethanol/acetone, 1:1) was added at a constant rate of 1 mL/min under stirring of 550 rpm, until turbidity just appeared. Finally, the formed ANPs were cross-linked by 8% glutaraldehyde (GA) overnight at room temperature. The unbound drug in the nanoparticle dispersion was removed by three cycles of washing and centrifugation at 14,000 rpm for 30 min each using a cooling centrifuge at 4 °C (Sigma Laboratory centrifuges, Osterode am Harz, Germany). The supernatant was collected for further analysis. After each cycle, 5 min sonication was used for the re-dispersion of the formulation.

4.2.2. Characterizations of Albumin Nanoparticles

The average particle size (P.S.) and polydispersity (PDI) of purified reconstituted nanoparticles were measured using dynamic light scattering (DLS) and utilizing a Malvern Zetasizer (Worcestershire, UK). The samples were diluted at a ratio of 1:10, with purified water. Thereafter, they were measured using the backscattered light detector operating at angle of 173° and the Zeta potential values were measured by laser Doppler anemometry. All samples were measured at 25 °C in triplicate to assess the reproducibility. Quantification of unbound SML in the supernatant was performed using a Dionex Ultimat 3000 UHPLC system (Thermo Scientific, Waltham, MA, USA) equipped with HPG-3200 RS pump, a DAD-3000 RS detector, a WPS-3000TRS analytical autosampler, and a Hypersil BDS C-18 column with the dimensions of (5 µm, 4.6 × 150 mm). A reversed-phase technique was proceeded using a mobile phase consisted of acetonitrile and 0.3 M KH2PO4, pH 3.5, in the volume ratio 70:30, respectively. The mobile phase flow rate was 1 mL/min, the injection volume was 20 µL, and the eluent was quantified by Diode-Array Detection (DAD) detector at 294 nm wavelength. The method accuracy was determined to be 99.99% with a limit of quantification (LoQ) of 100 ng/mL. Then, encapsulation efficiency (% EE) was calculated according to Equation (1);

$$\% \ EE = \frac{\text{Initial amount of SML} - \text{amount of unloaded SML}}{\text{Amount of drug initially added}} \times 100, \quad (1)$$

while to determine the percent of ANPs yield, the unbounded HSA concentration in the supernatant was determined spectrophotometrically at 595 nm, using a pre-constructed calibration curve (10–80 µg/mL), based on the method of Bradford [46]. The percentage of drug loading capacity (% LC) and the yield (% Y) of the nanoparticles were calculated according to Equations (2) and (3), respectively;

$$\% \ Yield = \frac{\text{Initial amount of HSA} - \text{amount of unbounded HSA}}{\text{Initial amount of HSA}} \times 100 \quad (2)$$

$$\% \ LC = \frac{\text{Amount of encapsulated SML}}{\text{Total weight of SML} - \text{ANPs}} \times 100. \quad (3)$$

For the interpretation of Fourier transform-infrared spectroscopy (FT-IR) and differential scanning calorimetry (DSC) thermograms of lyophilized SML, HAS, SML/HSA physical mixture, SML/HSA mixture after incubation, and SML-ANPs see supplementary material, Figures S1 and S2.

4.2.3. Design of Experiments (DOE) for Studying Critical Factors

Three levels for each of the investigated factors were chosen to generate an experimental design, namely, the D-optimal design (DOD) (Table 4). The concentration of HSA, pH of albumin-drug solution, and the type of the desolvating agent were treated as three independent variables affecting the SML-ANPs formulation. The design matrices comprised 18 experimental runs (see supplementary material, Table S1).

Table 4. Factors controlling SML-ANPs preparation and their levels in D-optimal design.

Independent Variable	Level (−1)	Level (0)	Level (+1)
PH	7	8	9
HSA (mg/mL)	25	50	100
D.A	Ethanol	-	Ethanol/acetone

Abbreviations: D.A: Desolvating agent; HSA: Humane serum albumin; SML-ANPS: Sesamol-loaded albumin nanoparticles.

4.2.4. In Vitro Drug Release of SML from Selected SML-ANPs

An optimal amount of selected SML-ANPs containing 5 mg of SML were suspended in phosphate buffered saline at pH 7.4 in a dialysis membrane (Molecular weight cut-off 12 kDa) and dialyzed against 50 mL of phosphate buffered saline. The medium was continuously stirred at 100 rpm and maintained at a temperature of 37 °C. Samples were withdrawn at predetermined time intervals and the same volume was replaced with pre-warmed fresh medium. The SML quantification was preformed, using HPLC as previously described in the encapsulation determination section.

Release Kinetic Studies

To study the release kinetics of SML, the data obtained from the in vitro release studies of selected SML-ANP were fitted to various kinetic models, such as zero-order, first-order, and the Higuchi, Korsmeyer–Peppas, and Hixson Crowell models [47]. Regression analysis was used to determine the constants and the corr4elation coefficients of the data (R^2) [48].

4.2.5. Morphological Characterizations

The morphology of selected SML-ANPs was visualized by Quanta FEG 250 scanning electron microscopes (SEM) at a magnification of 120,000× and an accelerated voltage of 20.0 kV. The sample was prepared by pipetting 10 µL of the SML-NPs suspension (2 mg/mL) onto copper tape and leaving it to dry.

4.2.6. Freeze Drying of the Selected SML-ANPs

Using CHRIST Alpha 2-4 LD plus freeze-dryer (Osterode am Harz, Germany), the ability of the selected SML-ANP to maintain their physiochemical characterizations under freeze drying conditions was studied in absence and in the presence of distinct types of cryoprotectants as trehalose, mannitol, and sucrose. The cryoprotectants were evaluated at three different concentrations of 1%, 2%, and 3%, in order to obtain a stable solid dosage form without negative impact on the product properties. In triplicate, samples and the respective control without cryoprotectants were frozen at −80 °C overnight prior to freeze drying process. The vacuum pressure was set at 0.011 mbar and the temperature was maintained at −60 °C for 48 h. After freeze drying, the samples were re-dispersed in distilled water. The particle size and the PDI were measured and compared with their respective characteristics before freeze-drying [49].

4.2.7. Evaluating the Reconstituted SML-ANPs Stability

To evaluate the stability of SML-ANPs, three batches of the selected formulation after freeze drying were stored in sealed Eppendorf tubes (1.5 mL) at 4 °C for 6 months and then reconstituted for analysis. The reconstituted freeze dried SML-ANP formulations were evaluated in terms of particle size and the polydispersity index. Besides, further experiments were performed to examine the stability in different biological media after a 2 h incubation. The nanoparticles were diluted 1 in 20 with purified water, phosphate buffered saline (PBS), and Dulbecco's Modified Eagle Medium (DMEM), and three readings were taken at after 2 h.

4.2.8. The Hepatoprotective Study of SML-ANPs

Sprague–Dawley male rats (200–250 g) were obtained from the Animals House in the Faculty of Science at Al-Azhar University, Cairo, Egypt and treated according to Helsinki's declaration of animals use (2008). Before performing liver biopsies on five rats, they were administered ether anesthesia. The hepatocyte isolation was performed according to the collagenase perfusion procedure which was previously described by Reese and Byard [50]. The hepatocytes (1×10^6 cells/mL) were placed in a Krebs–Henseleit buffer (pH 7.4) containing 12.5 mM HEPES and kept at 37 °C with 95% O_2 and 5% CO_2. The hepatocytes with a viability of more than 90%, which was measured with Trypan Blue, were used in the experiments [51]. Rat hepatocytes were exposed to a medium containing DOX (1µM). Then, the viability of cells was estimated by the MTT reduction assay [52]. The experimental groups tested were as follows: Control group: untreated rat hepatocytes; DOX-treated group: rat hepatocytes were treated with DOX (1 µM); SML treated group: rat hepatocytes were treated with DOX (1µM) and a nontoxic dose of free SML; and SML-ANPs treated group: rat hepatocytes were treated with DOX (1 µM) and a nontoxic dose of SML-ANPs. In case of tested formulations treatment, the hepatocytes were pretreated with either SML or SML-ANPs 24 h before adding the DOX. Each treatment was repeated four times (i.e., four wells for each treatment). The doses of DOX and SML were selected according to a preliminary cytotoxicity study and previous literature (supplementary file, Figure S3 and Table S6) [53,54].

4.2.9. Pharmacokinetic Study

Adult male healthy Wister albino rats (weighing in the range of 150 ± 20 g) were obtained from the animal house in the Faculty of Medicine, Assiut University, Assiut, Egypt. The rats were acclimatized for 7 days and maintained on a 12:12 h light/dark cycle, and they had free access to food and water. The protocol of the study (no. 155) was approved by the animal care and use committee of the Faculty of Pharmacy, Ain Shams University, Cairo, Egypt. A pharmacokinetic study was performed to assess SML sustained release from SML-ANPs and to estimate their ability as a drug carrier to modulate SML rapid clearance. Eight rats were randomly divided into two groups (four animals per group). The first group received a single dose of free SML solution (15 mg/kg), while the second received an SML-ANPs dispersion loaded with an equivalent amount to the injected SML solution. Blood samples were withdrawn via vein puncture from the caudal vein into heparinized tubes at predetermined time intervals (0.25, 0.5, 2, 4, 8, 12, and 24 h) after intravenous injection (IV). Then, plasma samples were separated by centrifugation at 3000 rpm for 10 min and stored at −20 °C for further analysis. Plasma SML concentrations were analyzed using a reversed phase-HPLC by the method described previously with some modifications [55,56]. The mobile phase composed of 70:30 v/v acetonitrile to 0.3 M orthophosphate buffer adjusted at pH 3.5 by phosphoric acid. The flow rate was set at 1.0 mL/min, the injection volume was 20 µL, and elute was analyzed with a DAD detector set at a wavelength of 294 nm. Acetonitrile (1 mL) was added to the plasma sample (200 µL) to precipitate the plasma proteins [57]. Then, plasma samples were vortexed for 10 min and then incubated and centrifuged at 4000 rpm for 15 min. The collected supernatants were filtered through a 0.45 µm syringe filter (Millipore, Billerica, MA, USA). Then, they were analyzed using the HPLC against a calibration curve of SML in the plasma that was constructed using blank plasma spiked and mixed with standard SML solutions to obtain a concentration range of 0.01–10 µg/mL. The spiked plasma samples were then subjected to the same extraction procedure as the tested plasma samples to avoid any quantitation error factor in sample preparation [55,57]. The pharmacokinetic parameters were calculated by fitting the plasma concentration–time data to a suitable model using WinNonlin Professional Edition software version 2.0 (Science Consulting, Apex, NC, USA). The maximum plasma concentration (C_{max}), the time of maximal concentration (T_{max}), the half-life ($T_{1/2}$), the area under the curve ($AUC_{0-\infty}$), and mean residence time ($MRT_{0-\infty}$) were calculated.

4.2.10. In Vivo Study of SML-ANPs

Acute administration of DOX in Wister rats, which normally induces a state of oxidative stress, is considered a widely used animal model to assess the protective ability of antioxidative agents. An optimal dose was chosen according to a preliminary study and following previous literature to be sufficient to induce a progressive oxidative state in rats. This study was carried out in adult male healthy Wister rats weighing in the range of 160 ± 30 g from the Animal Facility of the Faculty of Medicine, Assiut University, Egypt. The protocol of the study was approved by the Institutional Animals Ethics Committee of the College of Pharmacy, Ain Shams University (No. 155). Rats were acclimatized for 7–10 days before the initiation of the experiment to observe any sign of disease, they were maintained on a 25 ± 5 °C 12/12 h light/dark cycle, and they had free access to food and water.

Rats were randomized into four groups, each group containing 10 animals: the control group received saline four times per week, during three weeks (control group); the DOX group received a repeated dose of DOX (2.5 mg/kg, intraperitoneal injection (IP)) three times per week during the first two weeks and received just saline during the third week; the SML group received an SML solution 30 min before the administration of DOX during the first two weeks and before saline during the third week; and the SML-ANPs group received SML-ANPs 30 min before the administration of DOX during the first two weeks and saline during the third week. The body weights and the mortality rate of animals were recorded during the experiment. At the end of the study, the blood samples were collected and the animals were sacrificed to take samples from different organs for further examination, (see supplementary file).

Biochemical Assessment of the Selected SML-ANPs Formulations

Creatine kinase (CK) and lactate dehydrogenase (LDH) serum levels were detected as markers of cardiotoxicity with respective kits and with the help of an ELISA reader (Bio Tek; Santa Clara, USA) according to the manufacturer's protocols. Nevertheless, the liver injury was evaluated by measuring serum alanine aminotransferase (ALT) and aspartate transaminase (AST) levels as a specific biomarker using a specific kit following the manufacturer's protocol. Furthermore, the biochemical determination of malondialdehyde (MDA) serves to indicate lipid peroxide formation. MDA levels (marker of lipid peroxidation (LPO)) were assessed by reaction with thiobarbituric acid (TBA) at 100 °C. The reaction between MDA and TBA produces a pink pigment, which has a maximum absorption at 532 nm. Briefly, 50 µL of supernatant, 1 mL of TBA, and 1 mL of trichloroacetic acid (TCA) [0.75% TBA: 30% TCA] were mixed, placed in a boiling water bath for 60 min, and cooled and centrifuged for 15 min at 4000 rpm. The supernatant absorbance was measured against a reference blank at 532 nm by spectrophotometer; 1,1,3,3-Tetramethoxypropane (Sigma Chemicals, St. Louis, MO, USA) was used as a standard MDA. The results were expressed as n mol/mg protein.

Histopathological Analysis

Since the histological study of doxorubicin multi-organ toxicity is a wide topic, we focused on the toxicity of vital organs and a reproductive system that can be harmed by cancer and its associated treatments, and we evaluated the protective activity of our formulation against organ toxicity reported in previous literature [45,58–62]. Liver, kidney, heart, and testis specimens were cut and fixed in a 10% neutral buffered formalin. The formalin-fixed samples were routinely processed, embedded in paraffin, and sectioned. Serial 3 µm sections, serially dehydrated in an ethanol gradient, were stained with Mayer's hematoxylin (Merck, Darmstadt, Germany) and eosin (Sigma, St. Louis, MO, USA) and examined microscopically. The histological evaluation was performed by a histopathologist (Dr Mahmoud Soliman) in a blind fashion on coded samples, and a comparison was made with the sections from the control.

4.3. Statistical Analysis

All experiments were performed in triplicate and results were expressed as means ± standard deviations (SD) except for the in vivo study where the results were expressed as mean ± standard error (SE) for eight animals in each group (n = 8). Statistical analysis tests were performed using SPSS 21.0 software. For all results, the differences were considered significant when $p < 0.05$, and they were regarded as extremely significant when $p < 0.0001$ presented by * and ***, respectively. Comparisons between groups were performed using one-way multivariate ANOVA followed by a Tukey's post hoc test or Student t-test where appropriate.

5. Conclusions

Based on the findings presented in this study, it is possible to conclude that the desolvation method successfully produced SML-ANPs with promising physicochemical features, such as high stability, sustained release and high loading capacity, where the particle size, zeta potential, and loading capacity of the selected formulation were 127.24 nm, −26.21 mV, and 96.89 g/mg ANPs, respectively. In addition to the specific role of albumin molecules in cellular endocytosis, particles with diameters less than 200 nm improve cellular absorption. Albumin nanoparticles also enhanced pharmacokinetic characteristics. Sesamol suffer from low bioavailability, and they displayed a short half-life and a rapid elimination rate of 1.25 h and 0.53 L/h, respectively. However, albumin can act as an SML reservoir in the bloodstream with an extended half-life and slower elimination rates of 8.9 h and 0.11 L/h, respectively. SML-ANPS exhibited significant protective effects against hepatocytes pretreated with doxorubicin and the DOX-induced acute toxicity in albino rats as an oxidative stress animal model by down regulating the production of harmful free radicals and the LPO signaling pathway in serum and different organ tissues. Co-treatment with SML-ANPs significantly reduced the elevated serum CK and LDH by 59.3 and 64.5%, respectively, while AST and ALT were inhibited by 60.5 and 59% in comparison to the corresponding values of the free SML treated group: 35.6, 47.2, 49.9, and 41.2%, respectively. As a result, sesamol-loaded albumin nanoparticles may be considered a viable and potentially clinically applicable nano-based platform for the treatment of cancer and inflammatory illnesses in the future. However, more research into their medicinal potential is necessary before use in clinical application.

Supplementary Materials: The following supporting information can be downloaded at: https://www.mdpi.com/article/10.3390/ph15060733/s1, Figure S1: DSC thermograms of lyophilized SML, HAS, SML/HSA physical mixture, SML/HSA mixture after incubation, and SML-ANPs; Figure S2: FTIR spectra of HSA (A) SML (B) SML/HSA physical mixture (C) SML/HSA mixture after incubation (D), and SML-ANPS (E) together with the successful docking of sesamol on HSA (F); Table S1: Physicochemical characteristics of SML-ANPs; Table S2: The effect of the factors controlling SML-ANPs preparation and their levels in the D-optimal design, where pH is the most significant factor; Table S3: Release kinetics of SML-ANPs (F14); Table S4: Hepatoprotective effect of free SML and SML-ANPs on rat hepatocytes measured by the MTS assay; Table S5: The histopathological scores of the liver, kidney, heart, and testis in each groups [a]; Figure S3: Dose-response curve for sesamol effects on cell viability of rat hepatocytes to calculate the CC 50. The values are presented as mean ± SD (n in each group = 3); Table S6: Evaluation of sesamol cytotoxicity against Rat hepatocytes cell line after 48 h [50,63–65].

Author Contributions: Conceptualization, R.M.H.; data curation, S.Z., M.E.S., M.E. and R.M.H.; formal analysis, M.E.S. and R.M.H.; investigation, M.E.S. and M.E.; methodology, S.Z., M.E.S. and R.M.H.; project administration, R.M.H.; software, S.Z. and R.M.H.; supervision, M.E.S., M.E. and R.M.H.; validation, S.Z.; visualization, M.E.S., M.E. and R.M.H.; writing—original draft, S.Z.; writing—review and editing, M.E.S., M.E. and R.M.H. All authors have read and agreed to the published version of the manuscript.

Funding: This research received no external funding.

Institutional Review Board Statement: The animal study protocol was approved by the animal care and use committee of the faculty of Pharmacy, Ain shams University, Cairo, Egypt (no.155, 2017).

Informed Consent Statement: Not applicable.

Data Availability Statement: Data is contained within the article and supplementary materials.

Acknowledgments: The authors thank Hossam El-Din M Omar, Department of Zoology and Dean of Faculty of Science, Assiut University, Assiut, Egypt. The biochemical assessment and the preparation of histology slides were facilitated by the laboratory of the physiology of Zoology department, Faculty of Science, Assiut University under his supervision. The authors also would like to thank Mahmoud Soliman, department of Pathology and Clinical Pathology, Faculty of Veterinary Medicine, Assiut University, for the professional grading of the histology slides.

Conflicts of Interest: The authors declare no conflict of interest.

Abbreviations

ALT: Serum alanine aminotransferase; ANOVA: Analysis of variance; ANPs: albumin-based nanoparticles; AST: Aspartate transaminase; $AUC_{0-\infty}$: The area under the curve; CK: Creatine kinase; C_{max}: The maximum plasma concentration; CV%: Coefficient of variation; DAD: Diode-Array Detector; DL%: Percent of the drug loading; DOE: Design of experiments; DOD: D-optimal design; DOX: Doxorubicin; DLS: dynamic light scattering; DSC:

Differential scanning calorimetry; EE%: Entrapment efficiency; Fe^{2+}: iron; FT-IR: Fourier transform-infrared spectroscopy; GA: glutaraldehyde; GP: Group; HO•: hydroxyl radical; HSA: Human serum albumin; IV: intravenous injection; LDH: Lactate dehydrogenase; LoQ: Limit of quantification; LPO: Lipid peroxidation; MDA: Malondialdehyde; MRT0–∞: Mean residence time; MTT: 3-(4,5-Dimethyl-2-thiazolyl)-2,5-diphenyl-2H-tetrazolium bromide; USA: The United States of America; PBS: Phosphate buffered saline solution; PDI: Polydispersity index; PS: Particle size; ROS; reactive oxygen species; SD: Standard deviations; SE: Standard error; SEM: Scanning electron microscopes; SML: sesamol; SML-ANPS: Sesamol-loaded albumin nanoparticles; SPSS: Statistical Package for the Social Sciences; TBA: Thiobarbituric acid; TCA: Trichloroacetic acid; T1/2: the half-life; T_{max}: the time of maximal concentration; %Y: Yield; ZP: Zeta potential.

References

1. Pinto-Ribeiro, L.; Silva, C.; Andrade, N.; Martel, F. α-tocopherol prevents oxidative stress-induced proliferative dysfunction in first-trimester human placental (HTR-8/SVneo) cells. *Reprod. Biol.* 2022, 22, 100602. [CrossRef] [PubMed]
2. Sarmiento-Salinas, F.L.; Perez-Gonzalez, A.; Acosta-Casique, A.; Ix-Ballote, A.; Diaz, A.; Treviño, S.; Rosas-Murrieta, N.H.; Millán-Perez-Peña, L.; Maycotte, P. Reactive oxygen species: Role in carcinogenesis, cancer cell signaling and tumor progression. *Life Sci.* 2021, 284, 119942. [CrossRef]
3. Andreadi, A.; Bellia, A.; Di Daniele, N.; Meloni, M.; Lauro, R.; Della-Morte, D.; Lauro, D. The molecular link between oxidative stress, insulin resistance, and type 2 diabetes: A target for new therapies against cardiovascular diseases. *Curr. Opin. Pharmacol.* 2022, 62, 85–96. [CrossRef] [PubMed]
4. Songbo, M.; Lang, H.; Xinyong, C.; Bin, X.; Ping, Z.; Liang, S. Oxidative stress injury in doxorubicin-induced cardiotoxicity. *Toxicol. Lett.* 2019, 307, 41–48. [CrossRef]
5. Pisoschi, A.M.; Pop, A.; Iordache, F.; Stanca, L.; Predoi, G.; Serban, A.I. Oxidative stress mitigation by antioxidants—An overview on their chemistry and influences on health status. *Eur. J. Med. Chem.* 2021, 209, 112891. [CrossRef] [PubMed]
6. van der Zanden, S.Y.; Qiao, X.; Neefjes, J. New insights into the activities and toxicities of the old anticancer drug doxorubicin. *FEBS J.* 2021, 288, 6095–6111. [CrossRef] [PubMed]
7. Zhu, H.; Sarkar, S.; Scott, L.; Danelisen, I.; Trush, M.A.; Jia, Z.; Li, Y.R. Doxorubicin redox biology: Redox cycling, topoisomerase inhibition, and oxidative stress. *React. Oxyg. Species (Apex N.C.)* 2016, 1, 189. [CrossRef]
8. Phaniendra, A.; Jestadi, D.B.; Periyasamy, L. Free radicals: Properties, sources, targets, and their implication in various diseases. *Indian J. Clin. Biochem.* 2015, 30, 11–26. [CrossRef] [PubMed]
9. Varela-López, A.; Battino, M.; Navarro-Hortal, M.D.; Giampieri, F.; Forbes-Hernández, T.Y.; Romero-Márquez, J.M.; Collado, R.; Quiles, J.L. An update on the mechanisms related to cell death and toxicity of doxorubicin and the protective role of nutrients. *Food Chem. Toxicol.* 2019, 134, 110834. [CrossRef] [PubMed]
10. Zhou, S.; Zou, H.; Huang, G.; Chen, G. Preparations and antioxidant activities of sesamol and it's derivatives. *Bioorg. Med. Chem. Lett.* 2021, 31, 127716. [CrossRef] [PubMed]
11. Mohammed, H.S.; Hosny, E.N.; Khadrawy, Y.A.; Magdy, M.; Attia, Y.S.; Sayed, O.A.; AbdElaal, M. Protective effect of curcumin nanoparticles against cardiotoxicity induced by doxorubicin in rat. *Biochim. Biophys. Acta (BBA)-Mol. Basis Dis.* 2020, 1866, 165665. [CrossRef]
12. Di Cesare Mannelli, L.; Zanardelli, M.; Failli, P.; Ghelardini, C. Oxaliplatin-Induced Neuropathy: Oxidative Stress as Pathological Mechanism. Protective Effect of Silibinin. *J. Pain* 2012, 13, 276–284. [CrossRef] [PubMed]
13. Singh, T.G.; Singh, H.P.; Kaur, S.; Dhiman, S. Protective effects of sesamol against cisplatin-induced nephrotoxicity in rats: A mechanistic approach. *Obes. Med.* 2020, 19, 100269. [CrossRef]
14. Tian, H.; Guo, R. Cardioprotective potential of sesamol against ischemia/reperfusion injury induced oxidative myocardial damage. *Biomed. Res.* 2017, 28, 2156–2163.
15. Majdalawieh, A.F.; Mansour, Z.R. Sesamol, a major lignan in sesame seeds (Sesamum indicum): Anti-cancer properties and mechanisms of action. *Eur. J. Pharmacol.* 2019, 855, 75–89. [CrossRef]
16. Chu, P.-Y.; Chien, S.-P.; Hsu, D.-Z.; Liu, M.-Y. Protective effect of sesamol on the pulmonary inflammatory response and lung injury in endotoxemic rats. *Food Chem. Toxicol.* 2010, 48, 1821–1826. [CrossRef] [PubMed]
17. Abdelhamid, H.N.; El-Bery, H.M.; Metwally, A.A.; Elshazly, M.; Hathout, R.M. Synthesis of CdS-modified chitosan quantum dots for the drug delivery of Sesamol. *Carbohydr. Polym.* 2019, 214, 90–99. [CrossRef] [PubMed]
18. Jan, K.C.; Ho, C.T.; Hwang, L.S. Elimination and metabolism of sesamol, a bioactive compound in sesame oil, in rats. *Mol. Nutr. Food Res.* 2009, 53, S36–S43. [CrossRef] [PubMed]
19. Hou, Y.-C.; Tsai, S.-Y.; Liu, I.-L.; Yu, C.-P.; Chao, P.-D.L. Metabolic transformation of sesamol and ex vivo effect on 2, 2'-azo-bis (2-amidinopropane) dihydrochloride-induced hemolysis. *J. Agric. Food Chem.* 2008, 56, 9636–9640. [CrossRef] [PubMed]
20. Zhang, Y.; Sun, T.; Jiang, C. Biomacromolecules as carriers in drug delivery and tissue engineering. *Acta Pharm. Sin. B* 2018, 8, 34–50. [CrossRef] [PubMed]

21. Lamichhane, S.; Lee, S. Albumin nanoscience: Homing nanotechnology enabling targeted drug delivery and therapy. *Arch. Pharmacal Res.* **2020**, *43*, 118–133. [CrossRef] [PubMed]
22. Arroyo, V.; García-Martinez, R.; Salvatella, X. Human serum albumin, systemic inflammation, and cirrhosis. *J. Hepatol.* **2014**, *61*, 396–407. [CrossRef] [PubMed]
23. Naguib, S.S.; Hathout, R.M.; Mansour, S. Optimizing novel penetration enhancing hybridized vesicles for augmenting the in-vivo effect of an anti-glaucoma drug. *Drug Deliv.* **2017**, *24*, 99–108. [CrossRef] [PubMed]
24. Varshochian, R.; Jeddi-Tehrani, M.; Mahmoudi, A.R.; Khoshayand, M.R.; Atyabi, F.; Sabzevari, A.; Esfahani, M.R.; Dinarvand, R. The protective effect of albumin on bevacizumab activity and stability in PLGA nanoparticles intended for retinal and choroidal neovascularization treatments. *Eur. J. Pharm. Sci.* **2013**, *50*, 341–352. [CrossRef]
25. Abdel-Hafez, S.M.; Hathout, R.M.; Sammour, O.A. Towards better modeling of chitosan nanoparticles production: Screening different factors and comparing two experimental designs. *Int. J. Biol. Macromol.* **2014**, *64*, 334–340. [CrossRef]
26. Safwat, S.; Hathout, R.M.; Ishak, R.A.; Mortada, N.D. Augmented simvastatin cytotoxicity using optimized lipid nanocapsules: A potential for breast cancer treatment. *J. Liposome Res.* **2017**, *27*, 1–10. [CrossRef]
27. Karami, K.; Jamshidian, N.; Hajiaghasi, A.; Amirghofran, Z. BSA nanoparticles as controlled release carriers for isophethalaldoxime palladiacycle complex; synthesis, characterization, in vitro evaluation, cytotoxicity and release kinetics analysis. *New J. Chem.* **2020**, *44*, 4394–4405. [CrossRef]
28. Kayani, Z.; Firuzi, O.; Bordbar, A.-K. Doughnut-shaped bovine serum albumin nanoparticles loaded with doxorubicin for overcoming multidrug-resistant in cancer cells. *Int. J. Biol. Macromol.* **2018**, *107*, 1835–1843. [CrossRef]
29. Elmasry, S.R.; Hathout, R.M.; Abdel-Halim, M.; Mansour, S. In vitro transdermal delivery of sesamol using oleic acid chemically-modified gelatin nanoparticles as a potential breast cancer medication. *J. Drug Deliv. Sci. Technol.* **2018**, *48*, 30–39. [CrossRef]
30. Allison, A.C. *Structure and Function of Plasma Proteins*; Springer: New York, NY, USA, 1974; Volume 1.
31. Amighi, F.; Emam-Djomeh, Z.; Labbafi-Mazraeh-Shahi, M. Effect of different cross-linking agents on the preparation of bovine serum albumin nanoparticles. *J. Iran. Chem. Soc.* **2020**, *17*, 1223–1235. [CrossRef]
32. Sadeghi, R.; Moosavi-Movahedi, A.; Emam-Jomeh, Z.; Kalbasi, A.; Razavi, S.; Karimi, M.; Kokini, J. The effect of different desolvating agents on BSA nanoparticle properties and encapsulation of curcumin. *J. Nanopart. Res.* **2014**, *16*, 2565. [CrossRef]
33. Anhorn, M.G.; Mahler, H.-C.; Langer, K. Freeze drying of human serum albumin (HSA) nanoparticles with different excipients. *Int. J. Pharm.* **2008**, *363*, 162–169. [CrossRef] [PubMed]
34. Chang, L.; Shepherd, D.; Sun, J.; Ouellette, D.; Grant, K.L.; Tang, X.; Pikal, M.J. Mechanism of protein stabilization by sugars during freeze-drying and storage: Native structure preservation, specific interaction, and/or immobilization in a glassy matrix? *J. Pharm. Sci.* **2005**, *94*, 1427–1444. [CrossRef] [PubMed]
35. Llabot, J.M.; Luis de Redin, I.; Agüeros, M.; Dávila Caballero, M.J.; Boiero, C.; Irache, J.M.; Allemandi, D. In vitro characterization of new stabilizing albumin nanoparticles as a potential topical drug delivery system in the treatment of corneal neovascularization (CNV). *J. Drug Deliv. Sci. Technol.* **2019**, *52*, 379–385. [CrossRef]
36. Duarte, A.R.; Chenet, A.L.; de Almeida, F.J.S.; Andrade, C.M.B.; de Oliveira, M.R. The inhibition of heme oxigenase-1 (HO-1) abolishes the mitochondrial protection induced by sesamol in LPS-treated RAW 264.7 cells. *Chem.-Biol. Interact.* **2018**, *296*, 171–178. [CrossRef] [PubMed]
37. Nayak, P.G.; Paul, P.; Bansal, P.; Kutty, N.G.; Pai, K.S.R. Sesamol prevents doxorubicin-induced oxidative damage and toxicity on H 9c2 cardiomyoblasts. *J. Pharm. Pharmacol.* **2013**, *65*, 1083–1093. [CrossRef]
38. Patravale, V.; Dandekar, P.; Jain, R. *Nanotoxicology: Evaluating Toxicity Potential of Drug-Nanoparticles*; Elsevier: Amsterdam, The Netherlands, 2012; pp. 123–155.
39. Tremblay, A.R.; Delbes, G. In vitro study of doxorubicin-induced oxidative stress in spermatogonia and immature Sertoli cells. *Toxicol. Appl. Pharmacol.* **2018**, *348*, 32–42. [CrossRef]
40. Kumar, B.; Kuhad, A.; Chopra, K. Neuropsychopharmacological effect of sesamol in unpredictable chronic mild stress model of depression: Behavioral and biochemical evidences. *Psychopharmacology* **2011**, *214*, 819–828. [CrossRef]
41. Ren, B.; Yuan, T.; Diao, Z.; Zhang, C.; Liu, Z.; Liu, X. Protective effects of sesamol on systemic oxidative stress-induced cognitive impairments via regulation of Nrf2/Keap1 pathway. *Food Funct.* **2018**, *9*, 5912–5924. [CrossRef]
42. Mo, Y.; Barnett, M.E.; Takemoto, D.; Davidson, H.; Kompella, U.B. Human serum albumin nanoparticles for efficient delivery of Cu, Zn superoxide dismutase gene. *Mol. Vis.* **2007**, *13*, 746.
43. Fadel, M.; Fadeel, D.A.; Ibrahim, M.; Hathout, R.M.; El-Kholy, A.I. One-Step Synthesis of Polypyrrole-Coated Gold Nanoparticles for Use as a Photothermally Active Nano-System. *Int. J. Nanomed.* **2020**, *15*, 2605. [CrossRef] [PubMed]
44. Negrette-Guzmán, M. Combinations of the antioxidants sulforaphane or curcumin and the conventional antineoplastics cisplatin or doxorubicin as prospects for anticancer chemotherapy. *Eur. J. Pharmacol.* **2019**, *859*, 172513. [CrossRef] [PubMed]
45. Pugazhendhi, A.; Edison, T.N.J.I.; Velmurugan, B.K.; Jacob, J.A.; Karuppusamy, I. Toxicity of Doxorubicin (Dox) to different experimental organ systems. *Life Sci.* **2018**, *200*, 26–30. [CrossRef] [PubMed]
46. Bradford, M.M. A rapid and sensitive method for the quantitation of microgram quantities of protein utilizing the principle of protein-dye binding. *Anal. Biochem.* **1976**, *72*, 248–254. [CrossRef]
47. Bruschi, M.L. 5-Mathematical models of drug release. In *Strategies to Modify the Drug Release from Pharmaceutical Systems*; Woodhead Publishing: Cambridge, UK, 2015; pp. 63–86. [CrossRef]

48. Abdelkader, A.; El-Mokhtar, M.A.; Abdelkader, O.; Hamad, M.A.; Elsabahy, M.; El-Gazayerly, O.N. Ultrahigh antibacterial efficacy of meropenem-loaded chitosan nanoparticles in a septic animal model. *Carbohydr. Polym.* **2017**, *174*, 1041–1050. [CrossRef] [PubMed]
49. Dadparvar, M.; Wagner, S.; Wien, S.; Worek, F.; von Briesen, H.; Kreuter, J. Freeze-drying of HI-6-loaded recombinant human serum albumin nanoparticles for improved storage stability. *Eur. J. Pharm. Biopharm.* **2014**, *88*, 510–517. [CrossRef]
50. Reese, J.A.; Byard, J.L. Isolation and culture of adult hepatocytes from liver biopsies. *In Vitro* **1981**, *17*, 935. [CrossRef]
51. Shen, L.; Hillebrand, A.; Wang, D.Q.-H.; Liu, M. Isolation and primary culture of rat hepatic cells. *JoVE (J. Vis. Exp.)* **2012**, *64*, 3917. [CrossRef]
52. Safwat, S.; Ishak, R.A.H.; Hathout, R.M.; Mortada, N.D. Nanostructured lipid carriers loaded with simvastatin: Effect of PEG/glycerides on characterization, stability, cellular uptake efficiency and in vitro cytotoxicity. *Drug Dev. Ind. Pharm.* **2017**, *43*, 1112–1125. [CrossRef]
53. Chao, H.-H.; Liu, J.-C.; Hong, H.-J.; Lin, J.-W.; Chen, C.-H.; Cheng, T.-H. L-carnitine reduces doxorubicin-induced apoptosis through a prostacyclin-mediated pathway in neonatal rat cardiomyocytes. *Int. J. Cardiol.* **2011**, *146*, 145–152. [CrossRef]
54. Shabalala, S.C.; Dludla, P.V.; Muller, C.J.; Nxele, X.; Kappo, A.P.; Louw, J.; Johnson, R. Aspalathin ameliorates doxorubicin-induced oxidative stress in H9c2 cardiomyoblasts. *Toxicol. Vitr.* **2019**, *55*, 134–139. [CrossRef] [PubMed]
55. Geetha, T.; Singh, N.; Deol, P.K.; Kaur, I.P. Biopharmaceutical profiling of sesamol: Physiochemical characterization, gastrointestinal permeability and pharmacokinetic evaluation. *RSC Adv.* **2015**, *5*, 4083–4091. [CrossRef]
56. Gourishetti, K.; Keni, R.; Nayak, P.G.; Jitta, S.R.; Bhaskaran, N.A.; Kumar, L.; Kumar, N.; Krishnadas, N.; Shenoy, R.R. Sesamol-loaded PLGA nanosuspension for accelerating wound healing in diabetic foot ulcer in rats. *Int. J. Nanomed.* **2020**, *15*, 9265. [CrossRef] [PubMed]
57. Jan, K.-C.; Ho, C.-T.; Hwang, L.S. Bioavailability and tissue distribution of sesamol in rat. *J. Agric. Food Chem.* **2008**, *56*, 7032–7037. [CrossRef]
58. Ismail, D.I. Histological study on doxorubicin-induced testicular toxicity and the protective role of sesamol in rats. *Egypt. J. Histol.* **2016**, *39*, 38–49. [CrossRef]
59. Razavi-Azarkhiavi, K.; Iranshahy, M.; Sahebkar, A.; Shirani, K.; Karimi, G. The protective role of phenolic compounds against doxorubicin-induced cardiotoxicity: A comprehensive review. *Nutr. Cancer* **2016**, *68*, 892–917. [CrossRef]
60. Singh, N.; Khullar, N.; Kakkar, V.; Kaur, I.P. Sesamol loaded solid lipid nanoparticles: A promising intervention for control of carbon tetrachloride induced hepatotoxicity. *BMC Complementary Altern. Med.* **2015**, *15*, 142. [CrossRef]
61. El-Moselhy, M.A.; El-Sheikh, A.A. Protective mechanisms of atorvastatin against doxorubicin-induced hepato-renal toxicity. *Biomed. Pharmacother.* **2014**, *68*, 101–110. [CrossRef]
62. Safwat, S.; Ishak, R.A.; Hathout, R.M.; Mortada, N.D. Statins anti-cancer targeted delivery systems: Re-purposing an old molecule. *J. Pharm. Pharmacol.* **2017**, *69*, 613–624. [CrossRef]
63. Hassanzadeh, P.; Atyabi, F.; Dinarvand, R.; Dehpour, A.R.; Azhdarzadeh, M.; Dinarvand, M. Application of nanostructured lipid carriers: The prolonged protective effects for sesamol in in vitro and in vivo models of ischemic stroke via activation of PI3K signalling pathway. *DARU J. Pharm. Sci.* **2017**, *25*, 25. [CrossRef]
64. Li, J.; Chen, T.; Deng, F.; Wan, J.; Tang, Y.; Yuan, P.; Zhang, L. Synthesis, characterization, and in vitro evaluation of curcumin-loaded albumin nanoparticles surface-functionalized with glycyrrhetinic acid. *Int. J. Nanomed.* **2015**, *10*, 5475. [CrossRef] [PubMed]
65. Min, J.; Meng-Xia, X.; Dong, Z.; Yuan, L.; Xiao-Yu, L.; Xing, C. Spectroscopic studies on the interaction of cinnamic acid and its hydroxyl derivatives with human serum albumin. *J. Mol. Struct.* **2004**, *692*, 71–80. [CrossRef]

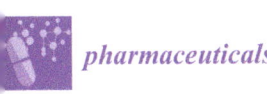

Article

Formulation and Characterization of Metformin-Loaded Ethosomes for Topical Application to Experimentally Induced Skin Cancer in Mice

Ibrahim A. Mousa [1], Taha M. Hammady [2], Shadeed Gad [2,*], Sawsan A. Zaitone [3,4,*], Mohamed El-Sherbiny [5,6] and Ossama M. Sayed [7]

1. General Authority of Health Care, Ismailia Governorate, Ismailia 11517, Egypt; ibrahim.201@pharm.suez.edu.eg
2. Department of Pharmaceutics and Industrial Pharmacy, Faculty of Pharmacy, Suez Canal University, Ismailia 41522, Egypt; taha_hamadi@pharm.suez.edu.eg
3. Department of Pharmacology & Toxicology, Faculty of Pharmacy, Suez Canal University, Ismailia 41522, Egypt
4. Department of Pharmacology & Toxicology, Faculty of Pharmacy, University of Tabuk, Tabuk 71491, Saudi Arabia
5. Department of Basic Medical Sciences, College of Medicine, AlMaarefa University, Riyadh P.O. Box 71666, Saudi Arabia; msharbini@mcst.edu.sa
6. Department of Anatomy, Faculty of Medicine, Mansoura University, Mansoura 3155, Egypt
7. Department of Pharmaceutics and Industrial Pharmacy, Faculty of Pharmacy, Sinai University, Kantra 41636, Egypt; osama.sayed@su.edu.eg
* Correspondence: shaded_abdelrahman@pharm.suez.edu.eg (S.G.); sawsan_zaytoon@pharm.suez.edu.eg or szaitone@ut.edu.sa (S.A.Z.); Tel.: +20-1003934422 (S.G.); Fax: +20-643230741 (S.G.)

Abstract: To achieve the best treatment of skin cancer, drug penetration inside the deepest layers of the skin is an important scientific interest. We designed an ethosome formulation that serves as a carrier for metformin and measured the in vitro skin permeation. We also aimed to measure the antitumor activity of the optimal ethosomal preparation when applied topically to chemically induced skin cancer in mice. We utilized a statistical Box–Behnken experimental design and applied three variables at three levels: lecithin concentration, cholesterol concentration and a mixture of ethanol and isopropyl alcohol concentrations. All formulations were prepared to calculate the entrapment efficiency %, zeta potential, size of the vesicles and drug release % after 1, 2, 4, 8 and 24 h. The size of the vesicles for the formulations was between 124 ± 14.2 nm and 560 ± 127 nm, while the entrapment efficiency was between $97.8 \pm 0.23\%$ and $99.4 \pm 0.24\%$, and the drug release % after 8 h was between $38 \pm 0.82\%$ and $66 \pm 0.52\%$. All formulations were introduced into the Box–Behnken software, which selected three formulations; then, one was assigned as an optimal formula. The in vivo antitumor activity of metformin-loaded ethosomal gel on skin cancer was greater than the antitumor activity of the gel preparation containing free metformin. Lower lecithin, high ethanol and isopropyl alcohol and moderate cholesterol contents improved the permeation rate. Overall, we can conclude that metformin-loaded ethosomes are a promising remedy for treating skin cancers, and more studies are warranted to approve this activity in other animal models of skin cancers.

Keywords: experimental skin cancer; entrapment efficacy; ethosomes; metformin; in vitro permeation; zeta potential

1. Introduction

Skin cancer is a rapidly increasing malignancy affecting humans worldwide [1]. Therapeutic options for skin cancer that include vemurafenib, vismodegib and cemiplimab-rwlc have been marketed [2,3]. These drugs are promising for treating skin cancer, as they enhance the overall survival and shrinkage of the primary tumors. These therapies appear promising but cannot treat 60% of patients. Further, patients develop a high tolerance to these therapies after a few weeks of treatment, enabling metastatic growth and relapse [4]. Hence, it is very important to discover new anti-skin cancer drugs and formulations [5].

Metformin is an important antidiabetic medication [6] that reduces the glucose level, leading to a reduction in the blood insulin level; thus minimizing its impact as a tumor growth factor [7]. Adenosine monophosphate-activated protein kinase (AMPK) is an energy central regulator that plays a crucial role in the restoration of energy balance within the cell in many metabolic pathways [8]. The direct effect of metformin is an activation of AMPK leading to the mammalian target of rapamycin (mTOR) signaling inhibition [9], which, in turn, plays a role in the proliferation of cancer stem cells [7,8,10].

Metformin was reported to suppress the growth of skin cancers in vitro [10]. Some in vivo studies declared that metformin either given in drinking water [11] or administered systemically [12] can mitigate skin cancer growth in animals. A recent study co-delivered a combination of metformin and the chemotherapeutic agent doxorubicin into melanoma tumors to trigger apoptosis and necrosis of the melanoma cells, leading to mitigation of the progression of melanoma growth [13]. One recent clinical trial showed that metformin provided a chemoprotective effect for patients at a high risk of basal cell carcinoma [14]. Additionally, metformin can inhibit skin cancer progression by other mechanisms, such as immune system activation, [15] increasing in autophagy and cell apoptosis by p53 and p21 activation, [16] inhibiting protein synthesis [17] and the destruction of cancer stem cells [14].

The oral administration of metformin produces adverse effects such as nausea, diarrhea and gastric upset, and some types of hepatotoxicity and pancreatitis have been reported. In addition, metformin is known to produce vitamin B12 deficiency, and lactic acidosis is also observed in patients with renal insufficiency [18]. Hence, the topical route should be preferred whenever appropriate.

There are many advantages in using transdermal drug delivery systems. For example, medications can avoid hepatic first-pass metabolism and factors that modify pharmacokinetics in the gastrointestinal tract; this can improve the systemic bioavailability while also lowering the risk of drug concentration-related side effects. Since the topically applied drugs are released in a predetermined range over a long time, this often increases patient compliance, because it is simple and convenient to apply them with a low-dose frequency [19]. Moreover, the topical route provides a large and varied surface of application, as well as ease of self-administration, and is an available alternative to both oral delivery and hypodermic drug injection.

Ethosomes are lipid-based nanovesicles with improved deformability, softness and elasticity and are the most investigated vesicular system. Ethosomes are multilamellar nanovesicles that are made up of phospholipid and ethanol [20,21]. Ethanol amends the phospholipid bilayer fluidity, breaks down the membrane barrier of the stratum corneum and, hence, improves the power of penetration [21]. Ethanol is a powerful penetration enhancer that gives vesicles special characteristics such as entrapment efficacy, size, negative electric potential, stability and better skin permeability [22]. The hair follicles and stratum corneum route allow ethosomes to permeate the epidermis, and the ethosomes are released into the upper skin layer, which results in the drug substances gradually penetrating while the phospholipids stay in the upper layer of the epidermis [23].

Selecting the type and concentration of phospholipid are important to prepare ethosomes, as they will affect the size of the vesicle, stability, percent of entrapment efficacy (EE%), electric potential, drug release % (DR%) and penetration of the vesicles into the skin [21]. Cholesterol is a rigid steroid molecule that enhances the drug stability and entrapment efficiency when used in ethosomal systems [24]. Isopropyl alcohol has a significant impact on the entrapment efficiency but a minor impact on DR% according to the transdermal drug–flux measurements through mice skin [25].

The current study aimed to formulate and characterize metformin-loaded ethosomal preparations and to select the best optimal formula to test its topical antitumor activity against experimentally induced skin cancer in mice. This study also aimed to deliver metformin to the skin layers for the treatment of skin cancer.

2. Results

The effects of different variables such as phospholipid, cholesterol and ethanol were evaluated through the evaluation of EE%, particle size, Zeta potential (ZP), vesicle size (VS) and DR%. Table 1 demonstrates the results of the 17 experiments.

Table 1. Effect of the independent variables on the EE%, VS, ZP and DR%.

Formula Number	Lecithin w/w% (X_1)	Cholesterol w/w% (X_2)	Ethanol and Isopropyl Alcohol w/w% (X_3)	EE% (Y_1)	VS (nm) (Y_2)	ZP (mV) (Y_3)	DR% (Y_4)
1	2	0	30	98.26 ± 0.52	203.00 ± 15.07	−54.05 ± 2.35	42.07 ± 0.34
2 *	3	0.5	30	98.08 ± 0.82	200.04 ± 11.21	−60.02 ± 2.21	66.31 ± 0.52
3	2	0.5	20	98.26 ± 0.41	245.11 ± 20.52	−47.31 ± 1.33	43.45 ± 0.45
4 *	3	0.5	30	98.08 ± 0.82	200.04 ± 11.21	−60.02 ± 2.21	66.31 ± 0.52
5	4	0.5	40	98.14 ± 0.92	223.02 ± 9.01	−50.23 ± 1.44	38.06 ± 0.41
6	4	1	30	98.01 ± 1.20	203.34 ± 11.30	−49.24 ± 0.87	53.14 ± 0.23
7	3	0	20	98.44 ± 0.35	414.01 ± 55.04	−51.01 ± 0.93	38.03 ± 0.82
8	3	0	40	98.26 ± 0.40	560.01 ± 127.14	−58.03 ± 1.20	45.47 ± 0.24
9	3	1	40	99.40 ± 0.24	161.03 ± 13.23	−57.04 ± 2.37	37.28 ± 0.64
10 *	3	0.5	30	98.08 ± 0.82	200.04 ± 11.21	−60.02 ± 2.21	66.31 ± 0.52
11	4	0	30	98.08 ± 0.52	173.13 ± 18.61	−53.17 ± 2.01	45.04 ± 0.62
12 *	3	0.5	30	98.08 ± 0.82	200.04 ± 11.21	−60.02 ± 2.21	66.31 ± 0.52
13	2	0.5	40	98.40 ± 0.35	124.01 ± 14.27	−60.08 ± 1.44	55.04 ± 0.98
14 *	3	0.5	30	98.08 ± 0.82	200.04 ± 11.21	−60.02 ± 2.21	66.31 ± 0.52
15	2	1	30	98.30 ± 0.44	192.41 ± 17.30	−54.31 ± 4.28	52.41 ± 0.45
16	3	1	20	98.11 ± 0.73	234.13 ± 20.63	−52.24 ± 1.81	70.02 ± 0.45
17	4	0.5	20	97.80 ± 0.23	380.06 ± 45.09	−50.06 ± 1.22	62.16 ± 0.45

EE%: entrapment efficacy %, VS: vesicle size, ZP: zeta potential and DR%: drug release % after 8 h. * Centred points. Data presented as the mean ± SD.

2.1. Influence of the Independent Variables on Entrapment Efficiency %

Table 1 shows the data of EE% for all the prepared formulations. The model obtained a suitable fitting with a linear model, the calculated correlation coefficient (R^2) was 0.8388 and the predicted R^2 was 0.6639, while the adjusted R^2, which was 0.7948. The difference was less than 0.2. The ANOVA obtained a significant difference ($p < 0.0001$) between the preparations. Equation (1) describes the influence of the independent variables on the EE%, as follows:

$$EE\% = +98.13 - 0.15 A + 0.0037 B + 0.1062 C \qquad (1)$$

where A= lecithin, B = cholesterol and C = ethanol.

As shown in Figure 1, when the concentration of lecithin increased, the EE% of metformin decreased with a significant difference ($p < 0.0001$), where the EE% of formulas #6 and #11 were 98.14 ± 0.92 and 98.08 ± 0.5, respectively. Further, an increment in the concentration of cholesterol led to an increased EE% of metformin ($p < 0.05$), where the EE% of formulas #6 and #9 were 98 ± 1.2% and 99.4 ± 0.24, respectively. When the ethanol concentration increased, the EE% of metformin increased ($p < 0.033$), where the EE% of formulas #9 and #13 were 99.4 ± 0.24 and 98.4 ± 0.35, respectively (Figures 1A and 2A).

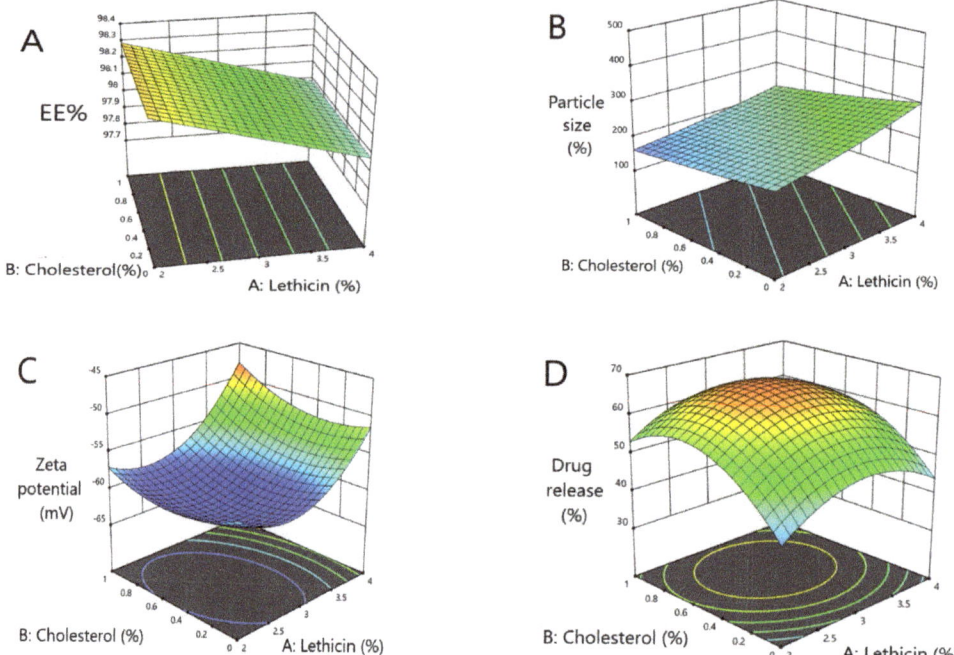

Figure 1. Three-dimensional response surface plots presenting the influence of the independent variables on (**A**) the EE%, (**B**) vesicles size, (**C**) ZP and (**D**) percent of drug released after 8 h.

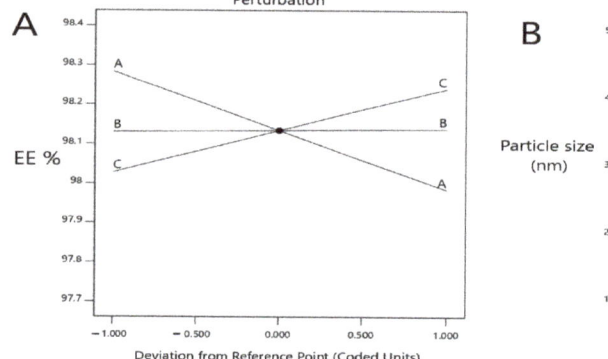
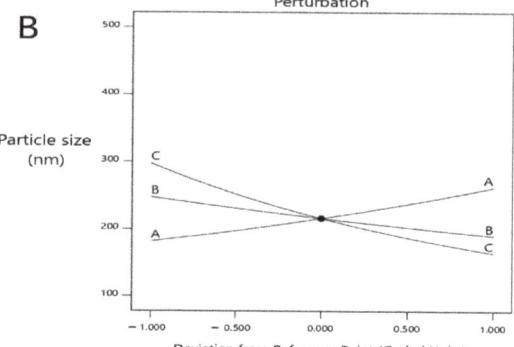

Figure 2. *Cont.*

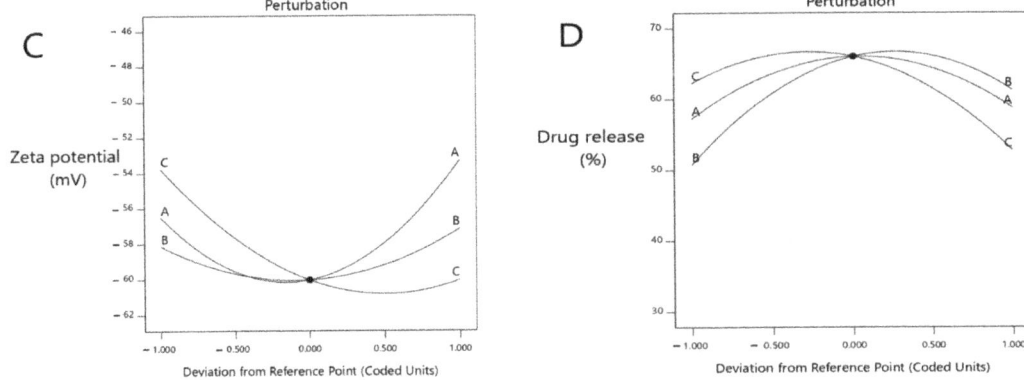

Figure 2. Perturbation explains the influence of the independent variables at (**A**) the EE%, (**B**) vesicles size, (**C**) ZP (mV) and (**D**) percent of drug release after 8 h.

2.2. Influence of the Independent Variables on the Vesicle Sizes

Data of the vesicle sizes for all the formulations are demonstrated in Table 1. The model obtained a suitable fitting with a linear interaction among the variables, and the correlation factor (R^2) was 0.8560. The ANOVA testing obtained a significant difference ($p < 0.0001$) between 0.0689 ± 0.0042 nm and the suggested equation (Inverse Sqrt transform), as follows:

$$1/\text{Sqrt (particle size} - 1.00) = +0.0528 - 0.0686\ A - 0.0045\ B + 0.0101\ C \quad (2)$$

As shown herein, by increasing the concentration of lecithin, the ethosomes vesicle size increased ($p < 0.0025$) where the vesicle sizes of formulas #17 and #5 were 380 ± 45 nm and 223 ± 9 nm, respectively. Further, by increasing the concentration of cholesterol, the ethosomes vesicle sizes increased ($p < 0.0306$); the vesicle sizes of formulas #16 and #6 were 234 ± 20.6 nm and 203 ± 11.3 nm, respectively. By increasing the concentration of ethanol, the ethosomes vesicle size decreased ($p < 0.0001$); the vesicle sizes of formulas #13 and #9 were 124 ± 14.2 nm and 161 ± 13.2 nm, respectively (Figures 1B and 2B).

2.3. Influence of the Independent Variables on ZP

Table 1 shows the ZP values for all the prepared formulations. The model obtained a quadratic equation, and the correlation factor (R^2) was 0.9935. The ANOVA test highlighted a significant difference in the ZP at $p < 0.05$, and the suggested equation was follows:

$$ZP = -60 + 1.62\ A + 0.5\ B - 3.13\ C + 1\ AB + 3.25\ AC + 0.5\ BC + 5.13\ A^2 + 2.38\ B^2 + 3.12\ C^2 \quad (3)$$

The ZP decreased with the increasing lecithin concentration, until a specific point, then increased the lecithin percentage from 2% to around 2.82%, which led to a decrease in ZP. When the lecithin percentage increased more than 2.82%, the ZP increased again (significant difference, $p < 0.0001$), where the ZP of formulas #13 and #17 were -60 ± 1.4 mv and -60 ± 1.4 mv, respectively. The ZP decreased as the cholesterol concentration increased until a specific point. Then, an increased cholesterol percentage from 0 to around 0.5 led to a decline in the ZP, and when the cholesterol percentage increased more than 0.5, this led to an increase in the ZP ($p < 0.0413$), where the ZP of formulas #13 and #6 were -60 ± 1.4 mv and -49 ± 0.8 mv, respectively. The ZP decreased with the increasing ethanol until a specific point, then increased the ethanol percentage from 20% to around 36%, which led to a decrease in the ZP, and when the ethanol percentage increased more than 36%, the ZP increased again. These results obtained a significant difference ($p < 0.0001$), where the ZP of formulas #13 and #3 were −60 ± 1.4 mv and −47 ± 1.3 mv, respectively (Figures 1C and 2C).

2.4. Influence of the Independent Variables at a Percent of Drug Release

The DR % data of the formulations are presented in Table 1. The model revealed a suitable fitting with a quadratic model, and the correlation factor (R^2) was 0.9870. The ANOVA highlighted a significant difference ($p < 0.0001$) at 53.53 ± 2.05%. Equation (4) describes the influence of the independent variables at the DR%:

$$DR\% = +66 - 0.75\,A - 5.25\,B + 4.75\,C - 0.5\,AB - 9\,AC - 10\,BC - 8\,A^2 - 10\,B^2 - 8.5\,C^2 \quad (4)$$

The model highlighted that the DR% significantly increased with decreasing lecithin ($p < 0.05$), while the DR% after 8 h of formulas #5 and #9 were 38 ± 0.41% and 37 ± 0.64%, respectively. In addition, the DR% increased upon decreasing the cholesterol amount significantly ($p < 0.05$), where the DR% after 8 h for formulas #5 and #9 were 38 ± 0.41% and 37 ± 0.64%, respectively. On the other hand, the DR% increased upon increasing the ethanol in a significant manner ($p < 0.05$), where the DR% after 8 h of formula numbers #13 and #11 were 55 ± 0.98% and 45 ± 0.62%, respectively (Figures 1D and 2D). A free drug solution was released completely throughout the dialysis bag within 10 min. The observed rapid drug release may be explained by the sink conditions provided through the experiment. Formula #13 showed the best cumulative release of the metformin percentage from the ethosomal formulations (Figure 3).

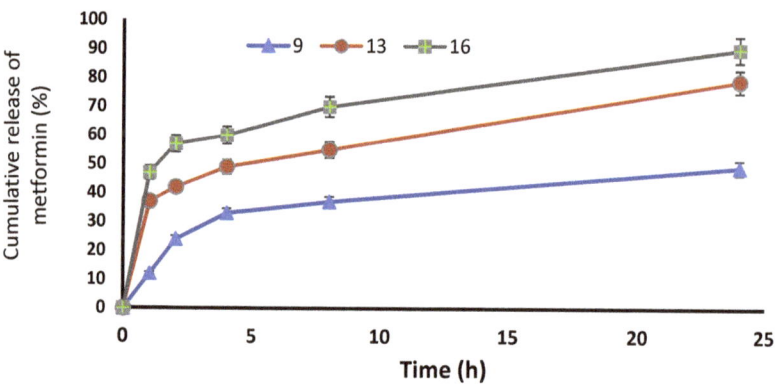

Figure 3. Cumulative release of metformin % from the ethosomal formulations #9, #13 and #16.

2.5. Selection of the Optimized Formula

We prepared ethosomes with a high percent of entrapment efficiency, small vesicle size, high ZP and high percent of DR% by using a three-level three-factor Box–Behnken design. The ANOVA test analyzed and evaluated all the data collected from each response; then, an optimized formula was obtained using the desirability method. The formula that contained 2.083% w/w lecithin, 0.524% w/w cholesterol and 37.495% v/v ethanol was selected as the optimized formula, as it showed the best desirability index value (0.811).

The chosen optimal formula, #13, displayed an EE% of 98.40 ± 0.35%, a vesicle size equal to 124.01 ± 14.27 nm and a release % equal to 55.04 ± 0.98 %. The ZP of the optimized formula #13 was 60.08 ± 1.44 mV, which provided good stability.

2.6. In Vitro Studies to Evaluate Skin Permeation

In formula #9, the amount of permeated metformin was 1224.27 ± 18.1 µg/cm², and the steady-state flux was 2.93 µg/cm²/h, while the percent of cumulative permeation was 72%. In the optimal formula, #13 showed an amount of permeated metformin equal to

1660 ± 32.4 µg/cm², while the steady-state flux was 3.61 µg/cm²/h; however, the percent of cumulative permeation was 97.6%. In addition, formula #16 showed an amount of permeated metformin equal to 1547 ± 21.7 µg/cm², the steady-state flux was 3.26 µg/cm²/h and the percent of cumulative permeation was 91%. Finally, the optimal formula #13 showed the best permeability at interval times with significance ($p < 0.05$), as this formulation had the highest ethanol and isopropyl alcohol concentration, lower lecithin concentration and moderate concentration of cholesterol (Table 2) (Figure 4). The TEER results of the measured electrostatic repulsion were above 30 ± 1.5 kΩ. That indicated a good state for the skin integrity [26].

Table 2. Skin permeation parameters after 24 h.

	The Amount of Permeated Metformin (µg/cm²)	The Steady-State Flux (µg/cm²/h)	The Percent of Cumulative Permeation (%)
Formula #9	1224.27 ± 18.1	2.93	72
The optimum formula #13	1660 ± 32.4	3.61	97.6
Formula #16	1547 ± 21.7	3.26	91

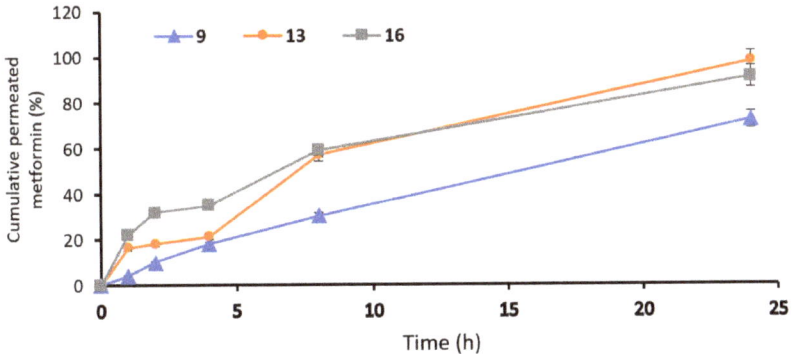

Figure 4. Permeation profiles of metformin from ethosomal formulations: #9, #13 and #16 ethosomal formulations.

2.7. Morphological Characterization of the Ethosomes

The morphology of the ethosomes was characterized by using a transmission electron microscope. The optimal formula was freshly prepared, then used for the transmission electron microscopy (TEM) images. The ethosomes showed in the TEM images as black dots (Figure 5). The TEM images showed ethosomes in well-identified spherical shapes and homogenous and non-aggregated vesicles, which confirmed their nanovesicular characteristics for the ethosomes.

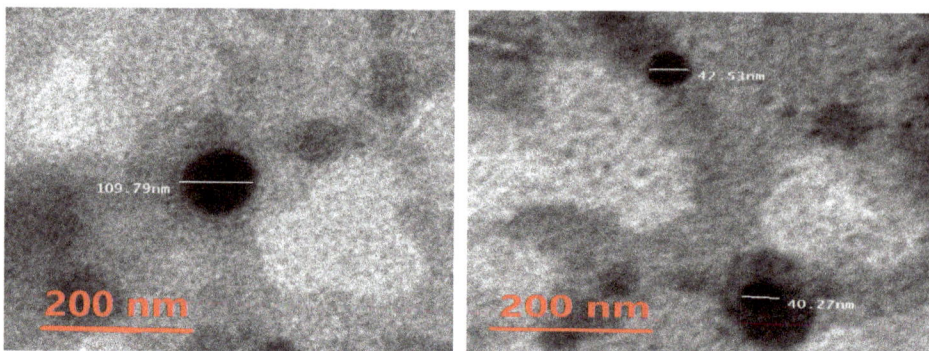

Figure 5. Photomicrograph of the optimal metformin-loaded ethosome formula as seen by the TEM.

2.8. Thermal Analysis of Optimal Metformin-Loaded Ethosomes Formula

The pure metformin curve revealed a sharp endothermic peak at 242 °C, while the optimal metformin-loaded ethosome formula (#13) showed a peak appearing at 135 °C, but the thermogram of the empty formula (excipient) revealed two endothermic peaks at 103 °C and 148 °C. Metformin in the optimal metformin-loaded ethosome formula (formula #13) did not show a characteristic peak. These findings highlight that metformin was dissolved within the ethosomes during the formulation process (Figure 6) [27].

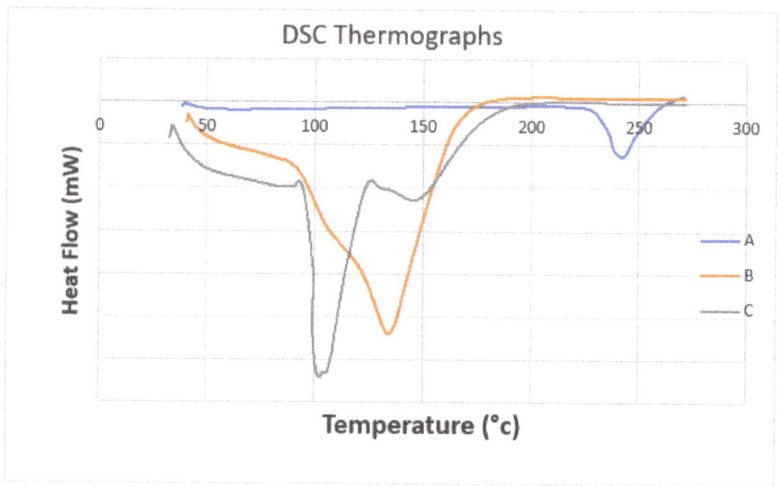

Figure 6. DSC thermograms of (**A**) pure metformin, (**B**) the optimal metformin-loaded ethosome formula and (**C**) an empty formula (excipient).

2.9. In Vivo Antitumoral Activity of the Optimized Metformin-Loaded Ethosomal Gel

The developed 7,12-dimethylbenz[α]-anthracene (DMBA)- induced lesions appeared at the back of each mouse and were monitored weekly, as shown in Figure 7. A specialized caliber was utilized to measure the width and length of each lesion (Figure 7A,B).

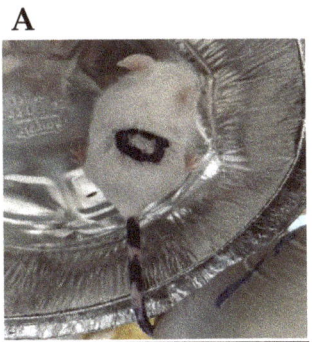 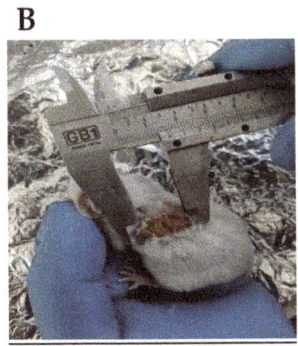 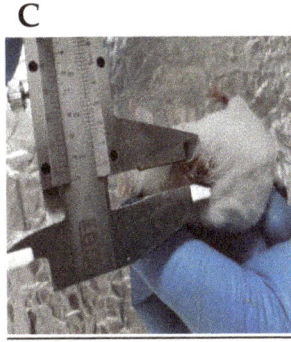

Figure 7. The skin lesions induced by DMBA in male mice. (**A**) A sample of the lesions in the vehicle group. (**B**,**C**) Measuring the dimensions of the lesions in a mouse from the DMBA + vehicle group. Dimensions were measured by a caliber adjusted at the edges of the lesion.

2.9.1. The Body Weight and Lesion Length and Width

The weight of the mice and diameters of the lesions were measured to evaluate the skin cancer progression [28]. The antitumor efficacy of the metformin-loaded ethosomes was evaluated in mice group #5. This metformin-loaded ethosome-containing gel produced a significant decrease in the lesion diameters compared with the other four gels over 28 days (Figure 8).

Figure 8A demonstrates the body weights of the mice during the course of the experiment. The ANOVA indicated no significant variations among the experimental groups at the four time points. Figure 8B illustrates the gross length of the skin lesions, and we found a significant increase in the length in the DMBA + empty gel group versus the vehicle + empty gel group at the four studied time points. Mice treated with free metformin gel or metformin ethosome gel showed significantly lower lesion lengths compared to the mice treated with the empty gel (Figure 8B). In Figure 8C, the lesion width in the DMBA + empty gel group was greater than that measured in the vehicle + empty gel group. The mice group treated with DMBA + metformin ethosome gel showed a smaller lesion width at all the study time points compared to the DMBA + empty gel group. Although the mice treated with DMBA + free metformin gel showed significantly smaller lesion widths compared to the DMBA + empty gel group at day 14, day 21 and day 28, the curative effect shown in the DMBA + metformin ethosome gel group was significantly enhanced (Figure 8C).

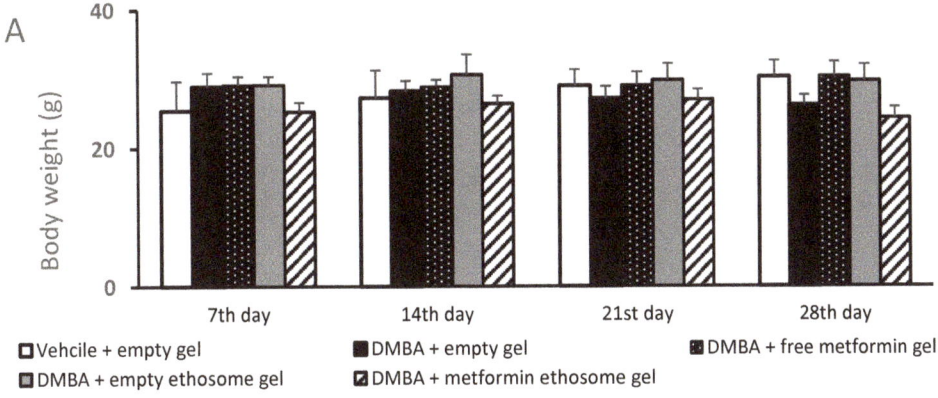

Figure 8. *Cont.*

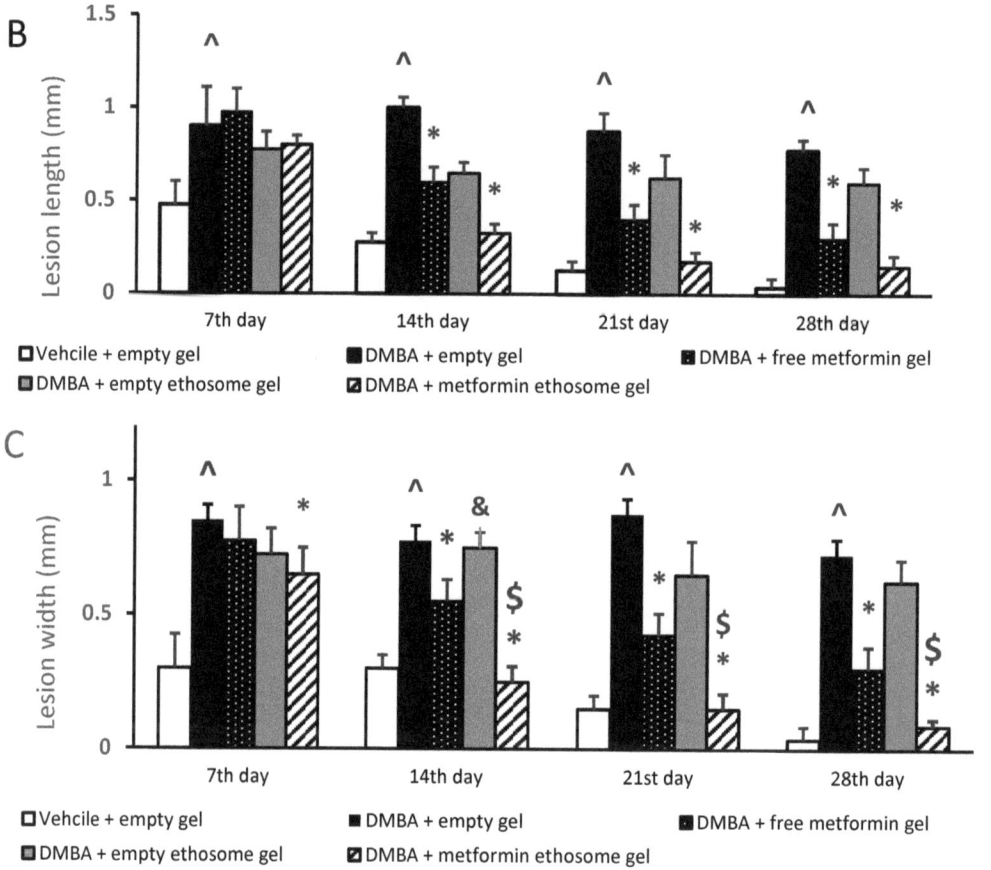

Figure 8. Body weights and dimensions of the skin lesions in the experimental groups. (**A**) Mice body weights, (**B**) lesion lengths (mm) and (**C**) lesion widths (mm). Data were the mean ± SD and analyzed using one-way ANOVA, followed by Bonferroni's pairwise comparison test ($p < 0.05$). ^: versus the vehicle + empty gel group, *: versus the DMBA + empty gel group, &: versus DMBA + free metformin gel. $: versus DMBA + empty ethosome gel.

2.9.2. The Thickness of the Hematoxylin and Eosin-Stained Skin Layers

We found that the vehicle + empty gel group displayed the normal morphological features of the mouse skin layers, with an apparent intact thin epidermal layer with intact keratinocytes and an intact dermal layer with well-organized collagen fibres and hair follicles without abnormal inflammatory cells infiltrates, as well as intact subcutaneous tissue (Figure 10A,A*). The DMBA + empty gel group showed a circumscribed raised, folded mass with non-keratinized epidermal layers hyperplasia with the adjacent ulcerated area covered with the scab of necrotic tissue depress; the underlying dermal layer showed severe diffuse inflammatory cell infiltrates from different populations accompanied with fibroblastic activation and a few records of keratin cysts, as well as abundant records of congested blood vessels (BVs) (Figure 10B,B*). Images from the DMBA + free metformin gel showed focal areas of moderate hyperplasia of non-keratinized epidermal layers without ulcerated lesion records associated with focal subepidermal fibroblastic activation with higher collagen fibres contents. The persistence of moderate-to-severe inflammatory cell infiltrates was shown, however, to have a less intense density compared with the model samples, accompanied with abundant records of subepidermal and subcutaneous congested BVs. The third group obtained healing in the damage of the epidermis and dermis layers and a decrease in the infiltrations of inflammatory cells (Figure 10C,C*). Images of the skin specimens from the DMBA + ethosome gel group showed circumscribed, raised non-ulcerated masses of skin with moderate epidermal thickening and folding covered with a mass of necrotic tissue to depress with focal subepidermal hemorrhagic patches and mild records of infiltrate of inflammatory cells, as well as fibroblastic activity with minimal records of congested subcutaneous BVs (Figure 10D,D*). Images of DMBA + metformin ethosome gel showing obvious improvements of histological organization epidermal/dermal layers with an almost apparent intact, mildly folded epidermal layer with apparent intact keratinocytes and abundant mature collagen formation in a mildly thick dermal layer with minimal inflammatory cells infiltrates. However, focal records of subcutaneous hemorrhagic patches with moderate inflammatory cell infiltrates, as well as congested and dilated BVs, were shown (Figure 10E,E*). In Figure 10, the DMBA + metformin-loaded ethosomes group showed an approximately normal structure in the epidermis and dermis layers and the nonexistence of inflammatory cells. The measured epidermal thickness was significantly decreased compared with the DMBA + empty gel group (Figure 10F).

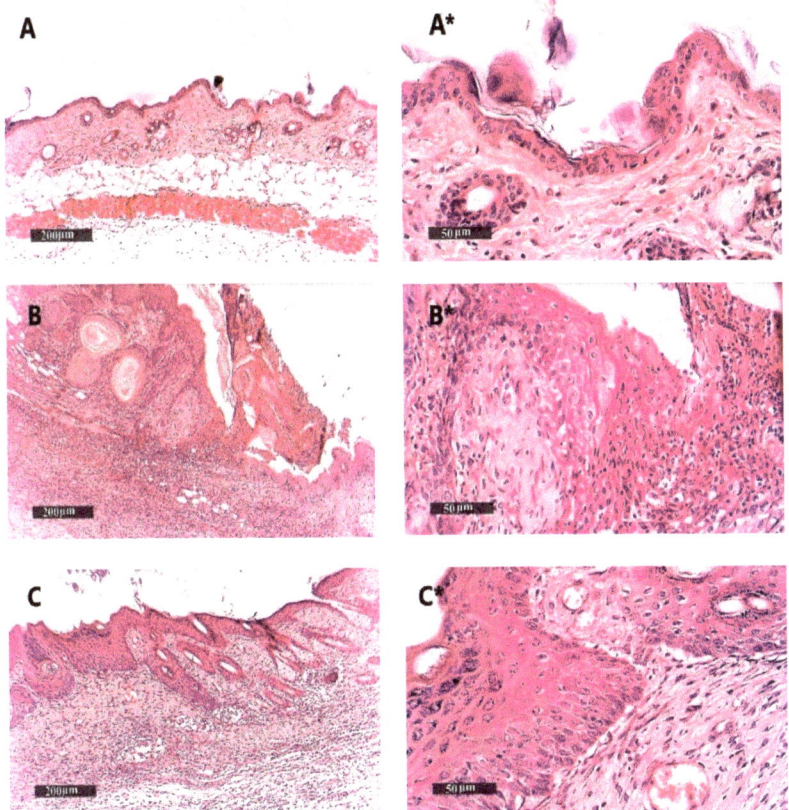

Figure 9. *Cont.*

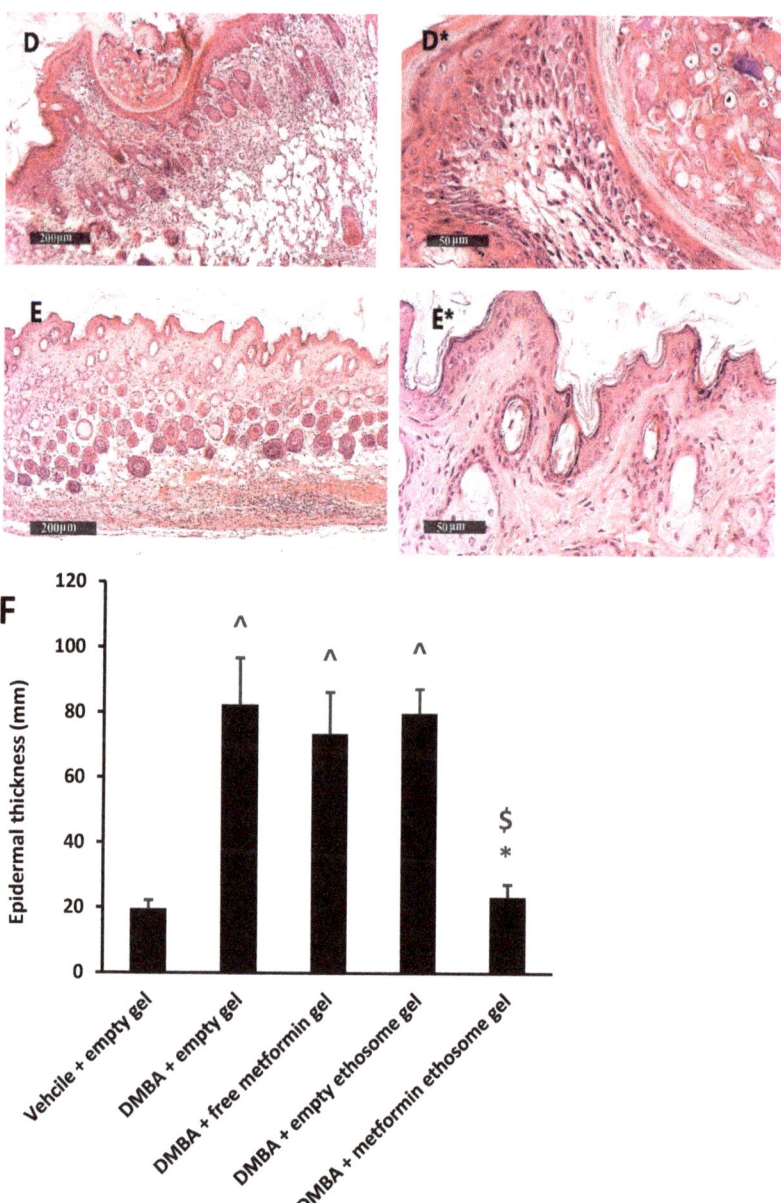

Figure 10. Histopathological picture of skin tissues stained with hematoxylin and eosin. (**A,A***) Images revealed normal morphological features of mouse skin layers with an apparent intact thin epidermal layer with intact keratinocytes and an intact dermal layer with well-organized collagen fibres and hair follicles without abnormal inflammatory cells infiltrates, as well as an intact subcutaneous tissue. (**B,B***) Images for DMBA + empty gel, showing a circumscribed raised, folded mass with non-keratinized epidermal layers of hyperplasia with the adjacent ulcerated area covered with the scab of necrotic tissue depress. The underlying dermal layer showed severe diffuse inflammatory cell infiltrates from different populations accompanied with fibroblastic activation and few records of keratin cysts, as well as abundant records of congested blood vessels (BVs). (**C,C***) Images from the

DMBA + free metformin group showing focal areas of moderate hyperplasia of non-keratinized epidermal layers without ulcerated lesion records associated with focal subepidermal fibroblastic activation with higher collagen fibres contents. The persistence of moderate-to-severe inflammatory cell infiltrates was shown; however, a less intense density compared with the model samples was accompanied by abundant records of subepidermal and subcutaneous-congested BVs. (**D,D***) Images for skin specimens from the DMBA + empty ethosome group showing a circumscribed, raised non-ulcerated mass of skin with moderate epidermal thickening and folding covered with a mass of necrotic tissue to depress with focal subepidermal hemorrhagic patches and mild records of infiltrate of inflammatory cells, as well as fibroblastic activity with minimal records of congested subcutaneous BVs. (**E,E***) Images for the DMBA + metformin-loaded ethosome group (optimal gel formula) showing obvious improvement of the histological organization epidermal/dermal layers with an almost apparent intact, mildly folded epidermal layer with apparent intact keratinocytes and an abundant mature collagen formation in a mildly thick dermal layer with minimal inflammatory cells infiltrates. However, there were also focal records of subcutaneous hemorrhagic patches with moderate inflammatory cell infiltrates, as well as congested and dilated BVs. (**F**) Epidermal thickness of the skin layers in all groups. Thicknesses of six regularly spaced skin parts were measured using ImageJ software (NIH, Bethesda, MD, USA). The average of the measured parts was calculated for every tissue specimen, and the mean of each group was then estimated. Data were the mean ± SD and analyzed using one-way ANOVA, while the pairwise comparison was estimated by Bonferroni's test at $p < 0.05$. ^: versus the vehicle + empty gel group, *: versus the DMBA + empty gel group, &: versus DMBA + free metformin gel. $: versus DMBA + empty ethosome gel, scale bar = 200 μm (left column) and scale bar = 50 μm (right column).

2.9.3. Histopathological Examination of Kidney Specimens Stained with H&E

The kidney samples from the vehicle + empty gel group demonstrated intact morphological features of renal parenchyma, including renal corpuscles and different nephron tubular segments, including tubular epithelium, with intact interstitial tissue, as well as vasculatures (Figure 11A). DMBA + empty gel or DMBA + ethosome gel showed a mild cystic dilatation of the renal tubular segments, accompanied by little interstitial mononuclear inflammatory cell infiltrates (Figure 11B,D). The DMBA + free metformin gel group showed mild focal records of tubular degenerative changes with intact renal corpuscles, as well as interstitial tissues with few sporadic inflammatory cell infiltrates (Figure 11C). The DMBA + metformin ethosome gel samples showed sporadic records of tubular degenerative changes with intact renal corpuscles, interstitial tissue and vasculatures (Figure 11E).

2.9.4. Histopathological Examination of Liver Specimens Stained with H&E

Liver samples from the vehicle + empty gel group showed the normal morphological structure of hepatic parenchyma (Figure 12A,A*). The DMBA + empty gel samples showed mild hepatocellular degenerative changes in the pericentral, as well as periportal, regions with diffuse mononuclear inflammatory cells infiltrating in the hepatic parenchyma (Figure 12B,B*). Samples from the DMBA + free metformin gel group showed mild hepatocellular vacuolar degenerative changes with the dilatation of hepatic BVs and minimal inflammatory cell infiltrates (Figure 12C,C*). Samples from the DMBA + ethosome gel group showed mild hepatocellular degenerative changes with intact hepatocytes and mild focal pericentral and periportal mononuclear inflammatory cells infiltrates (Figure 12D,D*). Samples from the DMBA + metformin ethosome gel group showed almost apparent intact hepatocytes all over the hepatic parenchyma and moderate dilation of the portal BVs with minor focal perivascular inflammatory cell infiltrates (Figure 12E,E*).

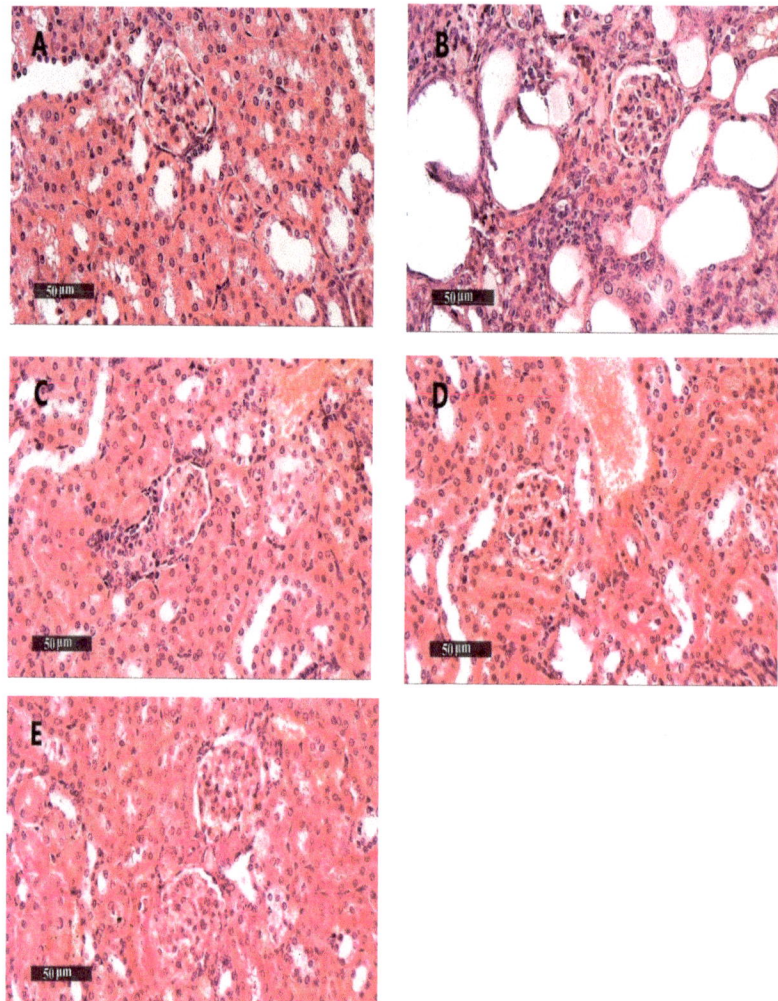

Figure 11. Kidney samples stained with H&E. (**A**) An image for a kidney specimen from the vehicle + empty gel group showing apparent intact morphological features of renal parenchyma, including renal corpuscles and different nephron tubular segments, including tubular epithelium, with intact interstitial tissue, as well as vasculatures. (**B,D**) Images for a kidney specimen from the DMBA + empty gel or DMBA + ethosome gel showing a mild cystic dilatation of renal tubular segments, with some flattening of the tubular epithelial lining. (**C**) An image for a kidney specimen from the DMBA + free metformin gel group showing mild focal records of tubular degenerative changes with intact renal corpuscles, as well as interstitial tissue with very few sporadic inflammatory cell infiltrates. (**E**) An image from DMBA + metformin ethosome gel samples showing little focal tubular degenerative changes with intact renal corpuscles, interstitial tissue and vasculatures, scale bar = 50 µm.

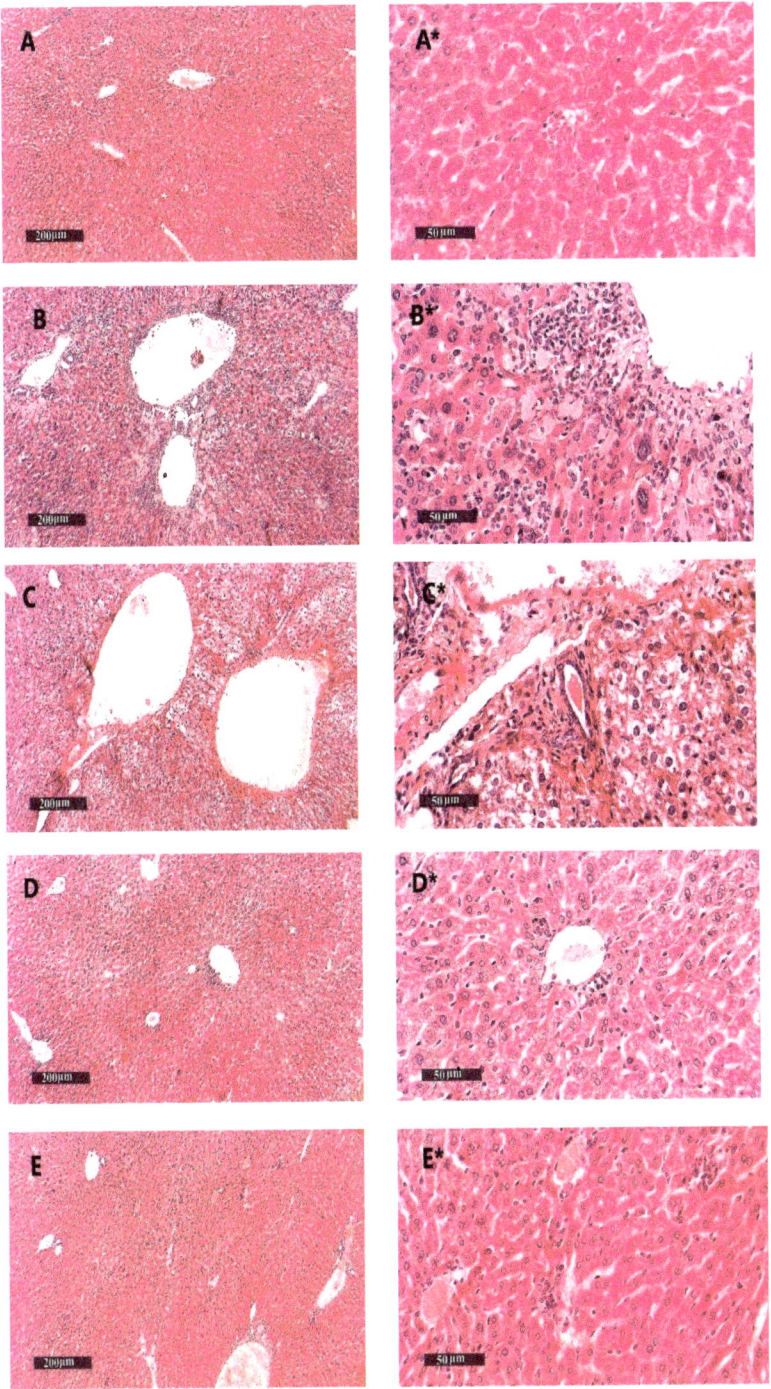

Figure 12. Liver samples stained with H&E. (**A**,**A***) Liver samples from the vehicle + empty gel group show the normal morphological structure of hepatic parenchyma. (**B**,**B***) DMBA + empty gel samples

show mild hepatocellular degenerative changes in the pericentral, as well as periportal, regions, with some mononuclear inflammatory cells infiltrating in the hepatic parenchyma. (**C,C***) Samples from the DMBA + free metformin gel group showing little hepatocellular vacuolar degenerative changes with minimal inflammatory cell infiltrate records. (**D,D***) Samples from the DMBA + ethosome gel group showing mild records of the hepatocellular degenerative changes with higher records of apparent intact hepatocytes, and mild focal mononuclear inflammatory cell infiltrates accompanied with the mild dilatation of hepatic BVs. (**E,E***) Samples from the DMBA + metformin ethosome gel group showing almost apparent intact hepatocytes all over hepatic parenchyma, and the moderate dilation of portal BVs with minor focal perivascular inflammatory cell infiltrates, scale bar = 200 µm (left column) and scale bar = 50 µm (right column).

2.9.5. Liver and Kidney Function Tests

We applied an ANOVA test on the data of the serum ALT, AST, albumin, urea and creatinine, but the data indicated nonsignificant differences among the study group (Figure 13A–E).

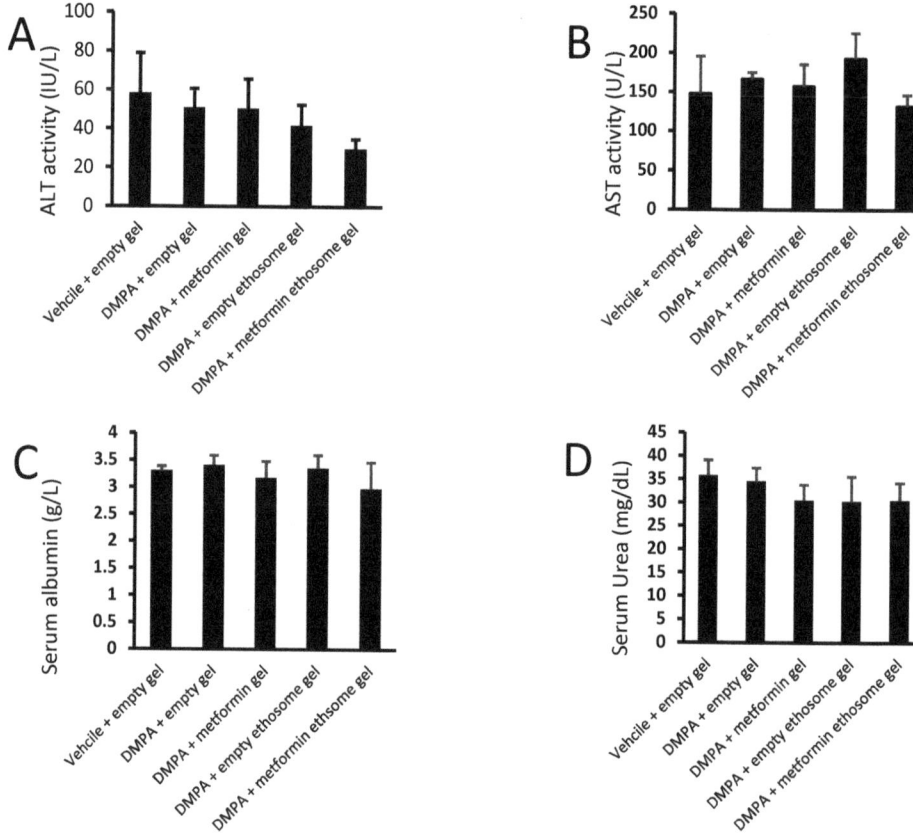

Figure 13. *Cont.*

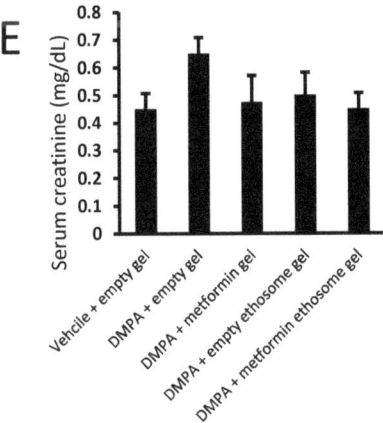

Figure 13. Liver and kidney function tests for mice from the experimental groups: (**A**) ALT, (**B**) AST, (**C**) albumin, (**D**) urea and (**E**) creatinine. Data were the mean ± SD, and the analysis was done by one-way ANOVA at $p < 0.05$.

3. Discussion

This study aimed to obtain the ability of ethosomes to raise the retained amount of metformin on the skin to improve skin cancer treatment. Ethosomes can penetrate the stratum corneum to the deep layers, as ethosomes contain a high alcohol content [29].

3.1. Influence of the Independent Variables on EE%

The concentrations of lecithin, ethanol and cholesterol are critical parameters to prepare ethosomes [20,30]. Lecithin builds lipid bilayer membranes in multilamellar vesicles of ethosomes [31]. Cholesterol is responsible for the stability and EE% of metformin [32].

Ethanol gives the vesicles more freedom and stability by providing softness and a negative charge [32]. Depending on the data collected from all formulations, a ethanol concentration of 40% was suitable to prepare the ethosomes that produced a high EE% and permeation [21,28,32]. However, increasing the concentration of ethanol above 40% will dissolve the ethosome membranes, causing a decrease in the EE% and increase in the vesicle sizes [32]. On the other hand, isopropyl alcohol is used with ethanol to prepare ethosomes as a skin penetration enhancer and to increase the EE% [25]. The high entrapment efficiency of the formulations is due to adding isopropyl alcohol with ethanol; isopropyl alcohol decreases the vesicle size and increases the ZP and EE%. Isopropyl alcohol can release metformin in the long term, which achieves the goal of our study [25,28,33].

Lecithin builds a phospholipid structure and is responsible for a multilamellar membrane of ethosomes [32]. Cholesterol has an important role in preventing leakage and reducing the permeability of drugs from vesicles [34]. Additionally, when the concentration of lecithin increases, this will lead to reducing the EE% because of the hydrophilic nature of metformin [35].

3.2. Influence of the Independent Variables on Vesicle Size and ZP

A concentration of 2–4% lecithin was used to prepare formulations of the ethosomes. Increasing the lecithin ratio will increase the vesicle sizes [36,37]. When the concentration of lecithin increases, this will lead to increasing the ethosome vesicle sizes, as lecithin molecules tend to coalesce and aggregate [38].

The negative charge of the vesicles was linked to high concentrations of ethanol, and this led to solubilizing some of the amount of lecithin inside the vesicles, which caused small multilamellar vesicles (SMLV), as ethanol has a high fluidizing effect [39]. Cholesterol had a positive effect on the vesicle size, which meant increasing the cholesterol range from 0.5% to 1%, leading to an increase in the vesicle sizes of the ethosomes [40].

A previous report indicated that a rise in ethanol concentration led to a decline in the ethosome vesicle sizes [41]. Ethanol plays a crucial role in skin penetration [42]. The concentration of ethosomes in most ethosomal formulations was 20–40% [37]. On the other hand, when the ethanol concentration increased, this resulted in a decline in the ethosome sizes [37]. Similarly, an incremental increase in the isopropyl alcohol concentration resulted in a decline in the ethosome vesicle sizes [25]. Due to the high value of the negative charge for the ZP, an electrostatic repulsion was formed and prohibited any aggregation between vesicles, which led to an increased stability of ethosomes [43,44].

Adding isopropyl alcohol and a high concentration of ethanol caused a high negative charge to the ethosomal formula, which led to a high penetration profile, and a high negative charge also caused a high EE%, as metformin is a cationic drug [28].

3.3. Influence of the Independent Variables on DR%

In our study, isopropyl alcohol and ethanol improved the metformin release from ethosomes, as they can increase the liquefaction and permeability that leads to an increased DR% [45]. Cholesterol and lecithin decrease the metformin release from ethosomes, as increasing concentrations of cholesterol and lecithin are incompatible with metformin solubility. Lecithin has a negative effect on DR%, as increasing the lecithin level will cause an increase in the vesicle rigidity and will cause a decrease in the DR% [46].

The optimal formula #13 showed the best DR% at the interval times, as this formulation has the highest ethanol and isopropyl concentration, lower lecithin concentration and moderate concentration from cholesterol. Using formulations with good penetrating and releasing properties produced an acceptable impression for the induction of a sustained releasing state.

3.4. In Vitro Skin Permeation Study

In our formulations, when the concentration of lecithin decreased, the permeation rate of metformin increased. Furthermore, decreasing the concentration of cholesterol caused an increase in the permeation rate of metformin. Similarly, one previous study found that, when the concentrations of lecithin and cholesterol increased, the rigidity of the ethosomal vesicle bilayer increased [32]. Ethanol enhanced the permeation rate of the drug as it interacted with the polar head group of the SC lipid molecules, lowering the melting point of the SC lipids and thereby increasing the lipid bilayer fluidity and cell membrane permeability [22,47]. The maximum permeability of the drug from the vesicles was due to a synergistic mechanism involving ethanol, vesicles and SC lipid molecules [29,48].

Carbopol has an anionic polymer and the best buffering capacity characters that keep the required pH and prevent skin irritation. When carbopol is mixed with ethosomes, it leads to reaching the required viscosity and the best bio-adhesion characteristics [49,50].

3.5. Thermal Analysis of Optimal Metformin-Loaded Ethosomes Formula

DSC has been used to show the physical state of metformin within the ethosomes, as well as the intermolecular interactions between metformin and ethosomes [27]. There was a lack for the characteristic metformin peaks, showing that metformin was fully solubilized in the ethosome system. On other hand, metformin was present in an amorphous state in the ethosomes; this can improve the release of the drug from the vesicles. The excipients and metformin showed no incompatibility state because of the absence of the characteristic melting point peak of the drug in the optimal formula [51].

3.6. In Vivo Antitumor Activity and Toxicology

The application of metformin-loaded ethosomes showed significant antitumor activity against the skin cancer compared to the application of free metformin. At the 14-days treatment point, the effect of the free metformin gel was better than the empty ethosome gel;

this may be linked to the anticancer effect of the free metformin. However, at the following time points (day 21 and day 28), there was no significant differences among the two groups.

In agreement with our study, a recent study highlighted that the application of metformin inhibits the promotion of experimental skin tumors in mice [52]. Several previous studies indicated that ethosomal preparations enhance topical anticancer drugs; for example, one research group documented that a gel preparation containing sonidegib-loaded ethosomes produced desirable therapeutic profits for treating skin cancer [28]. Another study indicated that ethosomes coloaded with evodiamine and berberine chloride showed a greater efficacy in the treatment of melanoma compared to the free forms [53]. Consistently, one more study confirmed that topically applied positively charged ethosomes of vismodegib was promising for the effective treatment of basal cell carcinoma, with a low incidence of adverse effects [28]. Regarding the toxicology study, we found that the liver and kidney histopathological changes were mild and did not indicate significant damages that would be reflected in a significant rise in the serum hepatic enzymes or kidney markers.

4. Material and Methods

4.1. Materials

Metformin hydrochloride (99.45% powder, BP 2012), 99.9% ethanol (v/v), isopropyl alcohol and carbopol 974p were obtained from Medical Union Pharmaceuticals (Ismailia, Egypt). Some 10× phosphate buffered saline was bought from Lonza Company (Verviers, Belgium). The 97% L-α-lecithin was granular, from soybean oil, CAS 8002-43-5, molecular weight = 750 g/mol and the method detection limit (MDL) number was MFCD00082428. The 97% cholesterol was bought from Acros Organics (Geel, Belgium).

4.2. Box–Behnken Experimental Design

By using the Box–Behnken (BB) three-level three-factor design shown in Table 3, we optimized and selected the formulation variables statistically for the preparation of ethosomes that carry metformin to achieve the maximum EE%, small vesicle size, high ZP and the greatest DR% [28]. The experimental design was generated and evaluated by the aid of the Design-Expert software (Version 11, Stat-Ease Inc., Minneapolis, MN, USA).

Table 3. Evaluation of the independent variables in the Box–Behnken design.

Factor	Levels of Independent Variables		
Independent Variables	Minimum (−1)	Moderate (0)	Maximum (+1)
X1 = L-α-Lecithin concentration (w/w%)	2%	3%	4%
X2 = Cholesterol concentration (w/w%)	0%	0.5%	1%
X3 = Ethanol and isopropyl alcohol concentration (w/w%)	20%	30%	40%
Y1 = Entrapment efficiency (%)		Maximum	
Y2 = Vesicle size (nm)		Minimum	
Y3 = Zeta Potential (mV)		Maximum	
Y4 = DR % (% of drug released after 8 h)		Maximum	

Seventeen experiments were prepared, and the 3 independent variables were studied: L-α-lecithin concentration (2–4 w/w%) (X1), cholesterol concentration (0 to 1 w/w%) (X2) and ethanol and isopropyl alcohol concentrations (20–40 w/w%) (X3). On other hand, the EE% (Y1: EE%), vesicle size (Y2: VS), ZP (Y3) and DR% (Y4) were chosen as the dependent variables.

A concentration of 2–4 w/w% lecithin was used to prepare formulations of ethosomes. [36,37]. The concentration of ethosomes in most ethosomal formulations was 20–40 w/w% [37]. A concentration of 0 to 1 w/w% cholesterol was used to prepare ethosomes in the most recent researches [32,54]. The optimal formula was chosen based on its desirability, which was then subjected to further examination [39].

4.3. Formulation of Metformin-Loaded Ethosomes

Formulation of the metformin-carrying ethosomes was designed depending on the method reported previously [21,33,34]. The aqueous and organic phases were prepared separately. Lecithin and cholesterol were dissolved in a mixture of ethanol and isopropyl alcohol to produce the organic phase, which was kept in a closed container. Metformin was insoluble in ethanol and isopropyl alcohol, so it was dissolved in distilled water to produce the aqueous phase. The aqueous phase was added to the organic phase drop by drop by a syringe pump. The mixture is stirred using a magnetic stirrer (Intilab, Cairo, Egypt) at a speed of 700 rpm for 5–30 min to obtain the required ethosomal formula at 30 °C. Finally, the ethosomal formulations were passed through a polytetrafluoroethylene (PTFE) filter with a pore size of 0.22 µm [39]. Then, the filtrates were stored in closed containers at 4 °C.

4.4. Characterization of the Metformin-Loaded Ethosomes

4.4.1. Determination of entrapment efficiency %

EE% is the percent of the total amount of metformin encapsulated in vesicles in the formulations. The unentrapped metformin was separated using a cooling centrifuge rotating at 16,000 rpm at 4 °C (Sigma cooling centrifuge, Sigma Laborzentrifugen GmbH, Germany) [39]. The supernatants were diluted in distilled water (10 mL, 3 min) [28]. The amount of entrapped metformin was estimated spectrophotometrically (Jasco UV–Vis spectrophotometer, Jasco, Japan), and the λmax of metformin was 234 nm; it was calculated using a standard calibration curve. By subtracting the amount of metformin in the supernatant from the initial amount and then dividing the result by the initial amount, the EE% can be calculated [55]:

$$EE\% = \frac{Total\ (50\ mg) - Free}{Total\ (50\ mg)} \times 100$$

4.4.2. Vesicle Size Analysis

Vesicle size is evaluated by using the dynamic light scattering method that is performed in the Malvern Zetasizer (Nano ZS, Malvern, UK) (DLS). Distilled water was utilized to dilute all formulations and mixed by shaking before the measurements to improve the scattering intensity and remove the multiple scattering phenomena. The particle size was measured after placing the samples in glass cuvettes [56]. Three replicates were done for each formulation and presented as the mean ± SD.

4.4.3. Zeta Potential Analysis

We measured the ZP using a computerized Malvern Zetasizer (Instrument at Manipal University, Manipal, India) based on the electrophoretic mobility. The particle charge is an important parameter to ensure the ethosomal suspension stability [42].

4.4.4. In Vitro Release Study

Some 1-mL samples from each formula (1.7 $w/w\%$ of metformin) were added to a dialysis bag (Mw cut-off = 14,000 Da). Forty millilitres of Sorensen phosphate buffer (pH = 6.5) was used as a release medium [39]. Then, the dialysis bag was immersed in the prepared release medium at 32 ± 0.5 °C in a dissolution apparatus (SR8, Hanson Research, Chatsworth, CA, USA) at 100 rpm. New 1-mL samples were withdrawn from the medium and replaced with the same volume from the fresh medium at 1, 2, 4, 8, 12 and 24 h. Estimation of the sample concentrations was done spectrophotometrically at a 234 nm [31,55].

$$DR\% = \frac{The\ amount\ of\ metformin\ released\ at\ time\ t}{The\ initial\ amount\ of\ entrapped\ metformin} \times 100$$

4.4.5. Optimization and Experimental Model Validation

Design-Expert® software chooses the model that gives statistically accepted polynomial equations [57,58]. These equations are utilized for demonstrating conclusions about each response after taking both the degree and sign of the calculated coefficients. "A positive sign indicates synergism, whereas a negative sign indicates antagonism" [31].

Design-Expert® software presents 3D response surface plots demonstrating the relation between each factor and the resultant response. The optimization process uses the desirability index (Di) to determine the suitable level of each response with an independent variable. When Di equal 0, this means an undesirable formula, while Di equal 1 means a desirable formula [31].

This study aimed to select the optimal formula that achieves the maximum EE% (Y1), ZP (Y3) and DR% (Y4) and minimum vesicle size (Y2). The model is accepted in case the range of the observations from the optimal formula occurs within the prediction interval of the confirmation node. The three optimized formulations were prepared 3 times for checking the optimal formula validity. Formulas with different release patterns (highest–lowest and middle values) were tested for the permeation study (Formulas 9, 13 and 16).

4.5. In Vitro Skin Permeation

The diffusible membranes were collected from abdominal rat skin in the Faculty of Pharmacy, Suez Canal University, Ismailia, Egypt. The skin of rats was used fresh, as reported previously [51]. Each diffusion membrane was mounted in a vertical diffusion cell (5 cm^2) as a donor compartment. Sorensen phosphate buffer (40 mL, pH = 6.5) was used as a receptor compartment [28]. The diffusion membrane containing 1 mL of each formula (1.7 w/w% of metformin) was immersed in the receptor compartment, which was stirred in a water bath at 600 rpm, and the temperature equaled 37 $\pm$ 0.5 °C. After that, 1-mL samples were taken from the medium and substituted by equal volumes from the fresh medium at 1, 2, 4, 8, 12 and 24 h. Finally, the samples were measured by a spectrophotometer at a wavelength of 234 nm [39,59]. The limit of quantitation (LOQ) was 0.84 µg, while the detection range was 1–20 µg/mL.

The animal skin model could provide higher permeation results than its human counterpart [60]. For checking the skin integrity, the trans-epidermal electrical resistance (TEER) test was applied. An aqueous NaCl solution (0.9%) was used for filling the diffusion cell's receptor, as well as the donor compartments. Each compartment was immersed in electrodes, and the resistance was determined utilizing an LCR bridge (LCR400, Thurlby Thandar Instruments, Cambridgeshire, England) at a frequency equal to 1 kHz. Various factors, including the instrument, applied frequency, resultant current, solution ionic strength and the surface area of the skin sample, are able to control the estimated resistance [26]. The standard limit value was set at 1 kΩ in the experiment.

4.6. Analysis of Permeation Study Data

jss is the steady-state flux that is calculated by the slope of the straight line of the cumulative amount of the permeated drug per unit area at a time (µg/cm^2/h) [39]. Kp is the permeability coefficient of metformin from each preparation (1/cm.h) that is calculated by dividing jss by the primary metformin concentration in the donor compartment (Co).

$$K_p = j_{ss}/C_o$$

4.7. Gel Formulation

The optimum formula gel was prepared by adding 0.7 g from carbopol 974p to the optimal formula under vigorous stirring; then, trimethylamine solution (5%) was used to neutralize the mixture, which was added drop by drop until the gel was formed [28,32].

4.8. Morphological Examination of the Optimal Metformin-Loaded Ethosomes Formula

The morphology of the optimal metformin-loaded ethosome formula (#13) in the gel preparation ensured that the vesicles were still formed. The gel was characterized by using TEM (TEM-1010, Tokyo, Japan) [61]. After sample preparation, it was dropped onto the surface of a copper grid coated with carbon. Each sample was left to dry in order to permit ethosomes to adhere to the carbon substrates. For staining, we applied a drop of 1% aqueous phosphotungestic acid dye to the grid, which was then air-dried for 2 min after removing excess dye with a piece of filter paper. The TEM was then used to examine and visualize the stained sample.

4.9. Thermal Analysis of Optimal Metformin-Loaded Ethosomes Formula

The thermal analysis of the optimal metformin-loaded ethosomes formula was studied by utilizing differential Scanning Calorimetry (Shimadzu, DSC 60, Kyoto, Japan). Five milligrams of each sample were added to an aluminum pan. Each sample was heated from room temperature to 300 °C at a heating rate equal to 10 °C/min under nitrogen flowing at a rate of 20 mL/min to prevent oxidation of the sample [62]. Pure metformin, optimal metformin-loaded ethosome formula and empty formula (excipient) thermograms have been compared.

4.10. In Vivo Mouse Study for Screening of Antitumor Activity and Toxicity

4.10.1. Mice Preparation and Ethical Approval

Thirty male Swiss albino mice (weight range equaled 25–30 g, 6–8 weeks of age) were purchased from VACSERA (Helwan, Egypt) and placed in groups of six in plastic cages. The experiment was done in the institutional animal house at the Faculty of Pharmacy, Suez Canal University, at a temperature range equal to 23 ± 5 °C, and the animals had free access to their normal diet and drinking water. The protocol of this study obtained approval from the institutional research ethics committee (#202004MA1).

4.10.2. Induction of Skin Lesions

A 2×2 cm^2 dorsal skin area was shaved on all animals using a hair clipper 48 h prior to the experiment. To induce skin lesions in mice, one dose of DMBA, which acts as an initiator for skin tumors (100 µg in 200 µL acetone) [63], was injected subcutaneously into each mice [28]. After one week, there was an increase in the number of epidermal lesions (the lesions > 1 mm in diameter for each mouse [63]. The skin lesions were assessed first by skin morphology (lesion width and lesion length) and, also, by histological methods (thickness of the epidermis).

4.10.3. Regimen of Applying Metformin-Loaded Ethosomes

Each group contained 6 animals, and the selected optimal formula was applied topically on the dorsal region of the skin (10 mg/cm^2 of the affected area) per week for a total of 4 weeks [27,48]. The experimental groups are shown in Table 4.

Table 4. Experimental groups for the in vivo mouse study.

Group 1	Received vehicle (acetone) and topical empty gel.
Group 2	Received DMBA and topical empty gel.
Group 3	Received DMBA and topical free metformin gel.
Group 4	Received DMBA and topical empty ethosomes gel.
Group 5	Received DMBA and metformin ethosomes gel.

The topical empty gel contained distilled water and carbopol 974 p only. On the other hand, the topical empty ethosome gel contained all the ethosome components (distilled water, ethanol, isopropyl alcohol, lecithin and cholesterol) and carbopol 974 p without metformin.

The measurements of the diameters of the skin cancer lesions were standardized for evaluating the efficacy of the selected optimal gel formula. Each mouse lesion more than 1 mm in diameter was measured weekly until the end of the study. At the end of the study protocol, the final lesion diameters were determined, and then, the mice were anaesthetized and slaughtered [64]. Blood samples were taken by cardiac puncture and settled for 30 min before centrifugation and separation of the serum samples.

4.10.4. Histopathological Methodology and Examination

Extracted skin specimens were fixed in 10% neutral-buffered formalin, then embedded in paraffin wax and sectioned by a microtome (at 4 µm) and processed for hematoxylin and eosin (H&E) staining (the sections were deparaffinized, rehydrated in alcohol, stained in Harris hematoxylin, rinsed in 95% ethanol, counterstained with eosin solution, dehydrated through 95% alcohol and cleared in xylene, followed by mounting). Light microscopy was used to examine the skin sections by an experienced pathologist (the nuclei, nucleolus and nuclear membrane were stained blue, and the cytoplasm and connective tissue were stained pink) [30]. Histopathological investigation for skin tumor specimens was performed to assess the efficacy of the different drug/vehicle formulations [63]. Thicknesses of six regularly spaced skin parts were measured using ImageJ software (NIH, Bethesda, MD, USA). The average of the measured parts was calculated for every tissue specimen.

4.10.5. Toxicological Screening

For testing any possibility of hepatic or renal toxicity due to the systemic absorption of the gel formula, a histopathological investigation was done for the liver and kidney specimens. The tissue samples were fixed in neutral-buffered formalin and processed for H&E staining and examination under light microscopy by an experienced blinded pathologist. In addition to the histopathological examination, the serum samples were directed for estimation of the liver enzymes (ALT and AST) and serum creatinine, urea and albumin.

4.11. Statistical Analysis

GraphPad prism was used to apply the statistical tests to the current data. Data were quantitative in nature and demonstrated in the form of the mean ± SD and analyzed using one-way ANOVA, as one factor (treatment regimen) was influencing the study groups. Bonferroni's test for multiple comparison analysis was at $p < 0.05$.

5. Conclusions

The topical application of ethosomal gel of metformin has a significant effect on treating chemically induced skin cancer in mice. This was shown by using the Box–Behnken design of "a three-level three-factor" to present a high percent of the EE%, minimum vesicle size, maximum ZP and high DR%.

Adding isopropyl alcohol with ethanol to form ethosomes increased the ability of ethanol to solubilize lecithin, which led to an increased stability and effectiveness of the ethosomes vesicles. Isopropyl alcohol also decreased the particle size of the vesicles, which increased the EE% and allowed the metformin to be released for an extended period. This is the goal of our research. Finally, a lower lecithin, high ethanol and isopropyl alcohol and moderate cholesterol obtained an enhancement of the permeation rate. Hence, the current findings may open up an avenue for future formulations for metformin as a therapeutic tool in fighting skin cancer.

Author Contributions: Conceptualization: O.M.S., T.M.H. and S.G.; Data Curation: I.A.M., T.M.H., S.G., S.A.Z., M.E.-S. and O.M.S.; Formal Analysis: I.A.M., S.A.Z. and O.M.S.; Software: I.A.M., T.M.H. and S.G.; Methodology: I.A.M. and O.M.S.; Resources: I.A.M. and O.M.S.; Validation: I.A.M. and O.M.S.; Visualization: T.M.H., S.G., S.A.Z., M.E.-S. and O.M.S.; Writing the Original Draft: I.A.M. and Writing, Review and Editing: T.M.H., S.G., S.A.Z., M.E.-S. and O.M.S. All authors have read and agreed to the published version of the manuscript.

Funding: This research was funded partly by the AlMaarefa University researchers supporting program, AlMaarefa University, Riyadh, Saudi Arabia, grant number MA-006.

Institutional Review Board Statement: The animal study protocol was approved by the Ethics Committee of Faculty of Pharmacy, Suez Canal University (protocol code 202004MA1 on 12 April 2020).

Informed Consent Statement: Not applicable.

Data Availability Statement: Data is contained within the article.

Acknowledgments: The authors are thankful to Medical Union Pharmaceuticals (Abu Sultan, Egypt) for kindly providing the metformin hydrochloride powder, and also, we thank Future Pharmaceutical Company for providing the carbopol 974p powder.

Conflicts of Interest: The authors declare no conflict of interest.

References

1. Neagu, M.; Caruntu, C.; Constantin, C.; Boda, D.; Zurac, S.; Spandidos, D.A.; Tsatsakis, A.M. Chemically induced skin carcinogenesis: Updates in experimental models (Review). *Oncol. Rep.* **2016**, *35*, 2516–2528. [CrossRef] [PubMed]
2. Jaune, E.; Rocchi, S. Metformin: Focus on melanoma. *Front. Endocrinol. (Lausanne)* **2018**, *9*, 472. [CrossRef] [PubMed]
3. Migden, M.R.; Chandra, S.; Rabinowits, G.; Chen, C.I.; Desai, J.; Seluzhytsky, A.; Sasane, M.; Campanelli, B.; Chen, Z.; Freeman, M.L.; et al. CASE (CemiplimAb-rwlc Survivorship and Epidemiology) study in advanced cutaneous squamous cell carcinoma. *Futur. Oncol.* **2020**, *16*, 11–19. [CrossRef] [PubMed]
4. Aplin, A.E.; Kaplan, F.M.; Shao, Y. Mechanisms of resistance to RAF inhibitors in melanoma. *J. Investig. Dermatol.* **2011**, *131*, 1817–1820. [CrossRef] [PubMed]
5. Brahmer, J.R.; Drake, C.G.; Wollner, I.; Powderly, J.D.; Picus, J.; Sharfman, W.H.; Stankevich, E.; Pons, A.; Salay, T.M.; McMiller, T.L.; et al. Phase I study of single-agent anti-programmed death-1 (MDX-1106) in refractory solid tumors: Safety, clinical activity, pharmacodynamics, and immunologic correlates. *J. Clin. Oncol.* **2010**, *28*, 3167–3175. [CrossRef]
6. Bridgeman, S.C.; Ellison, G.C.; Melton, P.E.; Newsholme, P.; Mamotte, C.D.S. Epigenetic effects of metformin: From molecular mechanisms to clinical implications. *Diabetes Obes. Metab.* **2018**, *20*, 1553–1562. [CrossRef]
7. Zeng, J.Y.; Sharma, S.; Zhou, Y.Q.; Yao, H.P.; Hu, X.; Zhang, R.; Wang, M.H. Synergistic activities of MET/RON inhibitor BMS-777607 and mTOR inhibitor AZD8055 to polyploid cells derived from pancreatic cancer and cancer stem cells. *Mol. Cancer Ther.* **2013**, *13*, 37–48. [CrossRef]
8. Karthik, G.M.; Ma, R.; Lövrot, J.; Kis, L.L.; Lindh, C.; Blomquist, L.; Fredriksson, I.; Bergh, J.; Hartman, J. mTOR inhibitors counteract tamoxifen-induced activation of breast cancer stem cells. *Cancer Lett.* **2015**, *367*, 76–87. [CrossRef]
9. Fu, Y.L.; Zhang, Q.H.; Wang, X.W.; He, H. Antidiabetic drug metformin mitigates ovarian cancer SKOV3 cell growth by triggering G2/M cell cycle arrest and inhibition of m-TOR/PI3K/Akt signaling pathway. *Eur. Rev. Med. Pharmacol. Sci.* **2017**, *21*, 1169–1175.
10. Mikhaylova, A.L.; Basharina, A.A.; Sorokin, D.V.; Buravchenko, G.I.; Samsonik, S.A.; Bogush, T.A.; Scherbakov, A.M. 48P Low glucose sensitizes A431 skin cancer cells to metformin treatments: A way forward to targeting PD-L1. *Ann. Oncol.* **2021**, *32*, S1360. [CrossRef]
11. Luo, Q.; Hu, D.; Hu, S.; Yan, M.; Sun, Z.; Chen, F. In vitro and in vivo anti-tumor effect of metformin as a novel therapeutic agent in human oral squamous cell carcinoma. *BMC Cancer* **2012**, *12*, 517. [CrossRef] [PubMed]
12. Tomic, T.; Botton, T.; Cerezo, M.; Robert, G.; Luciano, F.; Puissant, A.; Gounon, P.; Allegra, M.; Bertolotto, C.; Bereder, J.M.; et al. Metformin inhibits melanoma development through autophagy and apoptosis mechanisms. *Cell Death Dis.* **2011**, *2*, e199. [CrossRef] [PubMed]
13. Song, M.; Xia, W.; Tao, Z.; Zhu, B.; Zhang, W.; Liu, C.; Chen, S. Self-assembled polymeric nanocarrier-mediated co-delivery of metformin and doxorubicin for melanoma therapy. *Drug Deliv.* **2021**, *28*, 594–606. [CrossRef] [PubMed]
14. Adalsteinsson, J.A.; Muzumdar, S.; Waldman, R.; Wu, R.; Ratner, D.; Feng, H.; Ungar, J.; Silverberg, J.I.; Olafsdottir, G.H.; Kristjansson, A.K.; et al. Metformin is associated with decreased risk of basal cell carcinoma: A whole-population case-control study from Iceland. *J. Am. Acad. Dermatol.* **2021**, *85*, 56–61. [CrossRef] [PubMed]
15. Doan, H.Q.; Silapunt, S.; Migden, M.R. Sonidegib, a novel smoothened inhibitor for the treatment of advanced basal cell carcinoma. *Onco Targets Ther.* **2016**, *9*, 5671–5678. [CrossRef] [PubMed]
16. Song, Z.; Wei, B.; Lu, C.; Huang, X.; Li, P.; Chen, L. Metformin suppresses the expression of Sonic hedgehog in gastric cancer cells. *Mol. Med. Rep.* **2017**, *15*, 1909–1915. [CrossRef]

17. Niu, C.; Chen, Z.; Kim, K.T.; Sun, J.; Xue, M.; Chen, G.; Li, S.; Shen, Y.; Zhu, Z.; Wang, X.; et al. Metformin alleviates hyperglycemia-induced endothelial impairment by downregulating autophagy via the Hedgehog pathway. *Autophagy* **2019**, *15*, 843–870. [CrossRef]
18. Shurrab, N.T.; Arafa, E.S.A. Metformin: A review of its therapeutic efficacy and adverse effects. *Obes. Med.* **2020**, *17*, 100186. [CrossRef]
19. Ita, K. *Transdermal Drug Delivery: Concepts and Application*; Academic Press: Cambridge, MA, USA, 2020; ISBN 9780128225509.
20. Touitou, E.; Dayan, N.; Bergelson, L.; Godin, B.; Eliaz, M. Ethosomes-Novel vesicular carriers for enhanced delivery: Characterization and skin penetration properties. *J. Control. Release* **2000**, *65*, 403–418. [CrossRef]
21. Natsheh, H.; Touitou, E. Phospholipid vesicles for dermal/transdermal and nasal administration of active molecules: The effect of surfactants and alcohols on the fluidity of their lipid bilayers and penetration enhancement properties. *Molecules* **2020**, *25*, 2959. [CrossRef]
22. Ascenso, A.; Raposo, S.; Batista, C.; Cardoso, P.; Mendes, T.; Praça, F.G.; Bentley, M.V.L.B.; Simões, S. Development, characterization, and skin delivery studies of related ultradeformable vesicles: Transfersomes, ethosomes, and transethosomes. *Int. J. Nanomed.* **2015**, *10*, 5837–5851. [CrossRef] [PubMed]
23. Yang, L.; Wu, L.; Wu, D.; Shi, D.; Wang, T.; Zhu, X. Mechanism of transdermal permeation promotion of lipophilic drugs by ethosomes. *Int. J. Nanomed.* **2017**, *12*, 3357–3364. [CrossRef] [PubMed]
24. Zhu, X.; Li, F.; Peng, X.; Zeng, K. Formulation and evaluation of lidocaine base ethosomes for transdermal delivery. *Anesth. Analg.* **2013**, *117*, 352–357. [CrossRef] [PubMed]
25. Dave, V.; Kumar, D.; Lewis, S.; Paliwal, S. Ethosome for enhanced transdermal drug delivery of aceclofenac. *Int. J. Drug Deliv.* **2010**, *2*, 81–92. [CrossRef]
26. Guth, K.; Schäfer-Korting, M.; Fabian, E.; Landsiedel, R.; van Ravenzwaay, B. Suitability of skin integrity tests for dermal absorption studies in vitro. *Toxicol. Vitr.* **2015**, *29*, 113–123. [CrossRef] [PubMed]
27. Bouriche, S.; Alonso-García, A.; Cárceles-Rodríguez, C.M.; Rezgui, F.; Fernández-Varón, E. An in vivo pharmacokinetic study of metformin microparticles as an oral sustained release formulation in rabbits. *BMC Vet. Res.* **2021**, *17*, 315. [CrossRef]
28. Amr Gamal, F.; Kharshoum, R.M.; Sayed, O.M.; El-Ela, F.I.A.; Salem, H.F. Control of basal cell carcinoma via positively charged ethosomes of Vismodegib: In vitro and in vivo studies. *J. Drug Deliv. Sci. Technol.* **2020**, *56*, 101556. [CrossRef]
29. Goindi, S.; Dhatt, B.; Kaur, A. Ethosomes-based topical delivery system of antihistaminic drug for treatment of skin allergies. *J. Microencapsul.* **2014**, *31*, 716–724. [CrossRef]
30. Abdel Aziz, R.L.; Abdel-Wahab, A.; Abo El-Ela, F.I.; Hassan, N.E.H.Y.; El-Nahass, E.S.; Ibrahim, M.A.; Khalil, A.T.A.Y. Dose-dependent ameliorative effects of quercetin and L-Carnitine against atrazine- induced reproductive toxicity in adult male Albino rats. *Biomed. Pharmacother.* **2018**, *102*, 855–864. [CrossRef]
31. Salem, H.F.; Kharshoum, R.M.; El-Ela, F.I.A.; Gamal, A.F.; Abdellatif, K.R.A. Evaluation and optimization of pH-responsive niosomes as a carrier for efficient treatment of breast cancer. *Drug Deliv. Transl. Res.* **2018**, *8*, 633–644. [CrossRef]
32. Abdulbaqi, I.M.; Darwis, Y.; Khan, N.A.K.; Assi, R.A.; Khan, A.A. Ethosomal nanocarriers: The impact of constituents and formulation techniques on ethosomal properties, in vivo studies, and clinical trials. *Int. J. Nanomed.* **2016**, *11*, 2279–2304. [CrossRef] [PubMed]
33. Yang, F.; Kamiya, N.; Goto, M. Transdermal delivery of the anti-rheumatic agent methotrexate using a solid-in-oil nanocarrier. *Eur. J. Pharm. Biopharm.* **2012**, *82*, 158–163. [CrossRef] [PubMed]
34. Pathan, I.B.; Jaware, B.P.; Shelke, S.; Ambekar, W. Curcumin loaded ethosomes for transdermal application: Formulation, optimization, in-vitro and in-vivo study. *J. Drug Deliv. Sci. Technol.* **2018**, *44*, 49–57. [CrossRef]
35. Sandhiya, S.; Melvin, G.; Kumar, S.S.; Dkhar, S.A. The dawn of hedgehog inhibitors: Vismodegib. *J. Pharmacol. Pharmacother.* **2013**, *4*, 4–7. [CrossRef]
36. Limsuwan, T.; Amnuaikit, T. Development of Ethosomes Containing Mycophenolic Acid. *Procedia Chem.* **2012**, *4*, 328–335. [CrossRef]
37. Puri, R.; Jain, S. Ethogel topical formulation for increasing the local bioavailability of 5-fluorouracil: A mechanistic study. *Anticancer. Drugs* **2012**, *23*, 923–934. [CrossRef]
38. Ainbinder, D.; Godin, B.; Touitou, E. Ethosomes: Enhanced delivery of drugs to and across the skin. In *Percutaneous Penetration Enhancers Chemical Methods in Penetration Enhancement: Nanocarriers*; Springer: Berlin/Heidelberg, Germany, 2016; pp. 61–75. ISBN 9783662478622.
39. El-Menshawe, S.F.; Sayed, O.M.; Abou-Taleb, H.A.; El Tellawy, N. Skin permeation enhancement of nicotinamide through using fluidization and deformability of positively charged ethosomal vesicles: A new approach for treatment of atopic eczema. *J. Drug Deliv. Sci. Technol.* **2019**, *52*, 687–701. [CrossRef]
40. Vezočnik, V.; Rebolj, K.; Sitar, S.; Ota, K.; Tušek-Žnidarič, M.; Štrus, J.; Sepčić, K.; Pahovnik, D.; Maček, P.; Žagar, E. Size fractionation and size characterization of nanoemulsions of lipid droplets and large unilamellar lipid vesicles by asymmetric-flow field-flow fractionation/multi-angle light scattering and dynamic light scattering. *J. Chromatogr. A* **2015**, *1418*, 185–191. [CrossRef]
41. Zhang, Z.; Wo, Y.; Zhang, Y.; Wang, D.; He, R.; Chen, H.; Cui, D. In vitro study of ethosome penetration in human skin and hypertrophic scar tissue. *Nanomed. Nanotechnol. Biol. Med.* **2012**, *8*, 1026–1033. [CrossRef]
42. Umar, S. Development and Evaluation of Transdermal Gel of Lornoxicam. *Univers. J. Pharm. Res.* **2017**, *2*, 17–20. [CrossRef]

43. Verma, P.; Pathak, K. Nanosized ethanolic vesicles loaded with econazole nitrate for the treatment of deep fungal infections through topical gel formulation. *Nanomed. Nanotechnol. Biol. Med.* **2012**, *8*, 489–496. [CrossRef] [PubMed]
44. Chandra, A.; Aggarwal, G.; Manchanda, S.; Narula, A. Development of Topical Gel of Methotrexate Incorporated Ethosomes and Salicylic Acid for the Treatment of Psoriasis. *Pharm. Nanotechnol.* **2019**, *7*, 362–374. [CrossRef] [PubMed]
45. Elmoslemany, R.M.; Abdallah, O.Y.; El-Khordagui, L.K.; Khalafallah, N.M. Propylene glycol liposomes as a topical delivery system for miconazole nitrate: Comparison with conventional liposomes. *AAPS PharmSciTech* **2012**, *13*, 723–731. [CrossRef]
46. Florencia Martini, M.; Disalvo, E.A.; Pickholz, M. Nicotinamide and picolinamide in phospholipid monolayers. *Int. J. Quantum Chem.* **2012**, *112*, 3289–3295. [CrossRef]
47. Garg, B.J.; Garg, N.K.; Beg, S.; Singh, B.; Katare, O.P. Nanosized ethosomes-based hydrogel formulations of methoxsalen for enhanced topical delivery against vitiligo: Formulation optimization, in vitro evaluation and preclinical assessment. *J. Drug Target.* **2016**, *24*, 233–246. [CrossRef]
48. Chourasia, M.K.; Kang, L.; Chan, S.Y. Nanosized ethosomes bearing ketoprofen for improved transdermal delivery. *Results Pharma Sci.* **2011**, *1*, 60–67. [CrossRef]
49. Ahad, A.; Raish, M.; Al-Mohizea, A.M.; Al-Jenoobi, F.I.; Alam, M.A. Enhanced anti-inflammatory activity of carbopol loaded meloxicam nanoethosomes gel. *Int. J. Biol. Macromol.* **2014**, *67*, 99–104. [CrossRef]
50. Gamal, A.; Saeed, H.; Abo El-Ela, F.I.; Salem, H.F. Improving the antitumor activity and bioavailability of sonidegib for the treatment of skin cancer. *Pharmaceutics* **2021**, *13*, 1560. [CrossRef]
51. Shewaiter, M.A.; Hammady, T.M.; El-Gindy, A.; Hammadi, S.H.; Gad, S. Formulation and characterization of leflunomide/diclofenac sodium microemulsion base-gel for the transdermal treatment of inflammatory joint diseases. *J. Drug Deliv. Sci. Technol.* **2021**, *61*, 102110. [CrossRef]
52. Checkley, L.A.; Rho, O.; Angel, J.M.; Cho, J.; Blando, J.; Beltran, L.; Hursting, S.D.; DiGiovanni, J. Metformin inhibits skin tumor promotion in overweight and obese mice. *Cancer Prev. Res.* **2014**, *7*, 54–64. [CrossRef]
53. Lin, H.; Lin, L.; Choi, Y.; Michniak-Kohn, B. Development and in-vitro evaluation of co-loaded berberine chloride and evodiamine ethosomes for treatment of melanoma. *Int. J. Pharm.* **2020**, *581*, 119278. [CrossRef] [PubMed]
54. Nainwal, N.; Jawla, S.; Singh, R.; Saharan, V.A. Transdermal applications of ethosomes—A detailed review. *J. Liposome Res.* **2019**, *29*, 103–113. [CrossRef] [PubMed]
55. Journal, I.; Sciences, B.; Chappidi, S.R.; Education, P. Formulation and In Vitro evaluation of Liposomes containing Metformin Hydrochloride Formulation and In Vitro Evaluation of Liposomes Containing. *Int. J. Res. Pharm. Biomed. Sci.* **2016**, *4*, 479–485.
56. Gokhale, J.P.; Mahajan, H.S.; Surana, S.S. Quercetin loaded nanoemulsion-based gel for rheumatoid arthritis: In vivo and in vitro studies. *Biomed. Pharmacother.* **2019**, *112*, 108622. [CrossRef]
57. Olesen, U.H.; Clergeaud, G.; Lerche, C.M.; Andresen, T.L.; Haedersdal, M. Topical delivery of vismodegib using ablative fractional laser and micro-emulsion formulation in vitro. *Lasers Surg. Med.* **2019**, *51*, 79–87. [CrossRef]
58. Shen, L.N.; Zhang, Y.T.; Wang, Q.; Xu, L.; Feng, N.P. Enhanced in vitro and in vivo skin deposition of apigenin delivered using ethosomes. *Int. J. Pharm.* **2014**, *460*, 280–288. [CrossRef]
59. Salem, H.F.; Kharshoum, R.M.; Abou-Taleb, H.A.; AbouTaleb, H.A.; AbouElhassan, K.M. Progesterone-loaded nanosized transethosomes for vaginal permeation enhancement: Formulation, statistical optimization, and clinical evaluation in anovulatory polycystic ovary syndrome. *J. Liposome Res.* **2019**, *29*, 183–194. [CrossRef]
60. Bronaugh, R.L.; Stewart, R.F.; Simon, M. Methods for in vitro percutaneous absorption studies VII: Use of excised human skin. *J. Pharm. Sci.* **1986**, *75*, 1094–1097. [CrossRef]
61. Salem, H.F.; Kharshoum, R.M.; Sayed, O.M.; Abdel Hakim, L.F. Formulation design and optimization of novel soft glycerosomes for enhanced topical delivery of celecoxib and cupferron by Box–Behnken statistical design. *Drug Dev. Ind. Pharm.* **2018**, *44*, 1871–1884. [CrossRef]
62. Bhujbal, S.; Dash, A.K. Metformin-Loaded Hyaluronic Acid Nanostructure for Oral Delivery. *AAPS PharmSciTech* **2018**, *19*, 2543–2553. [CrossRef]
63. Dias, M.F.; de Figueiredo, B.C.P.; Teixeira-Neto, J.; Guerra, M.C.A.; Fialho, S.L.; Silva Cunha, A. In vivo evaluation of antitumoral and antiangiogenic effect of imiquimod-loaded polymeric nanoparticles. *Biomed. Pharmacother.* **2018**, *103*, 1107–1114. [CrossRef] [PubMed]
64. Praça, F.S.G.; Medina, W.S.G.; Eloy, J.O.; Petrilli, R.; Campos, P.M.; Ascenso, A.; Bentley, M.V.L.B. Evaluation of critical parameters for in vitro skin permeation and penetration studies using animal skin models. *Eur. J. Pharm. Sci.* **2018**, *111*, 121–132. [CrossRef] [PubMed]

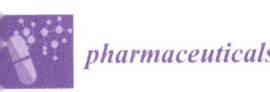

Article

Identification of Potential RBPJ-Specific Inhibitors for Blocking Notch Signaling in Breast Cancer Using a Drug Repurposing Strategy

Mengjie Rui, Min Cai, Yu Zhou, Wen Zhang, Lianglai Gao, Ke Mi, Wei Ji, Dan Wang and Chunlai Feng *

Department of Pharmaceutics, School of Pharmacy, Jiangsu University, Zhenjiang 212013, China; mjrui@ujs.edu.cn (M.R.); 2211915001@stmail.ujs.edu.cn (M.C.); 2221815020@stmail.ujs.edu.cn (Y.Z.); 2221915025@stmail.ujs.edu.cn (W.Z.); 2222015007@stmail.ujs.edu.cn (L.G.); 2212015010@stmail.ujs.edu.cn (K.M.); jinjian@ujs.edu.cn (W.J.); danwang@ujs.edu.cn (D.W.)
* Correspondence: feng@ujs.edu.cn

Abstract: Notch signaling is a key parameter in regulating cell fate during tissue homeostasis, and an aberrant Notch pathway can result in mammary gland carcinoma and has been associated with poor breast cancer diagnosis. Although inhibiting Notch signaling would be advantageous in the treatment of breast cancer, the currently available Notch inhibitors have a variety of side effects and their clinical trials have been discontinued. Thus, in search of a more effective and safer Notch inhibitor, inhibiting recombinant signal binding protein for immunoglobin kappaJ region (RBPJ) specifically makes sense, as RBPJ forms a transcriptional complex that activates Notch signaling. From our established database of more than 10,527 compounds, a drug repurposing strategy-combined docking study and molecular dynamic simulation were used to identify novel RBPJ-specific inhibitors. The compounds with the best performance were examined using an in vitro cellular assay and an in vivo anticancer investigation. Finally, an FDA-approved antibiotic, fidaxomicin, was identified as a potential RBPJ inhibitor, and its ability to block RBPJ-dependent transcription and thereby inhibit breast cancer growth was experimentally verified. Our study demonstrated that fidaxomicin suppressed Notch signaling and may be repurposed for the treatment of breast cancer.

Keywords: Notch signaling; RBPJ protein; drug repurposing; fidaxomicin; acarbose; schaftoside; breast cancer

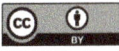

1. Introduction

The Notch signaling pathway is highly studied and is responsible for cellular communication and cell fate decision throughout a wide variety of developmental processes [1–3]. Notch signaling is initiated by ligand binding, followed by a series of cleavage events and the induced release of an intracellular domain (NICD). NICD then directly translocates into the cell nucleus and interacts with a transcription factor RBPJ (recombinant signal binding protein for immunoglobin kappaJ region) [4–6]. The resultant NICD/RBPJ complex further recruits transcriptional coactivators to activate the expression of Notch downstream target genes such as Hes1, Hes5, and Hey1 [7,8]. Aberrant activation of Notch signaling, which plays a critical role in cellular development, is linked to a number of diseases, including Alzheimer's disease, ischemic stroke, heart disease, and cancer [9–12]. Given its tumor-promoting role, selective inhibition of the Notch signaling pathway represents a valuable therapeutic target in cancer therapy.

A large number of Notch inhibitor candidates have been designed to inhibit γ-secretase, which mediates the cleavage of Notch receptors to liberate NICD. For example, a well-known small peptide inhibitor called DAPT {N-[N-(3,5-difluor-ophenacetyl)-l-alanyl]-S-phenylglycine tert-butyl ester} effectively inhibits the activity of γ-secretase (Supplementary Material Figure S1) [13]. These γ-secretase inhibitors developed in recent years have been found to cause a variety of toxic effects, including gastrointestinal bleeding, immunosuppression, cancerous skin lesions, and cognitive worsening in Alzheimer's Disease patients [14,15]. Therefore, more than half of the clinical trials of γ-secretase inhibitors have been halted [16,17]. Notch inhibitors should be further developed to avoid adverse effects, with an emphasis on increasing Notch selectivity. Another intriguing target in Notch signaling is the RBPJ protein, which is involved in both transcriptional activation and repression of Notch signaling [6,18]. Following its interaction with NICD and other coactivators, the activity of RBPJ shifts from repressing transcription to activating the transcription of Notch downstream genes. The rationale for developing an RBPJ inhibitor lies in the promise that disrupting the formation of the NICD–RBPJ–DNA complex provides a more specific means of modulating Notch function than γ-secretase inhibition.

The application of structure-based drug design in the search for novel RBPJ inhibitors benefits the translation of new drugs to the market. However, in spite of previous reports of novel RBPJ inhibitors [19,20], none has yet made significant progress clinically. RBPJ's structure indicates that it has various binding sites that are open for other molecules, including NICD, coactivators, and DNA [21–23]. As a result, small molecules are likely to occupy one of the RBPJ's binding sites to inhibit the formation of a transcriptional complex. It is theoretically possible to repurpose existing approved and investigational drugs as RBPJ inhibitors. Compared to de novo drug design, drug repurposing has numerous advantages: lower risk, reduced cost, and a shorter time to market [24–26].

In this study, we established a structure-based virtual screening strategy for identifying potential RBPJ-specific inhibitors from a database that collected compounds from a variety of sources. Following a molecular docking-based first-round screening, we performed molecular dynamic simulations to verify the hits and determine their binding free energies. Moreover, we experimentally demonstrated the inhibitory abilities of the selected compounds in vitro, as well as the anti-tumor efficacy in a tumor-bearing mice model.

2. Results

2.1. Strategic Overview of Drug Repurposing

For the first stage of drug repurposing, we used the crystal structure of NICD–MAML–RBPJ–DNA complex (PDB ID: 6PY8) to perform the RBPJ-based virtual screening. Crystal structure has revealed that RBPJ protein contains three domains: BTD (β-trefoil domain), NTD (the N-terminal domain), and CTD (the C-terminal domain) (Supplementary Material Figure S2). In this complex, the RBPJκ–associated module (RAM) domain of Notch intracellular domain (NICD) binds the BTD of RBPJ, showing that five residues (Val223, Phe221, Met243, Pro246, and Gln293) in BTD are important for the binding (Supplementary Material Table S1). Also, the Ankyrin repeat (ANK) domain of NICD binds the CTD of RBPJ, which identifies seven key residues of BTD (Gly350, Gln347, Leu348, Glu358, Glu385, Cys383, and Gly384). One transcriptional coactivator, MAML, interacts with the CTD-ANK interface and the NTD of RBPJ, revealing the key residues of RBPJ (Arg382, Arg378, Tyr381, Asn367, Arg369, Asn417, Lys130, Asp138, Phe88, Gly134, Ser136, Met98, and Cys86) (Supplementary Material Table S2). In light of the interaction between DNA and RBPJ, the crucial residues of RBPJ to maintain the interaction includes Lys44, Tyr46, Lys50, Arg51, Phe52, Ser151, Ser154, Gln158, Arg178, Arg180, Ser181, Gln182, and Lys271.

The virtual screening for RBPJ inhibitor was conducted using the docking module of MOE software(2020.09). We collected 10,527 compounds from various sources, including TCMSP, PubChem, DrugBank, and TOPSCIENCE Bioactive compound. Each compound in this collection was first subjected to blind docking, in which each one globally docked onto the entire surface of the RBPJ protein without any prior knowledge (PDB ID: 6PY8). 21 hits were selected from blind docking, and they exhibited docking scores less than −8 kcal/mol. These 21 molecules were further site-specifically docked into RBPJ based on the identified key amino acid residues of RBPJ. Three compounds, including fidaxomicin, schaftoside and acarbose, were identified to be the strongest RBPJ binder as they not only occupied the binding site strictly but also formed hydrogen bonds with multiple key RBPJ residues within the binding site (Figure 1). A positive control, RIN1 [19], was employed to further confirm the putative binding site of the RBPJ protein by molecule docking. The chemical structures of three hits and RIN1 were shown in Supplementary Material Figure S1. RIN1 has previously been shown to be capable of interrupting the formation of RBPJ-dependent transcriptional complex. The DNA-binding site of the RBPJ protein, as shown in Figure 1g,h, was also favored by RIN1, although only one molecule of RIN1 could not repel the DNA molecule from its binding site (Figure 1h). On the basis of the result of RIN1 docking investigation, it suggested that the selected three hits could potentially inhibit RBPJ-dependent transcription.

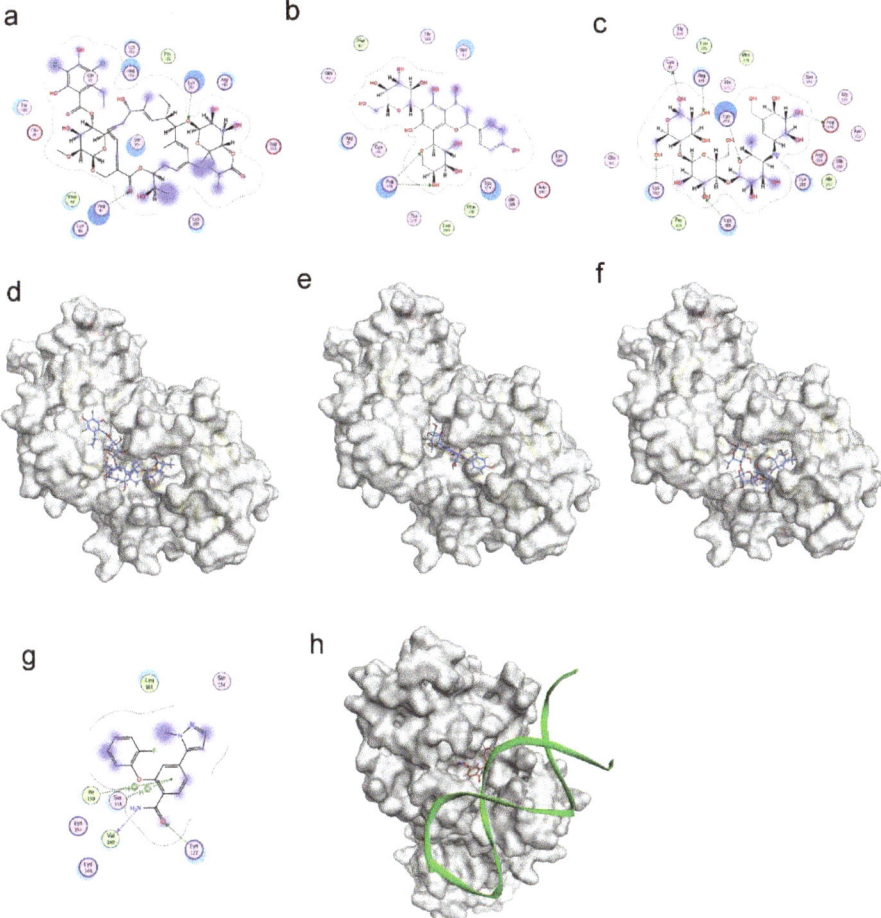

Figure 1. Molecular docking revealed binding modes of three hits and positive control with RBPJ protein by using MOE. Two-dimensional and three-dimensional docking poses of fidaxomicin (**a,d**), schaftoside (**b,e**), acarbose (**c,f**), and positive control RIN1 (**g,h**) at active sites of RBPJ were represented, respectively, showing the shape complementarity and the H-bonding with key contributing amino acids of RBPJ.

2.2. Evaluation of the Inhibitory Abilities of Three Selected Compounds

Following the screening results, we further investigated the potency of three hits to inhibit the formation of the NICD–MAML–RBPJ–DNA transcriptional complex. For each hit, docking was used to determine the maximum number of compound molecules that could simultaneously bind to the active site of RBPJ. The docking procedure began with the docking of a single molecule onto the RBPJ, resulting in the top scored pose in which the molecule bound to the active site. Then, using this resultant pose as the starting structure for the secondary round of docking, another molecule was docked onto this complex, yielding the top scored pose containing two molecules docked to the active site. This docking step was repeated several times until the nth input molecule was unable to bind to the RBPJ active site that was previously occupied by $n-1$ molecules. It is suggested that the more molecules bound to the active site, the more effective the compound would be at inhibiting the function of RBPJ. As shown in Figure 2a, three fidaxomicin molecules were positioned in such a way that all of them could simultaneously fit into the active site; this active site could hold up to four schaftoside (Figure 2b) or three acarbose molecules (Figure 2c).

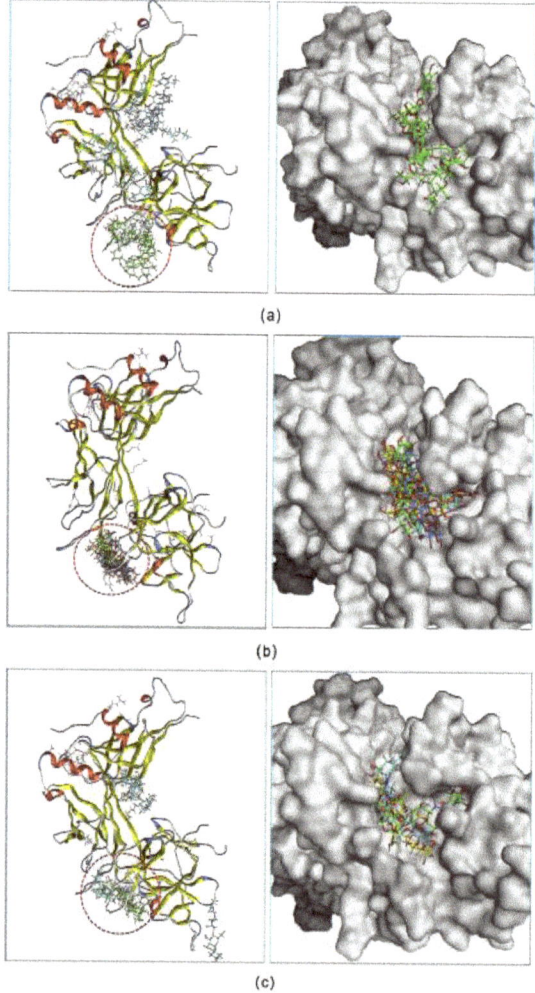

Figure 2. The inhibitory abilities of three hits were investigated in a docking experiment. Three fidaxomicin molecules (**a**), or four schaftoside molecules (**b**), or three acarbose molecules (**c**) could strictly occupy the active site of RBPJ that is indicated by a red dashed circle.

In addition, we investigated the DNA-competitive ability of each hit, which could further validate the potential of selected compounds as an RBPJ-specific inhibitor. To be specific, the obtained pose consisting of RBPJ and compounds was inputted as the docking receptor for the docking with the DNA molecule. As shown in Figure 3, the DNA molecule was pushed to dock onto other sites of RBPJ when various molecules of each hit occupied the active site, which confirmed the three hits to be DNA competitors and their ability to inhibit the formation of the NICD–MAML–RBPJ–DNA complex.

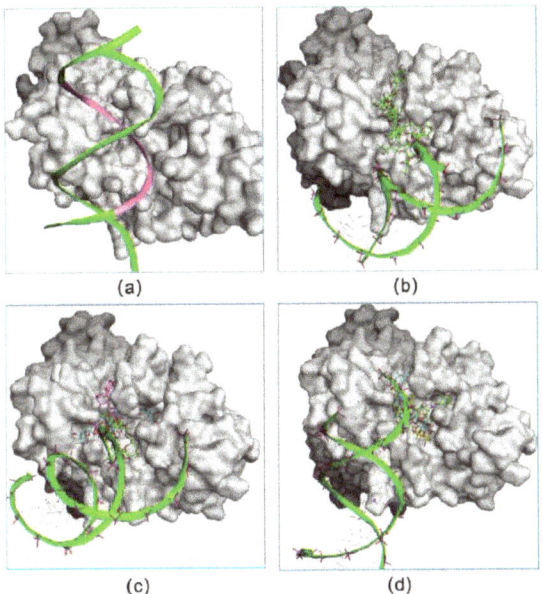

Figure 3. The verification on the abilities of small inhibitors to inhibit the formation of the NICD–MAML–RBPJ–DNA complex. The original DNA bound complex is shown (**a**). The occupancy of three fidaxomicin (**b**), four schaftoside (**c**) or three acarbose (**d**) molecules in the active site would inhibit the binding of DNA, indicating the DNA-competitive ability of the three hits.

2.3. Molecular Dynamic Simulations

At the second stage of drug repurposing, we further performed an all-atom molecular dynamic (MD) simulation to investigate the dynamic behavior of both selected hits and RBPJ and to assess their binding stability. The obtained poses consisting of each hit and RBPJ were subjected to 50 ns all-atom MD simulation. The stability profile of three hits in complex with RBPJ was examined by using their respective root mean square deviation (RMSD) values throughout all the simulation runs. As RMSD provides the degree of conformational variability of a protein, a ligand, or a ligand–protein complex, a high RMSD value for one ligand would indicate its incompatibility with the active site of the protein, as well as insufficient stability of the ligand–receptor complex across MD simulation timeframes. RMSD values for the Cα backbone of RBPJ and each compound were calculated and are shown in Figure 4. For the schaftoside–RBPJ complex, both RMSD curves of schaftoside and RBPJ exhibited relatively stable fluctuations with the fluctuation amplitude being less than 0.1 nm, suggesting that the MD simulations reached equilibrium after 10 ns and schaftoside bound tightly to the active site of RBPJ. Similarly, fidaxomicin and acarbose formed stable complexes with RBPJ because both systems were well equilibrated after 30 ns and yielded relatively steady RMSD values.

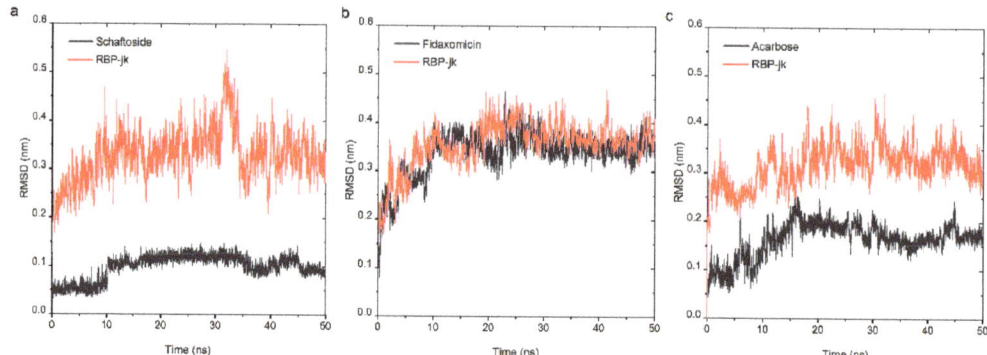

Figure 4. Analysis of RMSD trajectories for the complex of the RBPJ protein and selected hit throughout 50 ns all-atom MD simulation. RMSD plots for schaftoside (**a**), fidaxomicin (**b**), acarbose (**c**) in complex with RBPJ were illustrated, respectively. Each compound was shown in black and RBPJ protein shown in red. RMSD, root-mean-square deviation.

The MM-PBSA method was used to calculate the binding free energies of ligand-protein complex and to rank the binding affinity of three compounds [27–29]. The binding free energy in this method is decomposed into different components, including intermolecular van der Waals (ΔE_{vdW}), electrostatic interactions (ΔE_{elec}), non-polar solvation energy (ΔG_{np}), polar solvation free energy (ΔG_{pol}) and the configurational entropy ($-T\Delta S$). The components of the binding free energies of three complexes were listed in Table 1. The van der Waals (ΔE_{vdW}), electrostatic interactions (ΔE_{elec}) and non-polar solvation energy (ΔG_{np}) drove the complexation of each hit to RBPJ, while polar solvation free energy ($\Delta Gpol$) and the configurational entropy ($-T\Delta S$) worked against the binding. As shown, the calculated binding free energy of fidaxomicin was the lowest among the three, indicating that fidaxomicin could form the most stable complex with RBPJ. Schaftoside showed the second-ranked favorable binding energy. However, acarbose exhibited a positive binding free energy, which indicated an energetically unfavorable interaction between acarbose and the active site of RBPJ. Taken together, this finding further suggested fidaxomicin to be the strongest binder among the three.

Table 1. Energetic components of the binding energy for three hits in complex with RBPJ using MM-PBSA (kJ/mol).

Components	Fidaxomicin	Schaftoside	Acarbose
van der Waal energy (ΔE_{vdW})	−204.184	−182.001	−187.466
Electrostatic energy (ΔE_{elec})	−84.315	−106.519	−173.363
[a] ΔE_{MM}	−288.498	−288.52	−360.829
Polar solvation energy (ΔG_{pol})	141.176	210.695	307.811
Non-polar solvation energy (ΔG_{np})	−30.519	−24.261	−27.046
Configurational entropy ($-T\Delta S$)	101.286	58.367	126.046
Binding energy ([b] ΔG_{Bind})	−76.555	−43.72	45.982

Note: [a] $\Delta E_{MM} = \Delta E_{vdW} + \Delta E_{elec}$, [b] $\Delta G_{Bind} = \Delta E_{MM} + \Delta G_{pol} + \Delta G_{np} - T\Delta S$.

2.4. In Vitro Cytotoxicity Analysis and Intracellular Trafficking

Encouraged by the results of docking and molecular dynamic simulations, the inhibitory properties of three compounds were determined in different cell lines. As shown in Figure 5, fidaxomicin was active at micromolar concentrations to inhibit human breast cancer cell MCF-7 and mouse breast cancer cell 4T1, with IC$_{50}$ values of 53.4 and 32.3 µM, respectively. In comparison, schaftoside and acarbose did not exhibit significant antitumor effects against MCF-7 and 4T1 across the concentration range that was investigated

(Figure 5). Collectively, the anti-tumor efficacy of fidaxomicin was evidently superior to that of other two screened compounds in vitro.

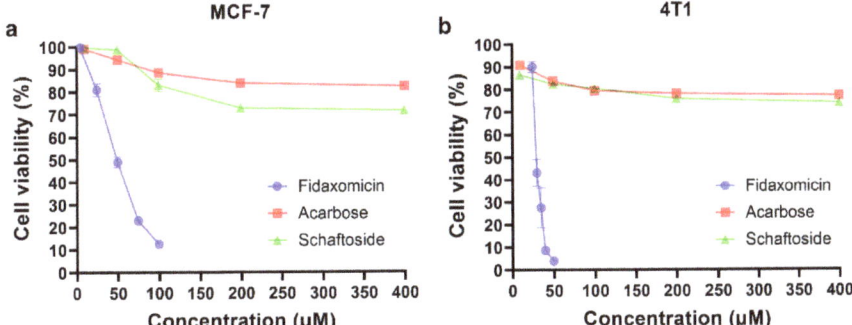

Figure 5. In vitro cytotoxicity analysis. (**a**) Cytotoxicity test in human breast cancer MCF-7 cells. (**b**) Cytotoxicity test in mouse breast cancer 4T1 cells. The cells were incubated with various concentrations of fidaxomicin, acarbose, or schaftoside for 48 h, and the viability of cells was examined by CCK-8 assay ($n = 5$ samples per group).

Next, to ensure that the anti-tumor ability of fidaxomicin resulted from inhibiting the formation of the transcriptional complex, effective internalization by tumor cells and intracellular nucleus targeting were of great importance. Here, CLSM was used to investigate the subcellular localization of fidaxomicin in 4T1 cells (Figure 6). The relatively weak fluorescence signal (green) of fidaxomicin was observed in the nuclei (red) of 4T1 cells after 0.5 h incubation, and enhanced fluorescence of fidaxomicin could be detected after 2 h and 4 h incubation, indicating that the fluorescence intensity of fidaxomicin in cell nuclei exhibited a time-dependent increase. These results confirmed that fidaxomicin was effectively taken up by 4T1 cells and then distributed into the cell nuclei. Furthermore, due to the nuclear location of the RBPJ protein, the intracellular trafficking behavior of fidaxomicin implied that this compound might inhibit the formation of the RBPJ complex, hence blocking the Notch signal pathway and eventually exerting the potential anti-tumor ability.

2.5. In Vitro Evaluation of RBPJ-Specific Inhibition

The ability of fidaxomicin to disrupt the interaction between NOTCH, RBPJ, and DNA was further confirmed by quantitative real-time PCR (qRT-PCR) analysis. The gene encoding Notch receptor Notch1 and Notch downstream target genes, including Hes1, Hes5, and Hey1 in 4T1 cells after incubation with fidaxomicin for 24 h and 48 h were analyzed (Figure 7). As a result, the 24-h treatment of fidaxomicin significantly repressed the amounts of Notch1, Hes1, Hes5, and Hey1 mRNAs. We observed that the expression of Hes1 was the most significantly repressed, and the repression of Notch1 and Hes1 responded to fidaxomicin treatment in a time-dependent manner. The decreases of Hes5 and Hey1 mRNA were less prominent than those of the other two genes, and they did not show a further decrease after 48 h incubation of fidaxomicin.

Additionally, the protein levels of Notch downstream targets Hes1 and Hes5 were analyzed by western blotting. Despite the decrease in mRNA levels, fidaxomicin did not appear to affect the expression of Hes1 and Hes5 proteins in 4T1 cells during the first 24-h incubation, as shown in Figure 8. However, following 48-h incubation with fidaxomicin, the protein levels of Hes1 and Hes5 were significantly reduced, which was consistent with the mRNA alterations in both genes after the same treatment. Combined with in vitro cytotoxicity and qRT-PCR results, these findings implied that fidaxomicin might effectively block the formation of the RBPJ-dependent transcriptional complex, leading to the inhibitory ability on Notch signaling and resulting in anti-tumor activity.

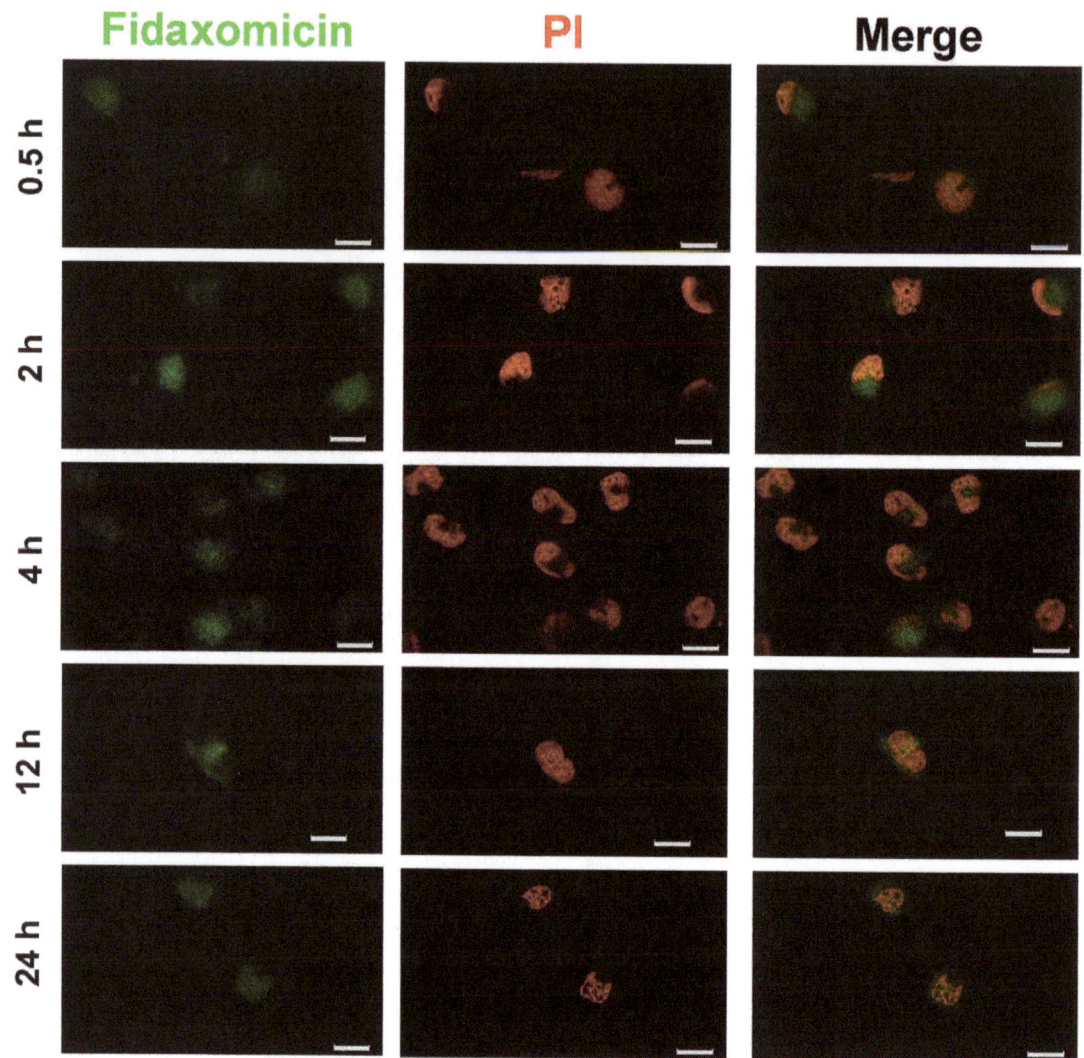

Figure 6. Cellular internalization of fidaxomicin in 4T1 cells. The confocal fluorescence images of 4T1 cells were obtained after incubation with fidaxomicin for 0.5, 2, 4, 12, and 24 h. Scale bar: 20 μm.

2.6. Antitumor Efficacy

Based on the in vitro cytotoxicity and the responses of inhibiting the Notch signaling, the antitumor efficacy of fidaxomicin in 4T1-tumor-bearing mice was then evaluated. When the average tumor volume reached about 100 mm^3, mice were treated with different groups of drugs by intratumoral administration every other day for three weeks, including 5, 25, and 50 mg/kg fidaxomicin, 25 mg/kg DAPT, 25 mg/kg 5-fluorouracil, and saline as a negative control. As shown in Figure 9a,b, the tumor volume of the saline group increased rapidly and reached 3000 mm^3 on the 28th day after the implantation.

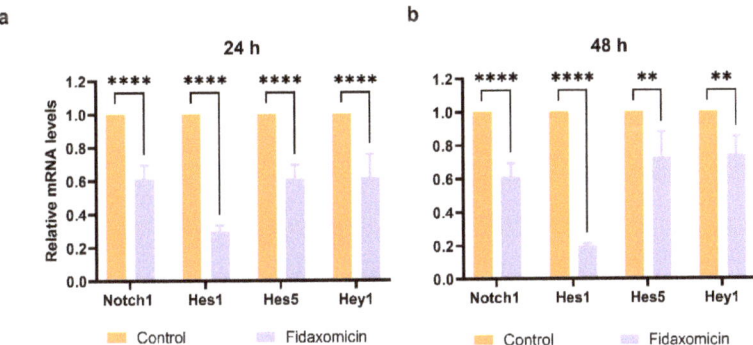

Figure 7. The mRNA levels of Notch target genes in 4T1 cells after incubation with fidaxomicin for a variety of times. (**a**) The results of a 24 h incubation with fidaxomicin; (**b**) the results of a 48 h incubation with fidaxomicin. qRT-PCR analysis revealed that the incubation of fidaxomicin significantly reduced the mRNA levels of Notch1, as well as Notch target genes Hes1, Hes5, and Hey1. Data shown represent the mean ± SD of triplicate experiments (** $p < 0.01$, and **** $p < 0.0001$ vs. control group).

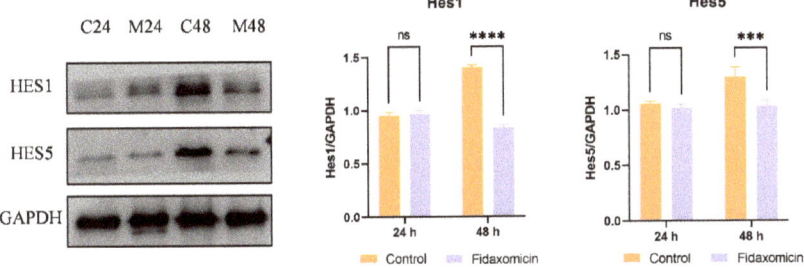

Figure 8. Western blot analysis of protein levels of Notch target molecules in 4T1 cells. C24 and C48 denote the protein levels in untreated 4T1 cells after culture for 24 h and 48 h, respectively. M24 and M48 indicate the protein levels in cells after fidaxomicin treatment for 24 h and 48 h, respectively. After incubation, whole-cell extracts were subjected to immunoblot analysis and incubated with antibodies to Hes1, Hes5, and GAPDH as a control. Data shown represent the mean ± SD of triplicate experiments (*** $p < 0.001$, and **** $p < 0.0001$ vs. control group, ns: no significance).

The growth curves of tumors revealed that the order of the inhibitory ability on tumor growth was fidaxomicin (50 mg/kg) > 5-fluorouracil (25 mg/kg) > fidaxomicin (25 mg/kg) > DAPT (25 mg/kg) > fidaxomicin (5 mg/kg) (Figure 9b). The low dose of fidaxomicin (5 mg/kg) exhibited a moderate tumor inhibition compared with the saline group. When the dose of fidaxomicin was further increased, stronger inhibitions were observed. As a result, fidaxomicin demonstrated potent anti-cancer activity, yielding 62.56% and 83.19% inhibitory efficacies on the growth of tumors at 25 and 25 mg/kg, respectively (Figure 9c). In comparison, DAPT, a well-known Notch inhibitor that inhibits the activity of gamma-secretase, exhibited an inhibition rate of 56.42% at a concentration of 25 mg/kg, whereas 5-fluorouracil, another extensively used chemotherapeutic drug, showed a better inhibition rate of 75.66% at the same dosage. The average tumor weight of mice treated with fidaxomicin was significantly lower than that of mice treated with DAPT or 5-fluorouracil at a dose of 25 mg/kg, indicating the greatest anti-tumor ability among the three treatment groups. In addition, there was no noticeable body weight change or obvious abnormalities in the three fidaxomicin groups, indicating that fidaxomicin was tolerable up to 50 mg/kg when administered 12 times (Figure 9d).

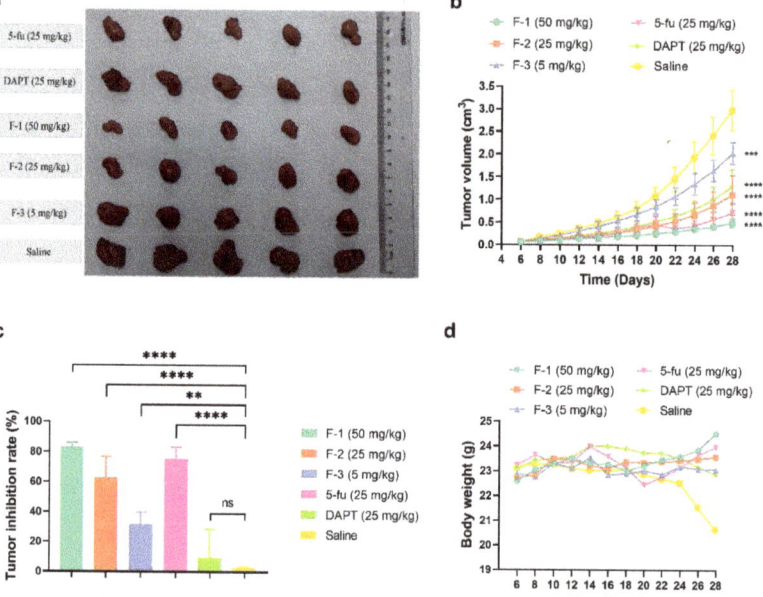

Figure 9. The in vivo antitumor effects of fidaxomicin in 4T1 tumor-bearing mice. (**a**) The photograph of tumors excised from sacrificed mice. (**b**) Tumor growth curve, (**c**) tumor inhibition rate, and (**d**) body weight profile were demonstrated after different treatments. Data shown represent the mean ± SD ($n = 5$, ** $p < 0.01$, *** $p < 0.001$, and **** $p < 0.0001$ vs. control group, ns: no significance).

We further verified the relationship between the in vivo anti-tumor efficacy of fidaxomicin and the inhibition of Notch signaling in 4T1 tumor-bearing mice. As shown in Figure 10, the protein levels of Hes5 were significantly reduced in the tumor grafts of mice treated with fidaxomicin in a dose-dependent manner in comparison with the saline control groups. The high dose of fidaxomicin could reduce the expression of Hes5 by 65.7%, implying that the anti-tumor activity of fidaxomicin was correlated with its possible inhibitory ability in Notch signaling. The positive control DAPT also reduced the expression of Hes5 at a dose of 25 mg/kg, showing that DAPT exerted its ability to block Notch signaling through the γ-secretase inhibitor.

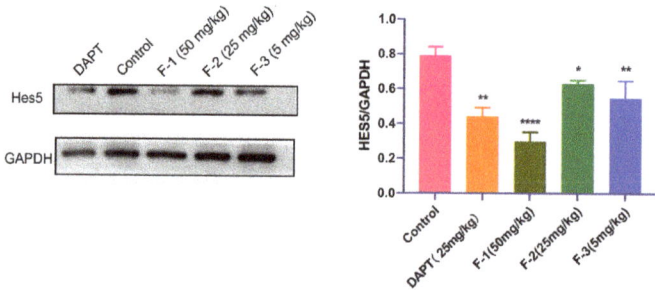

Figure 10. Relationship between in vivo anti-tumor activity of fidaxomicin and the inhibition in Notch signaling in 4T1 tumors. Western blot analysis of protein levels of Notch targets Hes5 in 4T1 tumors was performed after administration with saline, DAPT (25 mg/kg), fidaxomicin (50 mg/kg), fidaxomicin (25 mg/kg), and fidaxomicin (5 mg/kg). Data shown represent the mean ± SD of triplicate experiments (* $p < 0.05$, ** $p < 0.01$, and **** $p < 0.0001$ vs. control group).

3. Discussion

In this study, we demonstrated that fidaxomicin was identified as a potential small molecule inhibitor of RBPJ, eventually inhibiting Notch signaling in breast cancer cells. Since the Notch signal pathway regulates the differentiation of breast epithelial cells during normal development, aberrant Notch signaling, as seen by increased NICD release and target gene overexpression, is positively correlated with poor patient prognosis, such as aggressive, metastatic triple negative breast cancer (TNBC) and therapy resistance [30–32]. In light of these findings, the inhibition of overactive Notch signaling would be facilitated in the treatment of breast cancer. Regarding the function of RBPJ, the RBPJ–NICD–DNA complex induces transcription of Notch target genes including various Hairy/Enhancer of Split-related genes (Hes1, Hes5, and Hey1) [18,33]. In recent years, the involvement of these Hes/Hey canonical Notch target genes in breast cancer initiation and progression has been recognized. For example, Hes1, a basic helix–loop–helix (bHLH) transcriptional repressor, is an important direct RBPJ-dependent Notch target gene. The proliferation and invasion of TNBC cells were boosted by the overexpression of Hes1, while on the contrary, this effect was substantially abolished by silencing Hes1 gene expression [34]. Therefore, compared with GSIs, suppressing RBPJ-dependent gene transcription would confer advantages including direct mediation on Notch signaling as well as reduced side effects.

The drug repurposing strategy in this study was a combination of molecular docking and dynamic simulation. Molecular docking is a well-established method for screening potential compounds based on their complementarity with the target's binding site. We started by building a database of FDA-approved drugs, synthetic compounds, and natural extracts to be used in the initial screening study. The fact that RBPJ interacts with multiple components, including NICD, certain coactivators, and DNA, led us to first investigate the binding mode between each component and the RBPJ, identifying the possible binding sites and the key residues in these binding sites. After evaluating the docking scores of all compounds, 21 compounds with high docking scores were selected to dock onto the binding sites of RBPJ. Interestingly, we found that three hits preferred the sites where large molecule DNA binds rather than other coactivators and NICD, which suggested that the DNA binding site could be a possible target for the design of RBPJ inhibitors. To further prove that the three hits could effectively compete with DNA for RBPJ binding sites, we used docking to demonstrate how more than two molecules could fully occupy the DNA-binding site, causing DNA to weakly interact with the remaining sites. Based on these docking results, we were able to identify novel roles for the three hits as potential RBPJ-specific inhibitors.

Among the three hits, fidaxomicin is a first-in-class macrocyclic antibiotic for the treatment of *Clostridium difficile* infection. Regarding its mechanism of action, fidaxomicin primarily inhibits bacterial RNA polymerase at an early step in the transcription initiation stage. Specifically, fidaxomicin binds to the σ subunit of bacterial RNA polymerase, preventing the initial separation of DNA strands [35,36]. Other than the treatment of Gram-positive bacteria, fidaxomicin has not been found to be effective in any other application. In this study, we identified a novel role of fidaxomicin as a potential anti-tumor candidate. We further investigated the binding site for fidaxomicin by superimposing the complex docked with fidaxomicin over the RBPJ-dependent transcriptional complex. Interestingly, we discovered that the pocket of RBPJ that was occupied by fidaxomicin was open for DNA binding, whereas fidaxomicin had no effect on the interaction between RBPJ and NICD or other coactivators. As a result, the RBPJ transcriptional complex would not be formed, eventually inhibiting the expression of Notch downstream target genes. Another hit, acarbose, is an α-glucosidase inhibitor and is used to manage glycemic control in patients with type 2 diabetes mellitus [37,38]. As an oligosaccharide, acarbose inhibits the activities of several enzymes responsible for the hydrolysis of complex carbohydrates in the small intestines. The third hit schaftoside was a flavonoid that has been found in Chinese medicinal herbs. Previous studies have revealed that schaftoside has a variety of pharmacological activities, including anti-inflammatory [39,40], anti-melanogenic [41], anti-stress, and antioxidant capacities [39,42,43]. In light of the blind docking results, acarbose and schaftoside preferred to dock onto the DNA-binding pocket of RBPJ, which was also observed in top-ranked poses of a fidaxomicin–RBPJ complex. These docking poses implied that the two other hits would inhibit the formation of the RBPJ-related transcriptional complex in a similar manner to fidaxomicin.

Further docking experiments revealed that the highest number of molecules that could occupy the active site of RBPJ was three for fidaxomicin, four for schaftoside, and three for acarbose. Next, to investigate whether the compounds were DNA competitors, we studied the behavior of the selected compounds when DNA were docked to the pose of the RBPJ-selected compound complex. This result indicated that any of the three selected compounds could strictly occupy the DNA-binding site of RBPJ, thus causing DNA to interact weakly with another site of RBPJ. Taken together, our virtual screening and docking experiments revealed that the three identified compounds were potential RBPJ-specific inhibitors, interacting with the DNA-binding site of RBPJ and eventually exerting inhibitory ability on the expression of Notch target genes.

At the second stage of our drug repurposing strategy, dynamic simulation was employed to further refine the docking results by analyzing the binding properties of each identified compound, such as the binding free energy. Here we selected the molecular mechanism/Poisson–Boltzmann surface area (MM-PBSA) approach to obtain the binding free energy of each hit-RBPJ complex. However, although the computational cost of MM-PBSA is far lower than that of other approaches, which is a significant advantage, this method suffers from a higher number of computational errors and lower accuracy compared with other methods [44–46]. As a result, we used this approach to rank the binding free energies of the three hits in order to determine which one might be the most promising RBPJ inhibitor. The MM–PBSA results revealed that fidaxomicin performed the best, showing the lowest binding free energy of −76.555 kJ/mol. The binding free energy of schaftoside was −43.72 kJ/mol, which was ranked second. Surprisingly, acarbose revealed a positive binding free energy, which was not suitable for the interaction between acarbose and RBPJ. Because acarbose is a water-soluble oligosaccharide, its physicochemical properties might make it difficult to access the DNA-binding site of RBPJ, resulting in an unfavorable binding free energy. In addition, docking scores are assessed mainly based on the shape complementarity between candidate and target receptor, rather than the binding behavior of the candidate in a real situation with a given salt concentration, so the discrepancy between the docking experiment and dynamic simulation might be explained.

To validate the results of our drug repurposing, the anti-tumor activities of three hits were determined by cellular viability assay. Among them, fidaxomicin exhibited a potent anti-tumor effect against two breast cancer cell lines, with IC_{50} values in a micromolar range. When incubated with either the human breast cancer cell line MCF-7 or mouse breast cancer cell line 4T1 for 48 h, schaftoside was found to have negligible toxicity for both cell lines at concentrations up to 400 µM. Another hit, acarbose, showed poor anti-tumor effect against two cell lines, similar to that of schaftoside. Among the three hits, only fidaxomicin had the lowest IC50 values, i.e., 53.4 µM for MCF-7 and 32.3 µM for 4T1. Regarding the poor anti-tumor performance of schaftoside and acarbose, both compounds might not have good permeability that largely depends on their lipophilicity, molecular weight, and polarity [47]. For example, acarbose is a complex oligosaccharide and is soluble in aqueous solution [48], so it might not be able to penetrate across cellular membranes and subsequent nucleus membranes. Therefore, although the three hits could theoretically inhibit the formation of the RBPJ-dependent transcriptional complex, schaftoside and acarbose might not passively diffuse into the cell nucleus; on the contrary, fidaxomicin was proved to be distributed in the cell nucleus after incubation for 2 h by using CLSM, which met the requirement for the RBPJ-specific interaction. Further studies would be conducted to determine the cause of the poor performance of schaftoside and acarbose, and the application of appropriate delivery systems could help these compounds distribute to the nucleus, where they could then exert inhibitory effects on Notch signaling.

To establish whether fidaxomicin inhibits RBPJ in cells, the expressions of Notch target genes at the level of transcription and translation were assessed after compound treatment by using qRT-PCR and western blotting, respectively. Figure 7 summarized the results of qRT-PCR when 4T1 cells were incubated with fidaxomicin for either 24 h or 48 h. The reduced levels of Notch target genes, including Hes1, Hes5, and Hey1, were detected after fidaxomicin treatment, indicating that the RBPJ-mediated transcription was inhibited in cells. The protein levels of Notch targets Hes1 and Hes5 were significantly reduced after 48 h incubation of fidaxomicin, further confirming the fidaxomicin-induced inhibition of Notch signaling. Notably, the expressions of the two proteins were not significantly altered during the first 24 h incubation of fidaxomicin, which might be due to their functions. The Hes1 protein contains both DNA-binding and protein–protein interaction domains responsible for its role as a transcriptional regulator, which negatively regulates its own transcription [49,50]. Therefore, the already-existing Hes1 protein would still exert its activity and regulate the expression during the first 24-h incubation, resulting in a marginally declined protein level; when fidaxomicin exposure was extended to 24 h to 48 h, a significantly lower level of the Hes1 protein was observed. Hes5 is another transcriptional regulator, and the treatment with fidaxomicin caused a similar change in the level of the Hes5 protein to that observed with Hes1 level. This result could be explained by the fact that Hes5 has been reported to negatively control its transcription in neurogenesis and hepatocarcinogenesis [51–54]. Collectively, these results demonstrated that fidaxomicin might act as a potential RBPJ-specific inhibitor and effectively block Notch signaling.

Fidaxomicin's potential to inhibit the growth of 4T1 tumors was further demonstrated in a 22-day in vivo anticancer experiment. At the highest dose of 50 mg/kg, this compound was able to reduce tumor volume by 83.19%, and it also had a modest anti-tumor impact at a dose of 5 mg/kg, resulting in a decrease in tumor volume of 31.77%. To assess the anti-tumor potential, we used positive controls including a commonly used GSI (DAPT) and an established chemotherapeutic agent (5-fluorouracil). As a result, at a dose of 25 mg/kg, fidaxomicin had a better anti-tumor effect (62.56%) than DAPT (56.42%). On the other hand, fidaxomicin was not as effective against 4T1 tumor as 5-fluorouracil, which showed a reduction in tumor volume of 75.66% when given at the same dose.

The mechanism of action of fidaxomicin against tumors was elucidated by measuring Hes5 protein levels in tumor tissues. Since the levels of the Hes5 protein decreased more slowly than that of Hes1 in in vitro cellular studies, the changes in the Hes5 levels may better reflect the inhibitory effect of fidaxomicin on RBPJ-mediated transcription. In accordance with in vitro results, the levels of Hes5 proteins in tumor tissues were considerably decreased after mice received various doses of fidaxomicin, suggesting a possible RBPJ-dependent inhibitory mechanism of action. These findings matched the in vitro cellular assay results, indicating that the in vitro cytotoxicity was well translated into in vivo activity.

One limitation of our study is that we did not have the appropriate cell- or animal-based models to regulate the activity of the RBPJ protein at the time of our study, which would have allowed us to directly examine the inhibitory ability of selected hits on RBPJ function. Based on our findings, fidaxomicin has been proposed as a potential RBPJ-dependent inhibitor. However, further work is required to verify the binding mode of fidaxomicin with RBPJ as well as the precise mechanism of action. Another limitation of our study is that we did not investigate the phenotypes that were responsible for Notch signaling, such as the development of splenic marginal zone B (MZB) cells, thymic T cell development, generation of Esam$^+$ dendritic cells, sprouting of endothelial cells, and induction of goblet cell differentiation in the small intestine. CB-103 [20], a small molecule Notch inhibitor, was previously shown to reduce these phenotypes when administered orally. Although fidaxomicin in this study was injected intratumorally in this study, which might not have resulted in these phenotypes, we plan to leverage the potential systemic delivery of fidaxomicin and address this limitation in the future research.

In contrast to the widely used GSIs, our results suggested a promising future for the application of fidaxomicin. In spite of the fact that fidaxomicin is not as potent as currently available drugs, it represents a promising starting point for the development of a potential RBPJ-specific inhibitor, which might be further improved by using in silico design cycles.

4. Materials and Methods

4.1. Structure Preparation of the Screening Library

We built a virtual chemical library, a collection of 10,527 pharmacologically active compounds, by integrating four publicly available databases: (1) the DrugBank database (https://go.drugbank.com/, accessed on 1 June 2020); (2) the PubMed database (https://pubchem.ncbi.nlm.nih.go, accessed on 1 June 2020); (3) Traditional Chinese Medicine Systems Pharmacology (TCMSP) database (https://tcmspw.com/tcmsp.php, accessed on 1 June 2020) [55]; and (4) TOPSCIENCE Bioactive compound library (https://www.tsbiochem.com/ accessed on 1 June 2020). This library covered the major classes of compound candidates, including FDA-approved drugs, investigational new drugs, preclinical compounds, drug-like chemicals, and natural products with immunomodulating effects. The 3D structures of all these compounds were prepared, and in turn minimized using default parameters through Molecular Operating Environment (MOE 2019) software in terms of geometry and energy.

The three-dimensional crystal structure of the RBPJ–NOTCH1–NRARP ternary complex was downloaded from the Protein Data Bank (PDB) (PDB ID: 6PY8) and used as the target for the screening within this study. Next, we analyzed potential sites for the binding of ligand and DNA molecules to the RBPJ protein and restriction sets for rendering partial molecular surfaces, showing possible docking sites on the RBPJ protein. In turn, we removed all solvent molecules, ligands (NOTCH1 and NRARP) and DNA from the complex and refined the RBPJ protein by adding hydrogen atoms, filling in missing side chains and loops, and assigning hydrogen bonds through the Protein-Structure Preparation module of MOE 2019. The structure of RBPJ was then subjected to energy minimization using MOE with default parameters as mentioned above.

4.2. Docking Procedure

4.2.1. Blind Docking Studies to Screen Candidates

Molecular docking between RBPJ protein and each compound in the virtual screening library was performed using the docking module of MOE. A three-stage docking procedure was conducted to identify a potential Notch inhibitor. During the first stage, blind docking was employed to quickly dock the entire target surface with multiple binding sites.

The docking procedure at the first stage was applied for screening the significant candidates from the library. Briefly, selections of "Receptor" and "Ligand" in the MOE Dock module were assigned to corresponding structures, where "Site" was assigned to "All atom", which meant that each candidate was globally docked onto the RBPJ structure without any specified binding site, namely, blind docking. For each test compound, 100 different poses were generated and scored according to the default London dG scoring function, and in turn the best 10 poses were selected. During the screening, values of additional parameters remained unchanged. To select the potential candidate, the retention value was set as the binding energy less than −8 kcal/mol, and the location of the binding site was nearby the active binding sites.

Clustering of the generated poses was conducted to achieve the largest cluster, and in turn, each compound in the best possible cluster was evaluated on the basis of docking scores less than −8 kcal/mol, binding mode within the RBPJ active site, and molecular interactions with the key residues of the RBPJ. After completion of this stage of the docking process, 21 hits were selected.

4.2.2. Restricted Active Site Docking

The docking study at the second stage was a more directed screening which was carried out with the 21 obtained hits. Unlike the previous "blind docking", the docking search at this stage focused on the key residues of RBPJ that were involved in the interactions between the RBPJ protein and NICD or DNA. In addition to the docking score that should be less than −8 kcal/mol, the tested compound that could interact with more than three key residues of RBPJ and occupy a large binding space was retained for the next stage of the investigation. According to these screening criteria, three compounds were finally selected.

4.2.3. DNA-Competitive Docking Studies

To further verify the potent Notch-inhibiting ability of the obtained hits, a third-stage advanced docking study was performed. In this docking search, we examined the highest possible number of each tested compound that could simultaneously bind to the same active site of RBPJ. The docking parameters were as same as in blind docking that used in the first stage, but the receptor structure was different. In detail, one molecule, in the first blind docking cycle, bound to the target binding site and formed a complex, the best conformation of which was chosen as the receptor structure for the next blind docking cycle; as a result, a new complex containing an increasing number of tested compounds was generated in each blind docking cycle. Until an input compound could not stably bind to the active site of the complex from the previous cycle, the docking study finally came to an end. This docking study resulted in a top-ranked pose of the complex consisting of one RBPJ and several compound molecules. Clearly, the higher the number of compound molecules that occupied the active site of RBPJ, the stronger the ability of this compound to inhibit the Notch activity.

Next, to investigate the capacity of the selected compound to inhibit the formation of the RBPJ-dependent transcriptional complex, we carried out the DNA-competitive docking experiment. Briefly, the obtained pose of the complex, which contained one RBPJ and the maximum number of selected compound molecules, was used as receptor structure, and the DNA molecule was inputted in this round to dock onto the complex. Then, we studied the position of the DNA in the obtained pose, showing whether the selected compound could effectively occupy the DNA-binding site of RBPJ.

After completion of the three-stage docking study, the identified compounds were further evaluated by molecular dynamic simulations.

4.3. Molecular Dynamics (MD) Simulations

4.3.1. MD Simulation Procedure

The most promising compounds, fidaxomicin, schaftoside, and acarbose, in complex with the RBPJ protein were further evaluated using all-atom MD simulations, which were performed with the GROMACS software package (Version 2021.1, Royal Institute of Technology and Uppsala University, Sweden) using the AMBER99SB-ILDN forcefield parameter set. The topologies of three compounds in the GROMACS format were generated by the ACPYPE tool [56], where General Amber Force Field (GAFF) was used. For the MD simulation, the amber99SB-ILDN force field was used to parameterize the RBPJ protein. The complex consisting of the ligand and RBPJ protein was placed in a dodecahedron box, which was solvated with the TIP3P water model with a 10 angstrom padding region. Na^+ ions were added to neutralize the system. Energy minimization of the solvated system was performed by using the steepest descent method. After minimization, a series of equilibrium MD simulations were performed: 200 ps of NVT and 1 ns of NPT. The time step of the MD simulation was set to 2 fs with the LINCS algorithm to constraint hydrogen-connected covalent bonds [57]. The long-range electrostatic interaction was calculated by the fast smooth particle-mesh Ewald (PME) electrostatics method [58,59]. At each step, v-rescale temperature coupling and Parrinello–Rahman pressure coupling were applied to maintain the system at 300 K. Lastly, MD simulations were conducted for 50 ns with a time step of 2 fs.

4.3.2. Molecular Mechanics–Poisson Boltzmann Surface Area (MM-PBSA) Analysis

The binding free energies of the three hits were calculated with MM–PBSA analysis. We utilized the gmx_mmpbsa tool (https://github.com/Jerkwin/gmxtool/tree/master/gmx_mmpbsa, accessed on 10 August 2020) to analyze the binding free energy between each ligand and the RBPJ protein based on the trajectories obtained with GROMACS. For the dynamic trajectory of 50 ns, 50 frames were extracted at a time interval of 1000 ps and subsequently selected as input for MM–PBSA calculations. During the calculations, the binding free energy between ligand and RBPJ protein was decomposed into several terms: the gas-phase interaction energy (ΔE_{MM}), non-polar solvation energy (ΔG_{np}), polar solvation free energy (ΔG_{pol}), and the conformational entropy ($-T\Delta S$). ΔE_{MM} generally contains coulomb electrostatic energy (ΔE_{elec}) and van der Waals energy (ΔE_{vdW}).

4.4. Cell Culture

The mouse breast cancer 4T1 cell line and human breast cancer MCF-7 cell line were purchased from the Type Culture Collection of the Chinese Academy of Sciences (Shanghai, China). The 4T1 cells were cultured in RPMI-1640 medium supplemented with 10% fetal bovine serum (FBS) and 1% penicillin/streptomycin, and the MCF-7 cells were cultured in DMEM supplemented with 10% FBS and 1% penicillin/streptomycin.

4.5. In Vitro Anticancer Activity

The 4T1 and MCf-7 cells were seeded in 96-well plates (5000 cells/well) in 5% CO_2 at 37 °C and cultured for 24 h. Then, the cells were incubated with fresh media containing either fidaxomicin, schaftoside, or acarbose at various concentrations for 48 h. After further incubation with fresh media containing Cell Counting Kit-8 (CCK-8) solution for 2 h, the absorbance of each well was determined at 450 nm by a microplate reader.

4.6. Studies on the Mechanism of Anti-Tumor Action of Fidaxomicin

4.6.1. Cellular Uptake and Intracellular Localization

The 4T1 cells were seeded in 15 mm confocal microscope dishes (2×10^4 cells/dish) and incubated for one day. The stock fidaxomicin solution (53 mM) was diluted with complete RPMI-1640 medium to prepare working solutions (53 μM). The cells were incubated with working solutions for 0.5, 2, 4, 12, and 24 h. After incubation, cells were washed with PBS buffer and further fixed by using paraformaldehyde. Then, nuclei of all cells were stained with propidium iodide (PI) for about 10 min at 37 °C. Eventually, the dye solution was descanted, followed by washing three times with PBS and mounted with an anti-fluorescence quenching sealant.

The cells were then observed using a confocal laser scanning microscope (TCS SP5 II, Leica, Wetzlar, Germany). For fidaxomicin, the excitation wavelength was 351 nm, and the emission wavelength was 450 nm. For PI, the excitation wavelength was 488 nm, and the emission wavelength was 620 nm.

4.6.2. Quantitative Real-Time PCR (qRT-PCR)

Cultured 4T1 cells were treated with fidaxomicin at a concentration of 32.3 μM for 24 h and 48 h. After washing with PBS buffer, total RNA was extracted from cells by using an RNA-Quick Purification Kit (ES-RN001, YiShan Biotech, Shanghai, China) and reverse-transcribed using a Fast All-in-One RT Kit (ES-RT001, YiShan Biotech, Shanghai, China). Quantitative PCR for mRNA was performed using qPCR Master Mix (ES-QP002, YiShan, Shanghai, China) according to the manufacturer's protocol. The expression of mRNA was normalized to GAPDH. The primer sequences used in qRT-PCR are listed in Supplementary Material Table S3.

4.6.3. Western Blot Assay

Cultured 4T1 cells were treated with fidaxomicin as mentioned above. After washing with PBS buffer, total cell extracts were prepared by using a Cell Total Protein Extraction

Kit (Sangon Biotech, Shanghai, China) according to the manufacturer's protocol. Protein concentration was measured by using a BCA kit. Each sample containing 2 mg/mL protein was separated by using sodium dodecyl sulfate–polyacrylamide gel electrophoresis (SDS–PAGE) and transferred onto a PVDF membrane, which was incubated overnight at 4 °C with primary antibodies. The primary antibodies used were rabbit anti mouse Hes1 (11988; Cell Signalling Technology, Danvers, MA, USA), rabbit anti mouse Hes5 (EPR15578; Abcam, Cambridge, UK), and rabbit anti mouse GAPDH (AF7021; Affinity Biosciences, Cincinnati, OH, USA). The membranes were next incubated with secondary antibodies (Goat Anti-Rabbit IgG (H + L) HRP, S0001; Affinity Biosciences) at room temperature for 2 h. According to the western blot chemiluminescence detection method, protein bands on the membrane were observed by using a chemiluminescent imaging system.

4.7. In Vivo Anti-Tumor Activity

Eight-week-old female BALB/c mice were purchased from the laboratory animal center of Jiangsu University. Animal studies were conducted under the guidelines of an approved protocol from the Institutional Animal Care and Use Committee at Jiangsu University (Protocol ID: 2021031202). To establish the tumor-bearing mouse model, 0.2 mL of 4T1 cell suspensions (2×10^7 cells/mL) was inoculated to the mammary fat pad of BALB/c mice. When the tumor volume reached approximately 50–100 mm^3, tumor-bearing mice were randomly assigned to six groups of five mice each. Fidaxomicin, DAPT, and 5-fluorouracil were first dissolved in DMSO as stock solutions and then administered after dilution with saline to achieve a final concentration of DMSO of less than 0.5%. Mice were treated with fidaxomicin-1 (50 mg/kg), fidaxomicin-2 (25 mg/kg), fidaxomicin-3 (5 mg/kg), DAPT (25 mg/kg), 5-Fluorouracil (25 mg/kg), and saline. Each formulation was injected intratumorally every other day. The anti-tumor efficiency was evaluated by monitoring the tumor volume. The tumor sizes were measured on two vertical axes using a caliper every other day and calculated as (width^2 × length)/2. After 24 days, mice were sacrificed, and tumor tissues were excised and weighted.

The expressions of the Hes5 protein in tumor grafts were examined using Western blot assay. Total cell extracts were also prepared using a Cell Total Protein Extraction Kit (Sangon Biotech, Shanghai, China), as mentioned in the above Western blot method. The primary and secondary antibodies involved were the same as those used in the previous Western blot assay.

5. Conclusions

In summary, we identified fidaxomicin as a potential RBPJ-specific inhibitor through the use of a drug repurposing strategy. The antitumor activity of fidaxomicin was evaluated both in vitro and in vivo. It was shown that fidaxomicin could effectively inhibit the growth of two different breast cancer cell lines at micromolar concentrations. Furthermore, the administration of fidaxomicin resulted in a practical tumor inhibition in 4T1 tumor-bearing mice. Regarding the possible mechanism of action, the treatment of fidaxomicin lowered the expression of Notch downstream target genes at both transcriptional and translational levels, showing that fidaxomicin might potentially inhibit the formation of the RBPJ-dependent transcriptional complex. These results suggest that fidaxomicin might have potential for the treatment of RBPJ-dependent cancers. Additionally, this study represented an important step towards the repurposing of this FDA-approved drug for the treatment of breast cancer.

Supplementary Materials: The following supporting information can be downloaded at: https://www.mdpi.com/article/10.3390/ph15050556/s1, Figure S1: The chemical structures of compounds used in this study; Figure S2: Schematic diagram of the interaction between Notch, MAML, DNA, and RBPJ; Table S1: Interactions between human transcription factor RBPJ and NICD; Table S2: Interactions between human transcription factor RBPJ and coactivator MAML; Table S3: Primer sequence.

Author Contributions: Conceptualization, M.R. and C.F.; methodology, Y.Z., M.C. and W.Z.; investigation, Y.Z., M.C., L.G. and K.M.; validation, D.W. and W.J.; writing-original draft preparation, Y.Z.; writing-review and editing, M.R., D.W. and C.F.; visualization, M.R., Y.Z. and D.W.; supervision, M.R. and C.F.; project administration, M.R.; funding acquisition, M.R. and C.F. All authors have read and agreed to the published version of the manuscript.

Funding: This work was supported, in part, by the National Natural Science Foundation of China (No. 82074286), Natural Science Foundation of Jiangsu Province (Nos. BK20191428, BK20181445), Six Talent Peak Project from Government of Jiangsu Province (No. SWYY-013), the Science and Technology Innovation Fund of Zhenjiang-International Cooperation Projects (GJ2021012), Natural Science Foundation of the Higher Education Institutions of Jiangsu Province (21KJB350023), and Jiangsu University Foundation (20JDG075).

Institutional Review Board Statement: The animal study protocol was approved by the Ethics Committee of Animal Experimentation of Jiangsu University with ethics approval clearance certificate no.2021031202.

Informed Consent Statement: Not applicable.

Data Availability Statement: Data are contained within the article.

Conflicts of Interest: The authors declare no conflict of interest. The funders had no role in the design of the study; in the collection, analyses, or interpretation of data; in the writing of the manuscript, or in the decision to publish the results.

References

1. Yuan, X.; Wu, H.; Xu, H.; Xiong, H.; Chu, Q.; Yu, S.; Wu, G.S.; Wu, K. Notch signaling: An emerging therapeutic target for cancer treatment. *Cancer Lett.* **2015**, *369*, 20–27. [CrossRef] [PubMed]
2. Aster, J.C.; Pear, W.S.; Blacklow, S.C. The Varied Roles of Notch in Cancer. *Annu. Rev. Pathol. Mech. Dis.* **2017**, *12*, 245–275.
3. Misiorek, J.O.; Przybyszewska-Podstawka, A.; Kalafut, J.; Paziewska, B.; Rolle, K.; Rivero-Muller, A.; Nees, M. Context Matters: NOTCH Signatures and Pathway in Cancer Progression and Metastasis. *Cells* **2021**, *10*, 94. [CrossRef] [PubMed]
4. Borggrefe, T.; Oswald, F. The Notch signaling pathway: Transcriptional regulation at Notch target genes. *Cell. Mol. Life Sci.* **2009**, *66*, 1631–1646. [CrossRef] [PubMed]
5. Kopan, R.; Ilagan, M.X.G. The canonical Notch signaling pathway: Unfolding the activation mechanism. *Cell* **2009**, *137*, 216–233. [CrossRef] [PubMed]
6. Castel, D.; Mourikis, P.; Bartels, S.J.J.; Brinkman, A.B.; Tajbakhsh, S.; Stunnenberg, H.G. Dynamic binding of RBPJ is determined by Notch signaling status. *Genes Dev.* **2013**, *27*, 1059–1071. [CrossRef]
7. Bolós, V.; Grego-Bessa, J.n.; de la Pompa, J.L. Notch Signaling in Development and Cancer. *Endocr. Rev.* **2007**, *28*, 339–363. [CrossRef]
8. Guiu, J.; Shimizu, R.; D'Altri, T.; Fraser, S.T.; Hatakeyama, J.; Bresnick, E.H.; Kageyama, R.; Dzierzak, E.; Yamamoto, M.; Espinosa, L. Hes repressors are essential regulators of hematopoietic stem cell development downstream of Notch signaling. *J. Exp. Med.* **2013**, *210*, 71–84. [CrossRef]
9. Siebel, C.; Lendahl, U. Notch Signaling In Development, Tissue Homeostasis, And Disease. *Physiol. Rev.* **2017**, *97*, 1235–1294. [CrossRef]
10. Sanchez-Vega, F.; Mina, M.; Armenia, J.; Chatila, W.K.; Luna, A.; La, K.C.; Dimitriadoy, S.; Liu, D.L.; Kantheti, H.S.; Saghafinia, S.; et al. Oncogenic Signaling Pathways in The Cancer Genome Atlas. *Cell* **2018**, *173*, 321–337.e310. [CrossRef]
11. Louvi, A.; Artavanis-Tsakonas, S. Notch and disease: A growing field. *Semin. Cell Dev. Biol.* **2012**, *23*, 473–480. [CrossRef]
12. Janghorban, M.; Xin, L.; Rosen, J.M.; Zhang, X.H.-F. Notch signaling as a regulator of the tumor immune response: To target or not to target? *Front. Immunol.* **2018**, *9*, 1649. [CrossRef] [PubMed]
13. Dovey, H.; John, V.; Anderson, J.; Chen, L.; de Saint Andrieu, P.; Fang, L.; Freedman, S.; Folmer, B.; Goldbach, E.; Holsztynska, E. Functional gamma-secretase inhibitors reduce beta-amyloid peptide levels in brain. *J. Neurochem.* **2001**, *76*, 173–181. [CrossRef] [PubMed]
14. Imbimbo, B.P.; Giardina, G.A.M. γ-secretase inhibitors and modulators for the treatment of Alzheimer's disease: Disappointments and hopes. *Curr. Top. Med. Chem.* **2011**, *11*, 1555–1570. [CrossRef] [PubMed]
15. Li, T.; Wen, H.; Brayton, C.; Das, P.; Smithson, L.A.; Fauq, A.; Fan, X.; Crain, B.J.; Price, D.L.; Golde, T.E.; et al. Epidermal growth factor receptor and notch pathways participate in the tumor suppressor function of gamma-secretase. *J. Biol. Chem.* **2007**, *282*, 32264–32273. [CrossRef]
16. Jia, H.; Wang, Z.; Zhang, J.; Feng, F. gamma-Secretase inhibitors for breast cancer and hepatocellular carcinoma: From mechanism to treatment. *Life Sci.* **2021**, *268*, 119007. [CrossRef]
17. De Strooper, B. Lessons from a failed gamma-secretase Alzheimer trial. *Cell* **2014**, *159*, 721–726. [CrossRef]
18. Bray, S.J. Notch signalling in context. *Nat. Rev. Mol. Cell Biol.* **2016**, *17*, 722–735. [CrossRef]

19. Hurtado, C.; Safarova, A.; Smith, M.; Chung, R.; Bruyneel, A.A.N.; Gomez-Galeno, J.; Oswald, F.; Larson, C.J.; Cashman, J.R.; Ruiz-Lozano, P.; et al. Disruption of NOTCH signaling by a small molecule inhibitor of the transcription factor RBPJ. *Sci. Rep.* **2019**, *9*, 10811. [CrossRef]
20. Lehal, R.; Zaric, J.; Vigolo, M.; Urech, C.; Frismantas, V.; Zangger, N.; Cao, L.; Berger, A.; Chicote, I.; Loubery, S.; et al. Pharmacological disruption of the Notch transcription factor complex. *Proc. Natl. Acad. Sci. USA* **2020**, *117*, 16292–16301. [CrossRef]
21. Nam, Y.; Weng, A.P.; Aster, J.C.; Blacklow, S.C. Structural requirements for assembly of the CSL·intracellular Notch1·Mastermind-like 1 transcriptional activation complex. *J. Biol. Chem.* **2003**, *278*, 21232–21239. [CrossRef]
22. Collins, K.J.; Yuan, Z.; Kovall, R.A. Structure and function of the CSL-KyoT2 corepressor complex: A negative regulator of Notch signaling. *Structure* **2014**, *22*, 70–81. [CrossRef] [PubMed]
23. Yuan, Z.; VanderWielen, B.D.; Giaimo, B.D.; Pan, L.; Collins, C.E.; Turkiewicz, A.; Hein, K.; Oswald, F.; Borggrefe, T.; Kovall, R.A. Structural and functional studies of the RBPJ-SHARP complex reveal a conserved corepressor binding site. *Cell Rep.* **2019**, *26*, 845–854.e846. [CrossRef] [PubMed]
24. Pushpakom, S.; Iorio, F.; Eyers, P.A.; Escott, K.J.; Hopper, S.; Wells, A.; Doig, A.; Guilliams, T.; Latimer, J.; McNamee, C. Drug repurposing: Progress, challenges and recommendations. *Nat. Rev. Drug Discov.* **2019**, *18*, 41–58. [CrossRef] [PubMed]
25. Ng, Y.L.; Salim, C.K.; Chu, J.J.H. Drug repurposing for COVID-19: Approaches, challenges and promising candidates. *Pharmacol. Ther.* **2021**, *228*, 107930. [CrossRef]
26. Kumar, R.; Harilal, S.; Gupta, S.V.; Jose, J.; Uddin, M.S.; Shah, M.A.; Mathew, B. Exploring the new horizons of drug repurposing: A vital tool for turning hard work into smart work. *Eur. J. Med. Chem.* **2019**, *182*, 111602. [CrossRef] [PubMed]
27. Genheden, S.; Ryde, U. The MM/PBSA and MM/GBSA methods to estimate ligand-binding affinities. *Expert Opin. Drug Discov.* **2015**, *10*, 449–461. [CrossRef]
28. Wang, E.; Sun, H.; Wang, J.; Wang, Z.; Liu, H.; Zhang, J.Z.; Hou, T. End-point binding free energy calculation with MM/PBSA and MM/GBSA: Strategies and applications in drug design. *Chem. Rev.* **2019**, *119*, 9478–9508. [CrossRef]
29. Poli, G.; Granchi, C.; Rizzolio, F.; Tuccinardi, T. Application of MM-PBSA methods in virtual screening. *Molecules* **2020**, *25*, 1971. [CrossRef]
30. Zhong, Y.; Shen, S.; Zhou, Y.; Mao, F.; Lin, Y.; Guan, J.; Xu, Y.; Zhang, S.; Liu, X.; Sun, Q. NOTCH1 is a poor prognostic factor for breast cancer and is associated with breast cancer stem cells. *OncoTargets Ther.* **2016**, *9*, 6865. [CrossRef]
31. Giuli, M.V.; Giuliani, E.; Screpanti, I.; Bellavia, D.; Checquolo, S. Notch Signaling Activation as a Hallmark for Triple-Negative Breast Cancer Subtype. *J. Oncol.* **2019**, *2019*, 8707053. [CrossRef]
32. Bolos, V.; Mira, E.; Martinez-Poveda, B.; Luxan, G.; Canamero, M.; Martinez, A.C.; Manes, S.; de la Pompa, J.L. Notch activation stimulates migration of breast cancer cells and promotes tumor growth. *Breast Cancer Res.* **2013**, *15*, R54. [CrossRef]
33. Contreras-Cornejo, H.; Saucedo-Correa, G.; Oviedo-Boyso, J.; Valdez-Alarcon, J.J.; Baizabal-Aguirre, V.M.; Cajero-Juarez, M.; Bravo-Patino, A. The CSL proteins, versatile transcription factors and context dependent corepressors of the notch signaling pathway. *Cell Div.* **2016**, *11*, 12. [CrossRef] [PubMed]
34. Li, X.; Cao, Y.; Li, M.; Jin, F. Upregulation of HES1 Promotes Cell Proliferation and Invasion in Breast Cancer as a Prognosis Marker and Therapy Target via the AKT Pathway and EMT Process. *J. Cancer* **2018**, *9*, 757–766. [CrossRef] [PubMed]
35. Zhanel, G.G.; Walkty, A.J.; Karlowsky, J.A. Fidaxomicin: A novel agent for the treatment of Clostridium difficile infection. *Can. J. Infect. Dis. Med. Microbiol.* **2015**, *26*, 305–312. [CrossRef] [PubMed]
36. Johnson, A.P.; Wilcox, M.H. Fidaxomicin: A new option for the treatment of Clostridium difficile infection. *J. Antimicrob. Chemother.* **2012**, *67*, 2788–2792. [CrossRef]
37. Laube, H. Acarbose. *Clin. Drug Investig.* **2002**, *22*, 141–156. [CrossRef]
38. Bischoff, B. Pharmacology of α-glucosidase inhibition. *Eur. J. Clin. Investig.* **1994**, *24*, 3–10. [CrossRef]
39. Liu, M.; Zhang, J.; Song, M.; Wang, J.; Shen, C.; Chen, Z.; Huang, X.; Gao, Y.; Zhu, C.; Lin, C.; et al. Activation of Farnesoid X Receptor by Schaftoside Ameliorates Acetaminophen-Induced Hepatotoxicity by Modulating Oxidative Stress and Inflammation. *Antioxid. Redox Signal.* **2020**, *33*, 87–116. [CrossRef]
40. De Melo, G.O.; Muzitano, M.F.; Legora-Machado, A.; Almeida, T.A.; De Oliveira, D.B.; Kaiser, C.R.; Koatz, V.L.; Costa, S.S. C-glycosylflavones from the aerial parts of Eleusine indica inhibit LPS-induced mouse lung inflammation. *Planta Med.* **2005**, *71*, 362–363. [CrossRef]
41. Kim, P.S.; Shin, J.H.; Jo, D.S.; Shin, D.W.; Choi, D.H.; Kim, W.J.; Park, K.; Kim, J.K.; Joo, C.G.; Lee, J.S.; et al. Anti-melanogenic activity of schaftoside in Rhizoma Arisaematis by increasing autophagy in B16F1 cells. *Biochem. Biophys. Res. Commun.* **2018**, *503*, 309–315. [CrossRef]
42. Kinjo, Y.; Takahashi, M.; Hirose, N.; Mizu, M.; Hou, D.X.; Wada, K. Anti-stress and Antioxidant Effects of Non Centrifuged Cane Sugar, Kokuto, in Restraint-Stressed Mice. *J. Oleo Sci.* **2019**, *68*, 183–191. [CrossRef] [PubMed]
43. Dang, J.; Paudel, Y.N.; Yang, X.; Ren, Q.; Zhang, S.; Ji, X.; Liu, K.; Jin, M. Schaftoside Suppresses Pentylenetetrazol-Induced Seizures in Zebrafish via Suppressing Apoptosis, Modulating Inflammation, and Oxidative Stress. *ACS Chem. Neurosci.* **2021**, *12*, 2542–2552. [CrossRef] [PubMed]
44. Sun, H.; Li, Y.; Tian, S.; Xu, L.; Hou, T. Assessing the performance of MM/PBSA and MM/GBSA methods. 4. Accuracies of MM/PBSA and MM/GBSA methodologies evaluated by various simulation protocols using PDBbind data set. *Phys. Chem. Chem. Phys.* **2014**, *16*, 16719–16729. [CrossRef] [PubMed]

45. Srivastava, H.K.; Sastry, G.N. Molecular dynamics investigation on a series of HIV protease inhibitors: Assessing the performance of MM-PBSA and MM-GBSA approaches. *J. Chem. Inf. Model.* **2012**, *52*, 3088–3098. [CrossRef]
46. Byun, J.; Lee, J. Identifying the Hot Spot Residues of the SARS-CoV-2 Main Protease Using MM-PBSA and Multiple Force Fields. *Life* **2022**, *12*, 54. [CrossRef]
47. Brandl, M.; Eide Flaten, G.; Bauer-Brandl, A. Passive Diffusion Across Membranes. In *Wiley Encyclopedia of Chemical Biology*; Wiley: Hoboken, NJ, USA, 2008; pp. 1–10.
48. PubChem Compound Summary for CID 444254, Acarbose. Available online: https://pubchem.ncbi.nlm.nih.gov/compound/Acarbose (accessed on 10 March 2022).
49. Iso, T.; Kedes, L.; Hamamori, Y. HES and HERP families: Multiple effectors of the Notch signaling pathway. *J. Cell. Physiol.* **2003**, *194*, 237–255. [CrossRef]
50. Coglievina, M.; Guarnaccia, C.; Pintar, A.; Pongor, S. Different degrees of structural order in distinct regions of the transcriptional repressor HES-1. *Biochim. Biophys. Acta* **2010**, *1804*, 2153–2161. [CrossRef]
51. Fior, R.; Henrique, D. A novel hes5/hes6 circuitry of negative regulation controls Notch activity during neurogenesis. *Dev. Biol.* **2005**, *281*, 318–333. [CrossRef]
52. Ivanov, D. Notch Signaling-Induced Oscillatory Gene Expression May Drive Neurogenesis in the Developing Retina. *Front. Mol. Neurosci.* **2019**, *12*, 226. [CrossRef]
53. Luiken, S.; Fraas, A.; Bieg, M.; Sugiyanto, R.; Goeppert, B.; Singer, S.; Ploeger, C.; Warsow, G.; Marquardt, J.U.; Sticht, C.; et al. NOTCH target gene HES5 mediates oncogenic and tumor suppressive functions in hepatocarcinogenesis. *Oncogene* **2020**, *39*, 3128–3144. [CrossRef]
54. King, I.N.; Kathiriya, I.S.; Murakami, M.; Nakagawa, M.; Gardner, K.A.; Srivastava, D.; Nakagawa, O. Hrt and Hes negatively regulate Notch signaling through interactions with RBP-Jκ. *Biochem. Biophys. Res. Commun.* **2006**, *345*, 446–452. [CrossRef] [PubMed]
55. Ru, J.; Li, P.; Wang, J.; Zhou, W.; Li, B.; Huang, C.; Li, P.; Guo, Z.; Tao, W.; Yang, Y.; et al. TCMSP: A database of systems pharmacology for drug discovery from herbal medicines. *J. Cheminform.* **2014**, *6*, 13. [CrossRef] [PubMed]
56. Sousa da Silva, A.W.; Vranken, W.F. ACPYPE—AnteChamber PYthon Parser interfacE. *BMC Res. Notes* **2012**, *5*, 367. [CrossRef] [PubMed]
57. Hess, B.; Bekker, H.; Berendsen, H.J.C.; Fraaije, J.G.E.M. LINCS: A linear constraint solver for molecular simulations. *J. Comput. Chem.* **1997**, *18*, 1463–1472. [CrossRef]
58. Darden, T.; York, D.; Pedersen, L. Particle mesh Ewald: An N·log(N) method for Ewald sums in large systems. *J. Chem. Phys.* **1993**, *98*, 10089–10092. [CrossRef]
59. Essmann, U.; Perera, L.; Berkowitz, M.L.; Darden, T.; Lee, H.; Pedersen, L.G. A smooth particle mesh Ewald method. *J. Chem. Phys.* **1995**, *103*, 8577–8593. [CrossRef]

Article

Adenosine Conjugated Docetaxel Nanoparticles—Proof of Concept Studies for Non-Small Cell Lung Cancer

Hibah M. Aldawsari [1,2,*], Sima Singh [3], Nabil A. Alhakamy [1,2], Rana B. Bakhaidar [1], Abdulrahman A. Halwani [1], Nagaraja Sreeharsha [4,5,*] and Shaimaa M. Badr-Eldin [1,2]

1. Department of Pharmaceutics, Faculty of Pharmacy, King Abdulaziz University, Jeddah 21589, Saudi Arabia; nalhakamy@kau.edu.sa (N.A.A.); rbakhaidar@kau.edu.sa (R.B.B.); aahalwani@kau.edu.sa (A.A.H.); smbali@kau.edu.sa (S.M.B.-E.)
2. Center of Excellence for Drug Research and Pharmaceutical Industries, King Abdulaziz University, Jeddah 21589, Saudi Arabia
3. IES Institute of Pharmacy, IES University Campus, Kalkheda, Ratibad Main Road, Bhopal 462044, India; simasingh87@gmail.com
4. Department of Pharmaceutical Sciences, College of Clinical Pharmacy, King Faisal University, Al-Ahsa 31982, Saudi Arabia
5. Department of Pharmaceutics, Vidya Siri College of Pharmacy, Off Sarjapura Road, Bangalore 560035, India
* Correspondence: haldosari@kau.edu.sa (H.M.A.); sharsha@kfu.edu.sa (N.S.)

Abstract: Non-small cell lung cancer, a molecularly diverse disease, is the most prevalent cause of cancer mortality globally. Increasing understanding of the clinicopathology of the disease and mechanisms of tumor progression has facilitated early detection and multimodal care. Despite the advancements, survival rates are extremely low due to non-targeted therapeutics and correspondingly increased risk of metastasis. At some phases of cancer, patients need to face the ghost of chemotherapy. It is a difficult decision near the end of life. Such treatments have the capability to prolong survival or reduce symptoms, but can cause serious adverse effects, affecting quality of life of the patient. It is evident that many patients do not die from burden of the disease alone, but they die due to the toxic effect of treatment. Thus, increasing the efficacy is one aspect and decreasing the toxicity is another critical aspect of cancer formulation design. Through our current research, we tried to uncover both mentioned potentials of the formulation. Therefore, we designed actively targeted nanoparticles for improved therapeutics considering the overexpression of adenosine (ADN) receptors on non-small cell lung cancer (NSCLC) cells. Docetaxel (DTX), an essential therapeutic as part of combination therapy or as monotherapy for the treatment of NSCLC, was encapsulated in biodegradable poly(lactic-co-glycolic acid) nanoparticles. ADN was conjugated on the surface of nanoparticles using EDC-NHS chemistry. The particles were characterized in vitro for physicochemical properties, cellular uptake, and biocompatibility. The size and zeta potential of DTX nanoparticles (DPLGA) were found to be 138.4 ± 5.45 nm and −16.7 ± 2.3 mV which were found to change after ADN conjugation. The size was increased to 158.2 ± 6.3 nm, whereas zeta potential was decreased to −11.7 ± 1.4 mV for ADN-conjugated DTX nanoparticles (ADN-DPLGA) indicative of surface conjugation. As observed from transmission electron microscopy (TEM), the nanoparticles were spherical and showed no significant change in encapsulation efficiency even after surface conjugation. Careful and systematic optimization leads to ADN-conjugated PLGA nanoparticles having distinctive characteristic features such as particle size, surface potential, encapsulation efficacy, etc., that may play crucial roles in the fate of nanoparticles (NPs). Consequently, higher cellular uptake in the A549 lung cancer cell line was exhibited by ADN-DPLGA compared to DPLGA, illustrating the role of ADN receptors (ARs) in facilitating the uptake of NPs. Further in vivo pharmacokinetics and tissue distribution experiments revealed prolonged circulation in plasma and significantly higher lung tissue distribution than in other organs, dictating the targeting potential of the developed formulation over naïve drug and unconjugated formulations. Further, in vivo acute toxicity was examined using multiple parameters for non-toxic attributes of the developed formulation compared to other non-targeted organs. Further, it also supports the selection of biocompatible polymers in the formulation. The current study presents a proof-of-concept for a multipronged formulation technology strategy

Citation: Aldawsari, H.M.; Singh, S.; Alhakamy, N.A.; Bakhaidar, R.B.; Halwani, A.A.; Sreeharsha, N.; Badr-Eldin, S.M. Adenosine Conjugated Docetaxel Nanoparticles—Proof of Concept Studies for Non-Small Cell Lung Cancer. *Pharmaceuticals* 2022, 15, 544. https://doi.org/10.3390/ph15050544

Academic Editor: Huijie Zhang

Received: 28 March 2022
Accepted: 24 April 2022
Published: 28 April 2022

Publisher's Note: MDPI stays neutral with regard to jurisdictional claims in published maps and institutional affiliations.

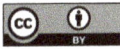

Copyright: © 2022 by the authors. Licensee MDPI, Basel, Switzerland. This article is an open access article distributed under the terms and conditions of the Creative Commons Attribution (CC BY) license (https://creativecommons.org/licenses/by/4.0/).

that might be used to maximize anticancer therapeutic responses in the lungs in the treatment of NSCLC. An improved therapeutic and safety profile would help achieve maximum efficacy at a reduced dose that would eventually help reduce the toxicity.

Keywords: docetaxel; adenosine receptors; PLGA; nanoparticles; lung cancer

1. Introduction

Lung cancer is the greatest cause of death and illness in the world (1.59 million deaths per year), followed by colon and liver cancer. NSCLC (non-small cell lung cancer) constitutes roughly 85% of all bronchogenic carcinomas [1] that pose a relentless threat to human health [2]. It is marked by a high proliferative rate, a strong predilection for metastasis, and a poor prognosis. More than 70% of NSCLC patients are elderly, current, or past heavy smokers, and the risk rises with increasing duration and intensity of smoking [3]. Although the disease is highly sensitive to chemotherapy and radiation, a higher dose of radiation causes severe damage to normal tissues around the tumor, causing poor patient compliance and therapeutic outcome [4]. On the other side, conventional chemotherapy has its shortcomings, such as nonspecific biodistribution, toxicity, etc. [5,6].

Cancer nanotherapeutics are rapidly evolving to solve several limitations of conventional drug delivery systems [7]. The ideal physicochemical characteristics that jointly confer molecular targeting, immune evasion, and controlled drug release have been a fundamental barrier to effective clinical translation of anticancer nanomedicines. Increasing understanding of the clinicopathology of the disease and mechanisms of tumor progression has proved that adenosine (ADN) receptors (ARs) are over-expressed on tumor cells of NSCLC [8]. There are multiple subtypes of ARs that are being explored, i.e., A1, A2A, A2B, and A3, for cancer research [9], though primarily A3ARs were found to be upregulated in multiple cancers including NSCLS [10]. This is the reason why the A3AR was considered to be the tumor marker. Extracellular ADN induces apoptosis in cancer cells via diverse signaling pathways linked to ARs. ADN and other AR agonists might be effective in preventing or slowing the progression of NSCLC and other cancers [11]. Although there are many studies on the role of ARs in cancer, the ligand potential of ADN in NSCLC is still superficially studied. Chung et al. illustrated the role of ADN, as a component of a polymer chain, in increasing the cellular uptake of the polymeric carrier in cancer cells and elucidated the reduction in cellular uptake of nucleic cargo when cells were pre-treated with free ADN [12]. However, they did not gain a deep understanding of the role of ARs in drug delivery. Later, Swami et al. profoundly reported improved efficacy of and-conjugated solid lipid nanoparticles in prostate and breast cancers vis-à-vis their native counterparts [7]. The results appear consistent with prior research but they need to be validated with NSCLC. Hence, it is mandatory to prove whether ADN ligand conjugated nanoparticles can assist in targeting NSCLC or not.

Poor prognosis in the early stages of cancer makes treatment of NSCLC difficult in later stages with monotherapy with platinum-based drugs. Therefore, Docetaxel (DTX) monotherapy is generally considered a standard line treatment when patients show progression after being treated with platinum-based chemotherapy [13]. DTX is a semisynthetic BCS Class IV, highly potent, water-insoluble taxol-derived broad-spectrum antineoplastic agent, with enhanced activity in malignant and cisplatin-resistant NSCLC. Clinically used DTX contains very high amounts of surfactants and alcohol that may preclude or limit their potential clinical application due to associated toxicities.

To elucidate the ligand potential of ADN in NSCLC, we designed ADN surface decorated PLGA nanoparticles encapsulating DTX. The Food and Drug Administration (FDA) and the European Medicines Agency (EMA) have authorized poly (lactic-co-glycolic acid) (PLGA) as a biodegradable and biocompatible polymer, raising the possibility of PLGA for sustained delivery systems. The polymer provides better control over release and degradation of the drug delivery system. There are many commercially available products based on PLGA such as Lupron Depot, Zoladex, etc. Their success rate proved the potential of using PLGA for the present research. Moreover, free carboxylic groups at flanking ends serve another advantage for conjugation of ADN without the need for any other excipient or linker. The literature supports many instances in which DTX was used in conjunction with PLGA nanoparticles, which dictate higher efficacy and less toxicity [14]. However, this study is the first-ever report on exploring the ADN-conjugated nanoparticles for effective management of NSCLC. We provided a proof-of-concept for systematically exploring DTX-loaded PLGA nanoparticles as a safe, improved, actively targeted therapeutic intervention for NSCLC using in vitro characterizations and in vivo evaluations.

2. Results and Discussion

2.1. Formulation and Characterization of DPLGA and ADN-DPLGA Nanoparticles

DTX encapsulation is responsible for increasing the mean particle size of the PLGA nanoparticles from 102.2 ± 3.23 nm to 138.43 ± 5.45 nm (Table 1).

Table 1. Mean particle size, surface potential, and entrapment efficiency among different formulations *.

Nanoparticle Formulation	Particle Size (nm)	Zeta Potential (mV)	Entrapment Efficiency (EE, %)
PLGA	102.2 ± 3.2	−17.0 ± 3.5	NA
DPLGA	138.4 ± 5.4	−16.7 ± 2.3	80.12 ± 1.98
ADN-DPLGA	158.2 ± 6.3	−11.7 ± 1.4	79.84 ± 2.66

* Data represent the mean of six determinations ± SD.

Upon conjugation, an additional increase in the mean particle size was evident owing to the attachment of multiple ADN molecules over the DPLGA nanoparticles surface (158.2 ± 6.3 nm). This is evident by the significant difference in the mean particle size of the two nanoparticles (Table 1). However, practiced peptide chemistry for the conjugation of free carboxylic groups on the surface of the DPLGA nanoparticles with the amine group of the ADN molecules resulted in decreased overall negative charge of ADN-DPLGA nanoparticles. Thus, the zeta potential of conjugated nanoparticles (ADN-DPLGA) was significantly lower (−11.7 ± 1.4) than that of non-conjugated particles (DPLGA, −16.7 ± 2.3 mV). Encapsulation efficiency expressed as % was observed as 80.12 ± 1.98 and 84.4 ± 2.61%, respectively, for DPLGA and ADN-DPLGA nanoparticles. An earlier report on multicomponent PLGA nanoparticles of docetaxel has shown entrapment efficiency of 69–75% [15]. There was no significant change in the DTX encapsulation after ADN decoration over the DPLGA nanoparticles, as illustrated in Table 1. TEM images of DPLGA Nanoparticles and ADN-DPLGA nanoparticles (Figure 1A,B) indicate that nanoparticles are spherical and have uniform size distribution. The conjugation did not affect the size and morphology of the particles.

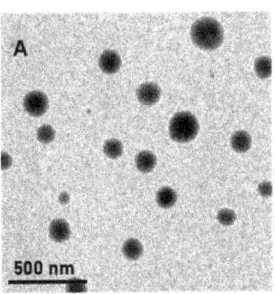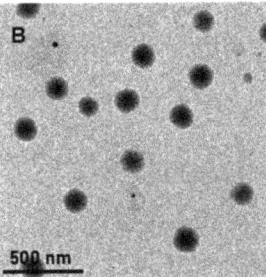

Figure 1. *Cont.*

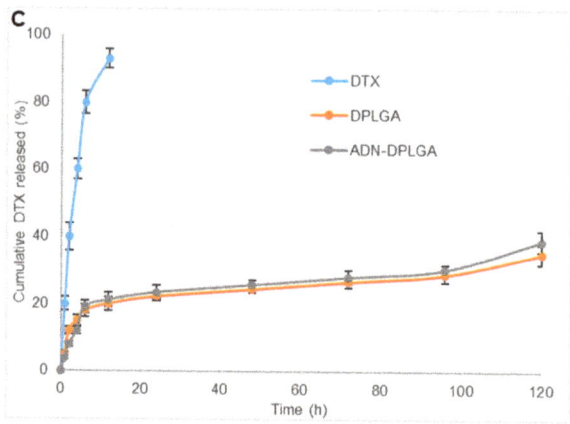
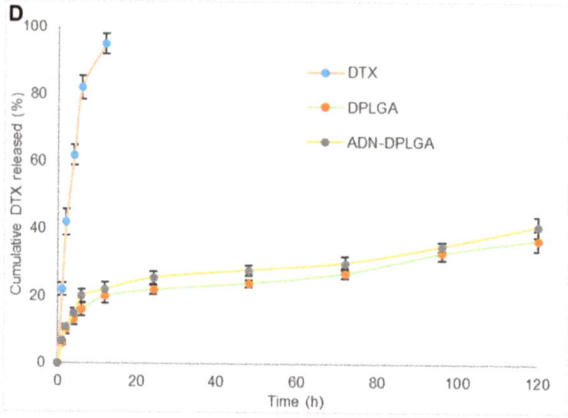

Figure 1. (**A,B**) The transmission electron microscopy (TEM) images of DPLGA and ADN-DPLGA nanoparticles, respectively. (**C,D**) The in vitro release profiles of DTX from pristine DTX, DPLGA, and ADN-DPLGA nanoparticles in phosphate buffer saline pH 7.4, and sodium acetate buffer (pH 5.0), respectively.

2.2. Conjugation Efficiency

The extent of conjugation of amine groups of ADN with free carboxylic groups of PLGA was assessed using the colorimetry method [7]. The results were very encouraging, presenting around 75% conjugation efficiency. Higher conjugation efficiency is also the cause of the larger size of ADN-DPLGA nanoparticles observed in size measurements and TEM images shown in earlier sections.

2.3. In Vitro Release Studies

In vitro release of DTX from pristine DTX suspension in two different pH media, namely pH 7.4 phosphate buffer saline and pH 5.0 sodium acetate buffer, was almost complete within 12 h (>95%) (Figure 1C,D). The developed PLGA nanoparticles showed a biphasic release pattern, indicated by initial burst release followed by sustained and slow release over a prolonged period. Approximately $20 \pm 2\%$ and $21.2 \pm 1.8\%$ of DTX were released from DPLGA and ADN-DPLGA nanoparticles, respectively. At the end of day 1, only 22.5 ± 1.3 and $23.5 \pm 1.2\%$ DTX was released in phosphate buffer saline. However, in the next 4 days, only an additional 13–16% of DTX was released. The initial rapid release of DTX can be attributed to the dissolution of DTX present on the surface of the nanoparticles. Similar phenomena were seen in sodium acetate buffer as well, for both nanoparticle formulations. However, the release in sodium acetate buffer was slightly faster than the release in phosphate buffer. This may facilitate the faster release of DTX from the nanoparticles once they are taken up by the cancer cells. However, the single-point measurement on 8th day denotes around 70% release, illustrating the degradation mechanism becoming the prominent mechanism of drug release. The findings were in accordance with the previously published reports [16,17]. An earlier report on lipid-based DTX particles showed around 80% release in 10 days [18]. When the release profile of DTX from pristine DTX suspension was compared with that of nanoparticles using the f_2 similarity factor, the release patterns were dissimilar as the value of f_2 was less than 50 ($f_2 = 15$ for DTX vs. DPLGA and $f_2 = 13.9$ for DTX vs. ADN-DPLGA in phosphate buffer saline pH 7.4 and $f_2 = 13.6$ for DTX vs. DPLGA and $f_2 = 14.2$ for DTX vs. ADN-DPLGA). The release profiles of DTX from DPLGA and ADN-DPLGA were similar as the f_2 similarity value was 87.8 and 82.9 for phosphate buffer saline pH 7.4 and sodium acetate buffer pH 5.0, respectively.

2.4. In Vitro Cell-Based Assays

2.4.1. In Vitro MTT Assay for Calculation of IC$_{50}$ (Half Maximal Inhibitory Concentration)

A concentration-dependent toxicity profile of the formulation was evident in the MTT assay on the A549 cell line. However, intraformational differences revealed higher activity, in terms of lower IC$_{50}$ values, in the case of PLGA nanoparticles compared to pristine DTX treatment (Figure 2).

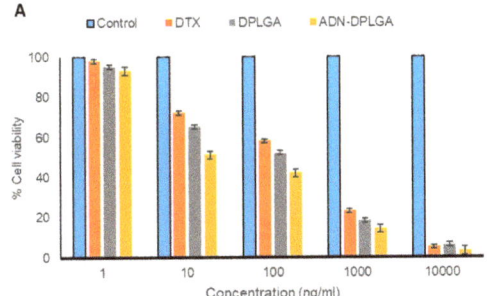
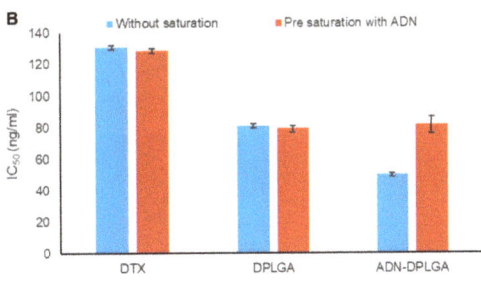

Figure 2. In vitro cell line studies. (**A**) Cell viability (%) of A549 cell lines treated with pristine DTX, DPLGA, and ADN-DPLGA nanoparticles. (**B**) Receptor competition assay outcomes showed an increase in the IC$_{50}$ of ADN-DPLGA nanoparticles after A549 cells were treated with free ADN (pre-saturation), causing blockage of ADN receptors on the cells. Thus, causing a reduction in the uptake of nanoparticles by the cells results in decreased efficacy. Values represent the mean of six determinations, and error bars indicate standard deviation.

IC$_{50}$ values were found to be 130.83, 80.72, and 49.50 ng/mL for pristine DTX, DPLGA, and ADN-DPLGA nanoparticles, respectively, after 48 h. The efficacy of DTX was significantly increased after being encapsulated in nanoparticles. We speculate that this might be due to the small particle size of nanoparticles resulting in higher internalization. Previous literature reported having 16-fold overexpression of ADN receptors in A549 [19]. This overexpression of the ADN receptor might be the reason for the higher retention of ADN-DPLGA nanoparticles in A549 cells due to ligand-mediated internalization. The higher efficacy in ADN-DPLGA was substantiated by the higher/rapid release of DTX in acidic pH, i.e., cancer cells (as presented in the release profile investigation in previous sections).

2.4.2. Receptor Competition Assay

The role of ADN receptors in the uptake of ADN-DPLGA nanoparticles was assessed using a receptor competition assay. Results were found to be in favor of the proposed hypothesis. It is observed that IC_{50} values were notably amplified ($p < 0.001$) after saturation of ADN receptors with free ADN, as shown in Figure 2B. Free ADN exposure to A549 cells caused blockage of ARs, causing a reduction in the receptor-mediated endocytosis of the ADN-DPLGA nanoparticles. These findings support the notion that uptake of the ADN-DPLGA nanoparticles is influenced by the overexpression of ADN receptors over A549 cells that represent an example of non-small cells causing lung cancer. Previously chen et al. also documented the effect of folic acid–folic acid receptor interaction

2.4.3. Cellular Uptake of Nanoparticles

A549, an epithelial carcinoma cell line, is commonly used as a model to study non-small-cell lung cancer [20]. Moreover, as already discussed in the previous results there is around 16-fold overexpression of ARs over A549 cell lines [19]. Following the literature evidence, we too observed higher uptake in the case of ADN-RhoPLGA nanoparticles due to selective uptake of ADN conjugated nanoparticles through highly specific and effective receptor-mediated endocytosis (Figure 3). These findings also corroborated our previous results obtained in the MTT assay. Similar inferences were drawn in several previous publications, where the authors illustrated the receptor–ligand interaction as the crucial factor for internalization of the nanoparticles to cancer cells [21,22]. Other than ARs, there are many receptors that were highlighted in previous research, assisting in cellular uptake of nanoparticles, i.e., transferrin, lactoferrin, sigma receptors, folic acid receptors, etc. [23–25].

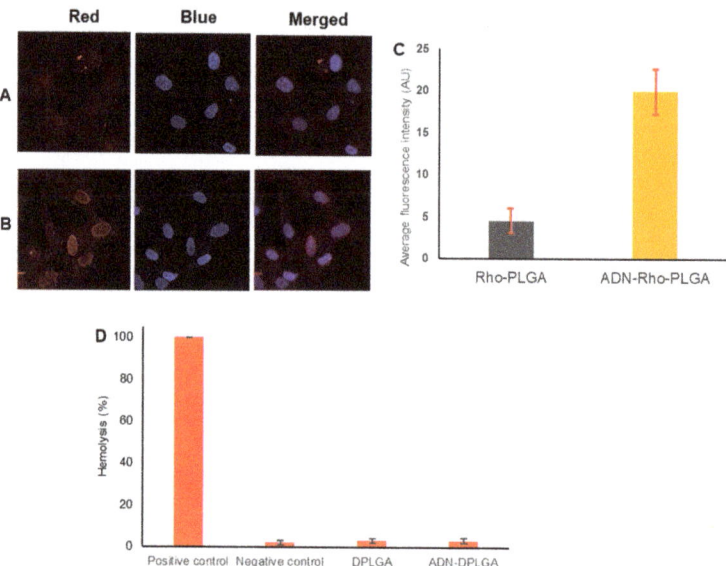

Figure 3. Cellular uptake and distribution of rhodamine 6G labeled DPLGA and ADN-DPLGA nanoparticles in A59 cells. (**A,B**) Representative CLSM images of A549 cells treated with rhodamine 6G labeled PLGA (Rho-PLGA) and ADN-RhoPLGA nanoparticles for 2 h. The cell nucleus was stained with Hoechst 33342. (**C**) Comparison of average fluorescence intensities for quantitative evaluation. The average fluorescence intensity of rhodamine was calculated using Image J software showing significantly higher uptake of ADN-PLGA nanoparticles by A549 cells. (**D**) represents the hemocompatibility analysis of DPLGA and ADN-PLGA nanoparticles when treated with red blood cells of rats. Positive control represents the treatment with Triton resulting in complete rupture of red blood cells causing maximum hemolysis. Negative control cells were treated with DMSO in phosphate buffer saline. The data represents the mean of 6 determinations, and error bars represent the standard deviation.

2.4.4. Hemocompatibility Analysis to Estimate Biocompatibility of Nanoparticles

Outlining the interaction of developed nanoparticles with red blood cells is an essential step toward establishing the safety of the product and the plausibility of utilizing the polymeric nanoparticles as delivery tools for several other therapeutic and biomedical applications. Formulations are composed of biocompatible and biodegradable. Therefore, we expect them to be safe for the blood cells. In the present investigation, the hemolytic effects of DPLGA nanoparticles and ADN-DPLGA nanoparticles were compared with Triton in PBS (1% w/v, positive control) and DMSO in PBS (0.1% v/v, negative control) (Figure 3D). In general, hemolysis less than 10% is considered non-hemolytic and, therefore, safe and biocompatible. In the present investigation, the DPLGA nanoparticle formulation and ADN-DPLGA nanoparticles showed 3.1 and 3.2% hemolysis. Therefore, the developed polymeric nanoparticles are considered safe for systemic administration for the treatment of NSCLC [26,27].

2.5. In Vivo Pharmacokinetics, Biodistribution, and Acute Toxicity Testing

2.5.1. Pharmacokinetic Studies

The mean plasma concentration vs. time profiles after single intravenous injection of DPLGA nanoparticles, ADN-DPLGA nanoparticles, and Docepar® (Parenteral Drugs India Ltd., Mumbai, India) in rats are shown in Figure 4.

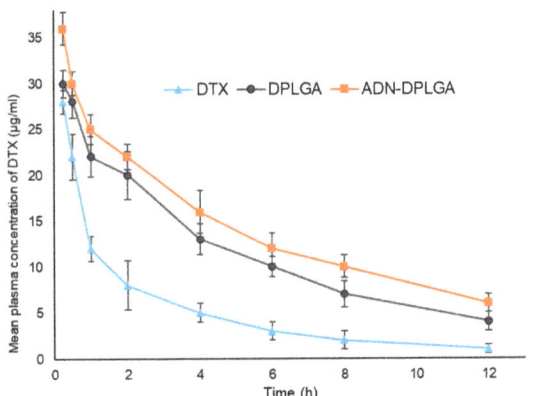

Figure 4. The mean plasma docetaxel concentration vs. time profile after a single intravenous injection of three different formulations, namely Docepar®, DPLGA, ADN-DPLGA nanoparticles equivalent to DTX (5 mg/kg). More retention and slower excretion were seen for PLGA formulations (DPLGA and ADN-DPLGA), thus, causing a larger area under curve (AUC).

It is presumed that hydrophobic surfaces tend to face early clearance from systemic circulation. Accordingly, in the present study, we observed much earlier clearance of the DTX compared to the ADN-DPLGA nanoparticles. Since ADN is a hydrophilic molecule containing sugar, it decreases RES uptake leading to reduced clearance and higher area under the curve (AUC). However, higher AUC in the case of unconjugated DPLGA nanoparticles is debatable. We speculate that it might be due to the negative charge on the surface of PLGA nanoparticles. The negative charge of the particles allows them to circumvent the RES uptake resulting in significantly prolonged systemic circulation compared to naïve drugs [28].

It can be seen that, compared with pure DTX, DTX nanoparticles, both DPLGA and ADN-DPLGA exhibited altered pharmacokinetic distribution of DTX in vivo and showed remarkably higher and prolonged plasma concentrations. The DPLGA nanoparticles exhibit almost ~3.38 times higher AUC (µg/mL·h) as compared to the pure drug (AUC_0^∞ DTX: 8.10

vs. AUC_0^∞ DPLGA: 27.41) while ADN-DPLGA nanoparticles show ~4.51 times higher AUC as compared to the pure drug (AUC_0^∞ DTX: 8.10 vs. AUC_0^∞ DPLGA: 36.63). Though, the insignificant difference in mean plasma concentration was evident among the two tested PLGA formulations. The findings were in agreement with the previous literature [7,29].

2.5.2. Tissue Distribution Analysis

In vivo biodistribution behavior of DTX post intravenous administration of the DTX nanoparticles (both ADN-DPLGA and DPLGA) in rats was investigated and compared with that of DTX commercially available injection as a control. The amounts of the drug distributed in the heart, liver, spleen, lung, and kidney were measured at different predetermined time points.

New and novel nanoparticulate drug delivery systems overcome nonspecific distribution hurdles by targeting the drug to the related organ/cells. Biodistribution studies help predict the fate of nanoparticulate formulations; consequently, one can determine the exposure of different drug titers in various organs. This is an important finding in understanding the toxicity profile of the formulation. The current study findings indicate that exposure to different tissues is minimal compared to native clinical formulation, i.e., Docepar®. There is an insignificant difference among the PLGA formulations owing to similar basic characteristics of the formulation (Figure 5). Swami et al. explained that through biodistribution, organs are exposed to elevated levels of drug concentrations leading to toxicity. Hence correlating the drug exposure with toxicity marker gives a holistic view of the targeting to toxicity potential of a formulation.

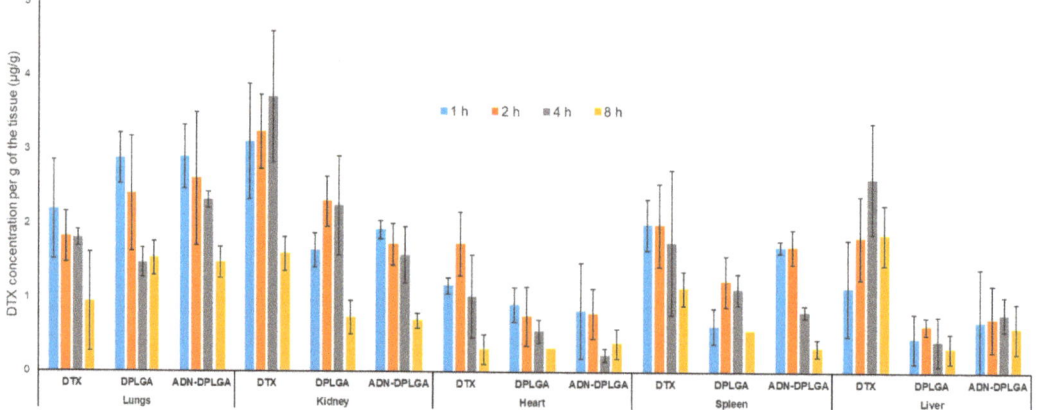

Figure 5. Tissue distribution studies. The concentration of DTX in various tissues after administration of three different formulations, namely, Docepar®, DPLGA, ADN-DPLGA nanoparticles equivalent to DTX (5 mg/kg) at four different time intervals, namely, 1, 2, 4, and 8 h. Data represents the mean of 6 determinations and error bars represent standard deviation.

To have a better understanding of the targeting efficiency (Te) of the DTX from both the nanoparticles, namely, DPLGA as well as ADN-DPLGA, parameter Te was calculated [30,31]. The Te demonstrates the ability of the delivery system to reach the target and non-target tissues. The Te values indicate preferential accumulation of nanoparticles in the lung tissues compared to the pristine DTX (Table 2).

These results indicate the accumulation of DTX nanoparticles in the lungs. However, there is an insignificant difference between the accumulation of ADN-DPLGA and DPLGA nanoparticles in the lungs. Though results of cell uptake studies clearly show a preferential uptake of ADN-DPLGA nanoparticles by the cancerous lung cells. ADN-DPLGA nanoparticles are the adenosine-conjugated nanoparticles that are expected to preferentially accumulate in the cancerous lung cells that exhibit over-expressed ARs.

However, the present study was carried out in non-cancerous, healthy animals with lung ARs. The absence of overexpressed adenosine receptors in healthy animals seems to be the reason for equivalent tissue accumulation of the ADN-DPLGA and DPLGA nanoparticles in the lungs. However, this study revealed a key component for designing future studies on disease/cancer models to understand adjoining effects of the ADN ligand (on nanoparticle surfaces) and overexpressed ARs (on lung cancer cells) on the migration of ADN-DPLGA nanoparticles.

Table 2. Comparative drug targeting efficiency of DTX form Docepar®, DPLGA, and ADN-DPLGA nanoparticles.

Organs	T_e DTX	T_e DPLGA	T_e ADN-DPLGA
Lung	0.24	3.23	3.87
Liver	2.35	0.25	0.18
Spleen	1.23	0.32	0.36
Kidney	2.08	0.92	0.98
Heart	1.06	0.65	0.54

2.5.3. In Vivo Toxicity Evaluations

Docepar®, a clinically used formulation of DTX, utilizes a cocktail of surfactant and alcohol to solubilize the hydrophobic DTX to avoid drug precipitation in vitro and the systemic circulation after intravenous administration. However, the formulation is known for its toxic effects, such as hypersensitivity reactions, tissue toxicity, etc., which coincide with the native side effects of the DTX. Hence, assessing our developed formulations' toxicities and comparing them with the clinically used formulation is of utmost necessity. Variations in serum toxicity markers to analyze the abnormality in the blood hepatobiliary system (ALT, AST) and kidney (BUN, creatinine) exemplified significant improvement ($p < 0.05$) when compared with the developed nanoparticles, as presented in Figure 6.

Docepar® showed significantly higher toxicity ($p < 0.001$) as compared to PLGA formulations due to already stated reasons. Though insignificant, ($p > 0.05$) a difference between the DPLGA and ADN-DPLGA nanoparticles was evident. The histology evaluations also corroborated higher toxicity. The histological evaluations of organ (kidney, liver, and spleen) specimens revealed a normal pattern of morphology in the case of the control group, DPLGA nanoparticles, and ADN-DPLGA nanoparticles. However, prominent characteristic features were perceived in the liver (hepatocytes degeneration and infiltrations), spleen (splenocytes damage), and kidney (necrotic tubules and debris).

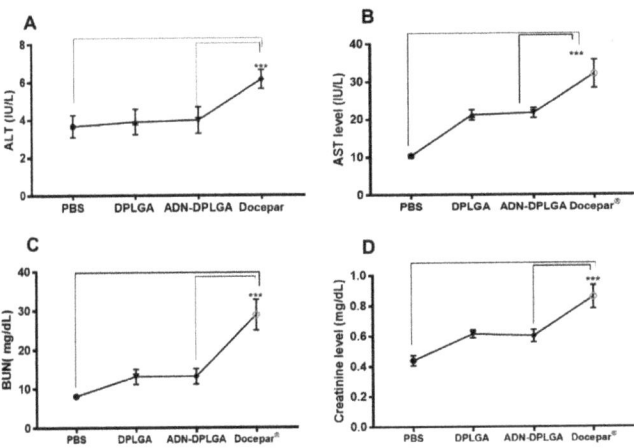

Figure 6. *Cont.*

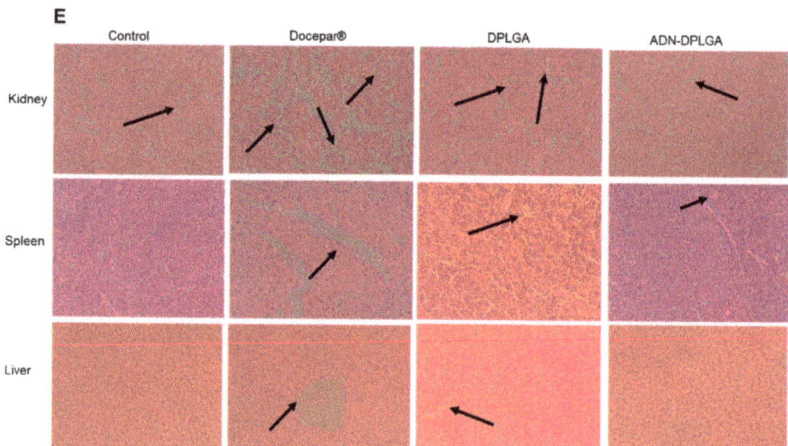

Figure 6. In vivo toxicity studies. (**A–D**) The serum biochemical markers levels representing ALT, AST, BUN, and creatinine, respectively, for four different groups of animals administered with untreated normal control (phosphate buffer saline, PBS), Docepar®, DPLGA, and ADN-DPLGA nanoparticles. Asterisk in biochemical studies signifies statistical limits in biochemical marker graphical representations: *** represents significant difference at $p < 0.001$, respectively, by Newman–Keuls analysis following ANOVA at 95% confidence limit. (**E**) Histological evaluations of different collected organs from the animals for toxicity investigations. Arrows indicate histological changes.

3. Materials and Methods

3.1. Materials

TherDose Pharma Pvt Ltd. generously provided docetaxel (DTX) and poly(d,l-lactic-co-glycolic acid) (PLGA) with a free carboxyl end group (uncapped) and an L/G molar ratio of 50:50, (Hyderabad, Andhra Pradesh, India) and Evonik (Mumbai, Maharashtra, India), respectively. ADN, Tween 80, 1-ethyl-3-(3-dimethylaminopropyl) carbodiimide hydrochloride (EDC), N-hydroxysuccinimide (NHS), Formaldehyde, Hoechst blue 33342 Rhodamine 6G, chloroform, methanol, acetone, dichloromethane, phosphotungstic acid, mannitol, dimethyl sulfoxide (DMSO), and acetonitrile were of HPLC grade (Merck, Mumbai, Maharashtra, India). The A549 cell line was obtained from the National Centre for Cell Science (NCCS, Pune, Maharashtra, India). Dulbecco's modified Eagle's Medium (DMEM), fetal bovine serum MTT (3-(4,5-dimethylthiazol- 2-yl)-2,5-diphenyl tetrazolium bromide), trypsin, EDTA, 2-(N-morpholino) ethanesulfonic acid (MES), Triton, and 96-well flat bottom tissue culture plates were purchased from Himedia (Mumbai, Maharashtra, India). Dialysis tubes were purchased from Spectrum (Float-A-Lyzer (G2, Spectrum, Repligen, MA, USA).

3.2. Preparation of DTX-Loaded PLGA Nanoparticles (DPLGA)

DTX (10 mg) was dissolved in 2 mL of acetone and dichloromethane mixture (1:1). PLGA (100 mg) was added to the DTX solution. This oil phase was emulsified for two minutes in an ice bath with an aqueous solution containing 0.25% Tween® 20 using a probe sonicator (VCX 130, Sonic and Materials, Newtown, CT, USA). After emulsification, the oil-in-water emulsion was magnetically stirred for eight hours to evaporate the organic solvent [32]. The dispersion of nanoparticles was centrifuged at 15,000 rpm for 20 min at 4 °C, then washed three times with deionized water, lyophilized (5% mannitol as a freeze-drying agent), and kept at 2–8 °C. The freeze-dried nanoparticles were characterized. Similarly, blank PLGA nanoparticles were also prepared.

3.3. Conjugation of ADN on the Surface of DPLGA Nanoparticles

Ten milligrams of DPLGA nanoparticles were distributed in five milliliters of 0.1 M MES buffer and incubated with NHS and EDC (1:5 w/w). The dispersion was kept under gentle stirring for 2 h at room temperature, protected from light to activate free carboxylic acid groups on the PLGA nanoparticles' surfaces. To this, 1 mg ADN was added, mixed well, and kept for further stirring for 4 h. ADN-conjugated DTX-loaded PLGA (ADN-DPLGA) nanoparticles were collected after centrifugation (Sigma Laborentrifugen GMBH, Osterode am Harz, Germany) at 15,000 rpm for 20 min and washed thrice with distilled water to remove unconjugated ADN in the supernatant. Prepared ADN–DPLGA pellets were recollected and freeze-dried (Lab Conco, Mumbai, Maharashtra, India). Freeze-dried nanoparticles were characterized further.

The conjugation efficiency of ADN to PLGA nanoparticles was quantified using phenol-sulphuric acid calorimetry assay as reported by Swami et al. [7] and expressed as a percentage of ADN bound to DPLGA nanoparticles. For cellular uptake, the nanoparticles were prepared using the same method along with rhodamine 6G as the fluorescent marker.

3.4. In Vitro Characterization of DPLGA and ADN-DPLGA Nanoparticles

The prepared nanoparticles, namely DPLGA and DTX-DPLGA, were characterized for several physicochemical parameters as stated below.

3.4.1. Analysis of Zeta Potential, Particle Size, and Transmission Electron Microscopy (TEM)

The developed nanoparticles, namely DPLGA and ADN-PLGA, were characterized for particle size using photon cross-correlation spectroscopy. The formulation sample was put in a clear polystyrene cuvette (path length = 1 cm) after being diluted with double distilled water to ensure that the light scattering intensity remained within the instrument's sensitivity range. Size measurements were performed using a nano-size analyzer (Nanophox, Sympatec India Pvt. Ltd., Mumbai, Maharashtra, India) at ambient temperature [33]. Zeta potential was measured on a zeta meter (Delsa Nano C, Beckman Coulter, Tokyo, Japan) [34]. For surface topography, images of nanoparticles were captured using high-resolution TEM (JEM 200, JEOL, Tokyo, Japan). The nanoparticle dispersion was put on a carbon-coated formvar grid and stained with neutralized phosphotungstic acid (1%) before being imaged under a microscope [35].

3.4.2. Entrapment Efficiency (EE, %)

EE corresponds to the percentage of DTX encapsulated within or/and adsorbed onto the DPLGA and DTX-DPLGA nanoparticles. The nanoparticles suspension was centrifuged at 5000 rpm for 5 min to settle down the precipitated drug [36]. The supernatant was collected and centrifuged (Sorvall benchtop centrifuge, ThermoScientific, Mumbai, Maharashtra, India) further at 21,000 rpm for 30 min at 4 °C to settle down the nanoparticles. The concentration of DTX in the supernatant and precipitate was calculated using the previously reported and validated RP-HPLC method [7].

3.4.3. In Vitro Release of DTX in Buffers

The release of DTX was studied from pristine DTX, DPLGA nanoparticles, and ADN-DPLGA nanoparticles by suspending in a Float-A-Lyzer (G2, Spectrum, Repligen, MA, USA) in two different release media, namely phosphate buffer saline pH 7.4 and sodium acetate buffer pH 5.0 containing Tween 80 to maintain sink condition and facilitate release [37]. The tests were performed at 37 °C (n = 6). The dialyzers were placed in sealed beakers with 100 mL release media and stirred on a magnetic stirrer at 100 rpm. DTX released at different time intervals was analyzed using the validated RP-HPLC method at pre-determined time intervals by withdrawing 0.5 mL of release media over 5 days. Immediately after sampling, the volume of release media was maintained at 100 mL by replacing equal amounts of release media. Release media samples were filtered through 0.22 μm

PVDF filters (Millex-VV, 13 mm, Merck, Mumbai, Maharashtra, India) and analyzed after appropriate dilution with a mobile phase of the RP-HPLC method. The dissolution profiles were compared using the f_2 similarity factor.

3.5. In Vitro Cell-Based Assays of DPLGA and ADN-DPLGA Nanoparticles

3.5.1. In Vitro Cell Toxicity (MTT Assay)

A549 (adenocarcinoma human alveolar basal epithelial cells) were selected due to the availability of overexpressed ARs. Cells were obtained from National Centre for Cell Sciences (NCCS, Pune, Maharashtra, India). Cell lines were maintained as prescribed by the ATCC guidelines. For cytotoxicity evaluation, different working dilutions of DTX in sterile phosphate buffer saline were created using a 10 mg/mL stock solution in DMSO. Cytotoxicity of all the formulations and naïve drugs was determined by MTT assay based on reduction of MTT dye (yellow) by the vital mitochondrial enzymes to blue-colored formazan product. A549 cells (1×10^4 cells/well) were seeded in 96-well plates and were allowed to attach overnight by incubating at 37 °C. For assessing the cytotoxicity, cells were exposed to different dilutions of DTX formulation and standard DTX and were incubated for 48 h at 37 °C in DMEM supplemented with a 10% FBS medium. After incubation, the media were aspirated, and the cells were washed twice with phosphate buffer saline (pH 7.4). The cells were processed for MTT assay [7]. The mean % of cell viability relative to untreated cells was estimated from data from multiple experiments (n = 6). The IC_{50} value was calculated using the curve fitting method.

3.5.2. Receptor Competition Assay

For competitive receptor assay, A549 cells were treated with free ligand before exposing cells with optimized formulations followed by the MTT assay as described earlier in the previous section [38]. Briefly, 1×10^4 cells were co-incubated with an excess of ADN. After 30 min of incubation, cells were washed twice with phosphate buffer saline (pH 7.4), followed by treatment of the cells with nanoparticle formulations and the pristine drug DTX. After incubation (48 h at 37 °C), cells were processed for MTT assay as reported earlier [21]. A comparison was completed between the IC_{50} values from the receptor competition assay and previously obtained IC_{50} values.

3.5.3. Investigations from Cellular Uptake Using Fluorescent Nanoparticles

The human non-small-cell lung cancer cell line A549 was obtained from the National Centre for Cell Sciences (NCCS, Pune, Maharashtra, India). The cells were grown in DMEM medium supplemented with 10% FBS at 37 °C with 5% CO_2 and 95% humidity. The media was replaced every 2–3 days, and the cells were detached from the culture flask using a 0.25% trypsin–0.02% EDTA solution after reaching a confluence level of 80–90%. For visualization of the cellular internalization by confocal laser scanning microscopy (CLSM, LSM 780, Carl Zeiss MicroImaging GmbH, Jena, Germany), A549 cells were seeded in a 24-well plate at a density of 1×10^5 cells per well along with a coverslip, allowed to adhere and grow for 24 h. Before the experiment, the cells were washed thrice with Dulbecco's buffer solution. Then, the cells were incubated with rhodamine 6G (Rho) loaded Rho-PLGA nanoparticles and ADN-RhoPLGA nanoparticles dispersed in the cell culture medium at 37 °C. After 2 h treatments, the cells were washed three times with cold phosphate buffer saline and treated with Hoechst blue 33342 (100 ng/mL) for 30 min. The media was removed, and cells were washed with phosphate buffer saline, fixed with 4% formaldehyde, and mounted on a coverslip. To preserve the samples, coverslips were placed on microscope slides. The CLSM apparatus was used to capture microscopy pictures. While recording the images, the microscopy gain and offset settings were kept constant throughout the study. Fluorescence in the cells was observed in CLSM with excitation wavelengths at 525 and 548 nm and emission wavelengths at 504 and 461 nm for rhodamine 6G and Hoechst blue 33342, respectively [27]. The mean fluorescence intensities were calculated from CLSM images using Image J software and plotted graphically.

3.5.4. In Vitro Hemocompatibility Assay

Biocompatibility was assessed using hemolysis testing. Biocompatibility of DPLGA and ADN-DPLGA was confirmed by incubating the formulations with red blood cells. Fresh blood was obtained from rats and centrifuged at 2500 rpm for 10 min at 4 °C in heparinized tubes. The pellet obtained after centrifugation was washed thrice with phosphate buffer saline, and cells were finally resuspended in phosphate buffer saline. In a 96-well plate, an equal volume of 100 µL of erythrocyte suspension and the nanoparticles' dispersion were combined. The plate was incubated at 37 °C for 1 h. After 1 h, the plate was centrifuged, and the supernatant was transferred to another 96-well plate. The absorbance was measured at 540 nm using a microplate reader (Erba LisaScan EM, Transasia, Mumbai, India). The supernatant generated from the centrifuged blood sample was used as a blank, and the supernatant derived from the blood sample treated with 1% Triton w/v was utilized as a positive control. Cells treated with 0.1% v/v DMSO in phosphate buffer saline were considered a negative control. All measurements were repeated (n = 6), and the percent hemolysis was calculated [26,27].

3.6. In Vivo Pharmacokinetics, Biodistribution, and Acute Toxicity Studies

The experimental protocol was approved by the Institutional Animals Ethics Committee (Vidya Siri College of Pharmacy, Bangalore, Karnataka, India). The experiment was carried out in accordance with the rules for experimental animal care established by the Committee for the Purpose of Control and Supervision on Experiments on Animals (CPCSEA). The protocol approval number is VSCP/EC/1405/2021/2, with a date of approval 14 May 2021. Female Sprague Dawley rats (150–200 g) were used for pharmacokinetic and biodistribution evaluations. Female Swiss albino mice (20–25 g) were utilized for toxicity evaluation. The animals were housed in normal wire mesh plastic cages in a room kept at 22 ± 0.5 °C with a 12 h light and 12 h dark cycle, and they were fed a standard pellet diet and provided water ad libitum. Experiments were carried out between 09:00 and 17:00 h.

3.6.1. Pharmacokinetic Studies

The rats were assigned to one of three treatment groups: Docepar® (commercially available product), DPLGA, or ADN-DPLGA nanoparticles. Each group had six animals (n = 6). The dose equivalent to 6 mg/kg of DTX was administered intravenously (IV) [22]. At different time intervals, blood samples were withdrawn and centrifuged at a fixed speed of 10,000 rpm for 5 min at 4 °C. The plasma samples were kept at −80 °C until they were processed. DTX concentrations were measured using the previously indicated verified and calibrated HPLC technique. Mean plasma concentration vs. time profile was represented graphically, and the area under the curve (AUC) was calculated [39] for comparison purposes.

3.6.2. Tissue Distribution Analysis

Animals were randomly divided into three treatment groups, namely, Docepar® (A commercially available product), DPLGA, and ADN-DPLGA nanoparticles. Individual groups had an equal number of animals. Each group received a single fixed dose of respective formulations equivalent to 5 mg/kg of DTX by IV route of administration. Mice (n = 6) were sacrificed at 1, 2, 4, and 8 h of post-dose and were dissected to isolate the heart, liver, spleen, kidney, and lungs. Tissues were weighed, homogenized in phosphate buffer saline, and were stored at −80 °C until further processing [40]. DTX concentration in each tissue was assessed after extracting in the organic phase and analyzing by validated RP-HPLC as described earlier. The lung targeting ability of the DTX nanoparticles was calculated using plasma concentration data. The tissue targeting ability of the delivery system was measured based on the drug targeting efficiency (T_e) calculated using the equation below.

$$T_e = \frac{(AUC_0^\infty) \, Target \, tissue}{(AUC_0^\infty) \, Non \, target \, tissue} \quad (1)$$

3.6.3. In Vivo Toxicity—Biochemical Analysis and Histopathology

To estimate drug-induced toxicities, mice were randomly divided into four different formulation groups, namely, untreated normal control (phosphate buffer saline, PBS), Docepar®, DPLGA, and ADN-DPLGA nanoparticles containing nanoparticles in an equal number of animals (n = 6). Formulations with a dose equivalent to 5 mg/kg of DTX were administered intravenously. The untreated normal group similarly received only normal saline [41]. Animals were humanly sacrificed after 7 days, followed by the collection of blood samples using cardiac puncture. Serum was separated, and several biochemical markers such as blood urea nitrogen (BUN), aspartate aminotransferase (AST), alanine aminotransferase (ALT), and creatinine levels were analyzed according to the instructions of the commercial kits (Sigma Aldrich, Bangalore, Karnataka, India). The vital organs, namely the liver, spleen, and kidney, were preserved in 10% formaldehyde in phosphate buffer saline, embedded in paraffin wax, and sliced into layers using a microtome (Leica, Wetzlar, Germany). The sections were observed in a light microscope (Olympus, Tokyo, Japan) after staining with Hematoxylin and Eosin (H&E).

3.7. Statistical Analysis

The statistical significance of the data was determined using a one-way analysis of variance (ANOVA) at a 95% confidence level. The Newman–Keul's test for statistical significance at the 95% confidence level was used to examine any significant differences between groups.

4. Conclusions

Lung cancer continues to be the most lethal form of cancer today. The present investigation is a proof-of-concept for developing targeted nanoparticulate interventions for non-small lung cancer (NSCLC) overexpressing adenosine (ADN) receptors (ARs). In the current investigation, an ADN ligand having a high affinity for ARs was postulated to develop ADN-conjugated PLGA nanoparticulate formulations containing docetaxel (DTX) as a chemotherapeutic agent. A series of investigations were conducted, and inferences were drawn in favor of the developed formulation. Planned comparisons between conventional clinically used formulations, i.e., Docepar® and tested formulations established the supremacy of the developed formulation over Docepar®.

Ligand-conjugated nanoparticulate systems offer a flexible and versatile technology that can be adapted to various drugs by modulating the process parameters to achieve the desired therapeutic response. When administered systemically, such ADN-conjugated nanoparticles can also serve as a platform technology for the active targeting of drugs to the cells with overexpressed ADN receptors with minimal non-target side effects.

Author Contributions: Conceptualization, H.M.A. and N.S.; data curation, S.S., N.A.A., R.B.B., A.A.H., N.S. and S.M.B.-E.; formal analysis, H.M.A., S.S., N.A.A., R.B.B., A.A.H., N.S. and S.M.B.-E.; funding acquisition, H.M.A., S.S., N.A.A., R.B.B., A.A.H., N.S. and S.M.B.-E.; investigation, H.M.A., S.S., N.A.A., R.B.B., A.A.H., N.S. and S.M.B.-E.; methodology, H.M.A., S.S., N.A.A., R.B.B., A.A.H., N.S. and S.M.B.-E.; project administration, H.M.A. and S.M.B.-E.; resources, A.A.H.; software, N.A.A.; supervision, S.S., R.B.B. and S.M.B.-E.; validation, S.M.B.-E.; visualization, H.M.A.; writing—original draft, H.M.A., S.S., N.A.A., R.B.B., A.A.H. and N.S.; writing—review and editing, H.M.A., N.A.A., R.B.B., A.A.H., N.S. and S.M.B.-E. All authors have read and agreed to the published version of the manuscript.

Funding: This project was funded by Institutional Fund Projects under grant no. (IFPRC-070-249-2020).

Institutional Review Board Statement: The experimental protocol was approved by the Institutional Animals Ethics Committee (Vidya Siri College of Pharmacy, Bangalore, Karnataka, India). The experiment was carried out in accordance with the rules for experimental animal care established by the Committee for the Purpose of Control and Supervision on Experiments on Animals (CPCSEA). The protocol approval number is VSCP/EC/1405/2021/2, with a date of approval 14 May 2021.

Informed Consent Statement: Not applicable.

Data Availability Statement: Data is contained within the article.

Acknowledgments: The authors extend their appreciation to the Deputyship for Research & Innovation, Ministry of Education in Saudi Arabia for funding this research work through the project number IFPRC-070-249-2020 and King Abdulaziz University, DSR, Jeddah, Saudi Arabia.

Conflicts of Interest: The authors declare no conflict of interest.

References

1. Board, P.A.T.E. Non-small cell lung cancer treatment (PDQ®). In *PDQ Cancer Information Summaries [Internet]*; National Cancer Institute: Bethesda, MD, USA, 2021.
2. Jain, A.; James, N.; Shanthi, V.; Ramanathan, K. Design of ALK Inhibitors for Non-Small Cell Lung Cancer–A Fragment Based Approach. *Indian J. Pharm. Educ. Res.* **2020**, *54*, 114–124. [CrossRef]
3. Herbst, R.S.; Morgensztern, D.; Boshoff, C.J.N. The biology and management of non-small cell lung cancer. *Nature* **2018**, *553*, 446–454. [CrossRef]
4. Gorain, B.; Choudhury, H.; Nair, A.B.; Dubey, S.K.; Kesharwani, P. Theranostic application of nanoemulsions in chemotherapy. *Drug Discov. Today* **2020**, *25*, 1174–1188. [CrossRef] [PubMed]
5. Woodman, C.; Vundu, G.; George, A.; Wilson, C.M. Applications and strategies in nanodiagnosis and nanotherapy in lung cancer. In *Seminars in Cancer Biology*; Academic Press: Cambridge, MA, USA, 2021; pp. 349–364.
6. Patil, R.Y.; More, H.N. Antioxidants with multivitamin and mineral supplementation attenuates chemotherapy or radiotherapy-induced oxidative stress in cancer patients. *Indian J. Pharm. Educ. Res* **2020**, *54*, 484–490. [CrossRef]
7. Swami, R.; Singh, I.; Jeengar, M.K.; Naidu, V.; Khan, W.; Sistla, R. Adenosine conjugated lipidic nanoparticles for enhanced tumor targeting. *Int. J. Pharm.* **2015**, *486*, 287–296. [CrossRef]
8. Inoue, Y.; Yoshimura, K.; Kurabe, N.; Kahyo, T.; Kawase, A.; Tanahashi, M.; Ogawa, H.; Inui, N.; Funai, K.; Shinmura, K.; et al. Prognostic impact of CD73 and A2A adenosine receptor expression in non-small-cell lung cancer. *Oncotarget* **2017**, *8*, 8738–8751. [CrossRef]
9. Polosa, R.; Holgate, S.T. Adenosine receptors as promising therapeutic targets for drug development in chronic airway inflammation. *Curr. Drug Targets* **2006**, *7*, 699–706. [CrossRef]
10. Mazziotta, C.; Rotondo, J.C.; Lanzillotti, C.; Campione, G.; Martini, F.; Tognon, M. Cancer biology and molecular genetics of A3 adenosine receptor. *Oncogene* **2022**, *41*, 301–308. [CrossRef]
11. Jafari, S.M.J.C. Role of Adenosine receptor in lung cancer. *Jorjani Biomed. J.* **2018**, *6*, 018–0360.
12. Chung, Y.C.; Cheng, T.Y.; Young, T.H. The role of adenosine receptor and caveolae-mediated endocytosis in oligonucleotide-mediated gene transfer. *Biomaterials* **2011**, *32*, 4471–4480. [CrossRef]
13. Fossella, F.V. Docetaxel in second-line treatment of non-small-cell lung cancer. *Clin. Lung Cancer* **2002**, *3* (Suppl. 2), S23–S28. [CrossRef] [PubMed]
14. Kulhari, H.; Pooja, D.; Shrivastava, S.; Naidu, V.G.M.; Sistla, R. Peptide conjugated polymeric nanoparticles as a carrier for targeted delivery of docetaxel. *Colloids Surf. B Biointerfaces* **2014**, *117*, 166–173. [CrossRef] [PubMed]
15. Conte, C.; Monteiro, P.F.; Gurnani, P.; Stolnik, S.; Ungaro, F.; Quaglia, F.; Clarke, P.; Grabowska, A.; Kavallaris, M.; Alexander, C. Multi-component bioresponsive nanoparticles for synchronous delivery of docetaxel and TUBB3 siRNA to lung cancer cells. *Nanoscale* **2021**, *13*, 11414–11426. [CrossRef]
16. Cui, Y.-N.; Xu, Q.-X.; Davoodi, P.; Wang, D.-P.; Wang, C.-H. Enhanced intracellular delivery and controlled drug release of magnetic PLGA nanoparticles modified with transferrin. *Acta Pharmacol. Sin.* **2017**, *38*, 943–953. [CrossRef] [PubMed]
17. Rafiei, P.; Haddadi, A. Docetaxel-loaded PLGA and PLGA-PEG nanoparticles for intravenous application: Pharmacokinetics and biodistribution profile. *Int. J. Nanomed.* **2017**, *12*, 935–947. [CrossRef] [PubMed]
18. da Rocha, M.C.O.; da Silva, P.B.; Radicchi, M.A.; Andrade, B.Y.G.; de Oliveira, J.V.; Venus, T.; Merker, C.; Estrela-Lopis, I.; Longo, J.P.F.; Báo, S.N. Docetaxel-loaded solid lipid nanoparticles prevent tumor growth and lung metastasis of 4T1 murine mammary carcinoma cells. *J. Nanobiotechnol.* **2020**, *18*, 43. [CrossRef] [PubMed]
19. Brown, R.; Clarke, G.; Ledbetter, C.; Hurle, M.; Denyer, J.; Simcock, D.; Coote, J.; Savage, T.; Murdoch, R.; Page, C.J.E.R.J. Elevated expression of adenosine A1 receptor in bronchial biopsy specimens from asthmatic subjects. *Eur. Respir. J.* **2008**, *31*, 311–319. [CrossRef] [PubMed]
20. Townsend, M.H.; Anderson, M.D.; Weagel, E.G.; Velazquez, E.J.; Weber, K.S.; Robison, R.A.; O'Neill, K.L. Non-small-cell lung cancer cell lines A549 and NCI-H460 express hypoxanthine guanine phosphoribosyltransferase on the plasma membrane. *OncoTargets Ther.* **2017**, *10*, 1921–1932. [CrossRef] [PubMed]

21. Nagaraja, S.; Basavarajappa, G.M.; Attimarad, M.; Pund, S. Topical Nanoemulgel for the Treatment of Skin Cancer: Proof-of-Technology. *Pharmaceutics* **2021**, *13*, 902. [CrossRef] [PubMed]
22. Nair, A.; Morsy, M.A.; Jacob, S. Dose translation between laboratory animals and human in preclinical and clinical phases of drug development. *Drug Dev. Res.* **2018**, *79*, 373–382. [CrossRef] [PubMed]
23. Yang, P.-H.; Sun, X.; Chiu, J.-F.; Sun, H.; He, Q.-Y. Transferrin-Mediated Gold Nanoparticle Cellular Uptake. *Bioconjug. Chem.* **2005**, *16*, 494–496. [CrossRef] [PubMed]
24. Loureiro, J.A.; Gomes, B.; Fricker, G.; Coelho, M.A.N.; Rocha, S.; Pereira, M.C. Cellular uptake of PLGA nanoparticles targeted with anti-amyloid and anti-transferrin receptor antibodies for Alzheimer's disease treatment. *Colloids Surf. B Biointerfaces* **2016**, *145*, 8–13. [CrossRef] [PubMed]
25. Chen, J.; Li, S.; Shen, Q.; He, H.; Zhang, Y. Enhanced cellular uptake of folic acid-conjugated PLGA-PEG nanoparticles loaded with vincristine sulfate in human breast cancer. *Drug Dev. Ind. Pharm.* **2011**, *37*, 1339–1346. [CrossRef]
26. Pund, S.; Pawar, S.; Gangurde, S.; Divate, D. Transcutaneous delivery of leflunomide nanoemulgel: Mechanistic investigation into physicomechanical characteristics, in vitro anti-psoriatic and anti-melanoma activity. *Int. J. Pharm.* **2015**, *487*, 148–156. [CrossRef]
27. Jagwani, S.; Jalalpure, S.; Dhamecha, D.; Jadhav, K.; Bohara, R. Pharmacokinetic and Pharmacodynamic Evaluation of Resveratrol Loaded Cationic Liposomes for Targeting Hepatocellular Carcinoma. *ACS Biomater. Sci. Eng.* **2020**, *6*, 4969–4984. [CrossRef] [PubMed]
28. Xiao, K.; Li, Y.; Luo, J.; Lee, J.S.; Xiao, W.; Gonik, A.M.; Agarwal, R.G.; Lam, K.S.J.B. The effect of surface charge on in vivo biodistribution of PEG-oligocholic acid based micellar nanoparticles. *Biomaterials* **2011**, *32*, 3435–3446. [CrossRef] [PubMed]
29. Singh, I.; Swami, R.; Jeengar, M.K.; Khan, W.; Sistla, R. p-Aminophenyl-α-D-mannopyranoside engineered lipidic nanoparticles for effective delivery of docetaxel to brain. *Chem. Phys. Lipids* **2015**, *188*, 1–9. [CrossRef] [PubMed]
30. Gupta, P.K.; Hung, C.T. Quantitative evaluation of targeted drug delivery systems. *Int. J. Pharm.* **1989**, *56*, 217–226. [CrossRef]
31. Harsha, S.; Al-Dhubiab, B.E.; Nair, A.B.; Al-Khars, M.; Al-Hassan, M.; Rajan, R.; Attimarad, M.; Venugopala, K.N.; Asif, A.H. Novel Drying Technology of Microsphere and Its Evaluation for Targeted Drug Delivery for Lungs. *Dry. Technol.* **2015**, *33*, 502–512. [CrossRef]
32. Nair, A.B.; Al-Dhubiab, B.E.; Shah, J.; Attimarad, M.; Harsha, S. Poly (lactic acid-co-glycolic acid) Nanospheres improved the oral delivery of candesartan cilexetil. *Indian J. Pharm. Educ. Res* **2017**, *51*, 571–579. [CrossRef]
33. Sreeharsha, N.; Rajpoot, K.; Tekade, M.; Kalyane, D.; Nair, A.B.; Venugopala, K.N.; Tekade, R.K. Development of Metronidazole Loaded Chitosan Nanoparticles Using QbD Approach-A Novel and Potential Antibacterial Formulation. *Pharmaceutics* **2020**, *12*, 920. [CrossRef]
34. Akrawi, S.H.; Gorain, B.; Nair, A.B.; Choudhury, H.; Pandey, M.; Shah, J.N.; Venugopala, K.N. Development and Optimization of Naringenin-Loaded Chitosan-Coated Nanoemulsion for Topical Therapy in Wound Healing. *Pharmaceutics* **2020**, *12*, 893. [CrossRef] [PubMed]
35. Shah, J.; Nair, A.B.; Shah, H.; Jacob, S.; Shehata, T.M.; Morsy, M.A. Enhancement in antinociceptive and anti-inflammatory effects of tramadol by transdermal proniosome gel. *Asian J. Pharm. Sci.* **2020**, *15*, 786–796. [CrossRef] [PubMed]
36. Nair, A.B.; Sreeharsha, N.; Al-Dhubiab, B.E.; Hiremath, J.G.; Shinu, P.; Attimarad, M.; Venugopala, K.N.; Mutahar, M. HPMC- and PLGA-Based Nanoparticles for the Mucoadhesive Delivery of Sitagliptin: Optimization and In Vivo Evaluation in Rats. *Materials* **2019**, *12*, 4239. [CrossRef]
37. Kotta, S.; Aldawsari, H.M.; Badr-Eldin, S.M.; Binmahfouz, L.S.; Bakhaidar, R.B.; Sreeharsha, N.; Nair, A.B.; Ramnarayanan, C. Lung targeted lipopolymeric microspheres of dexamethasone for the treatment of ARDS. *Pharmaceutics* **2021**, *13*, 1347. [CrossRef] [PubMed]
38. Kulhari, H.; Pooja, D.; Shrivastava, S.; Kuncha, M.; Naidu, V.G.M.; Bansal, V.; Sistla, R.; Adams, D.J. Trastuzumab-grafted PAMAM dendrimers for the selective delivery of anticancer drugs to HER2-positive breast cancer. *Sci. Rep.* **2016**, *6*, 23179. [CrossRef] [PubMed]
39. Satyavert; Gupta, S.; Choudhury, H.; Jacob, S.; Nair, A.B.; Dhanawat, M.; Munjal, K. Pharmacokinetics and tissue distribution of hydrazinocurcumin in rats. *Pharmacol. Rep. PR* **2021**, *73*, 1734–1743. [CrossRef] [PubMed]
40. Morsy, M.A.; Nair, A.B. Prevention of rat liver fibrosis by selective targeting of hepatic stellate cells using hesperidin carriers. *Int. J. Pharm.* **2018**, *552*, 241–250. [CrossRef]
41. Swami, R.; Kumar, Y.; Chaudhari, D.; Katiyar, S.S.; Kuche, K.; Katare, P.B.; Banerjee, S.K.; Jain, S. pH sensitive liposomes assisted specific and improved breast cancer therapy using co-delivery of SIRT1 shRNA and Docetaxel. *Mater. Sci. Eng. C* **2021**, *120*, 111664. [CrossRef] [PubMed]

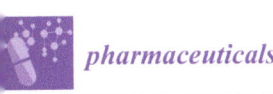

Article

A Theranostic Nanocomplex Combining with Magnetic Hyperthermia for Enhanced Accumulation and Efficacy of pH-Triggering Polymeric Cisplatin(IV) Prodrugs

Yang Qu [1,2], Zhiqi Wang [1], Miao Sun [1], Tian Zhao [3], Xuanlei Zhu [1], Xiaoli Deng [1], Man Zhang [1], Ying Xu [1,*] and Hongfei Liu [1,4,*]

[1] College of Pharmacy, Jiangsu University, Zhenjiang 212013, China; quyang@ujs.edu.cn (Y.Q.); 2211915014@stmail.ujs.edu.cn (Z.W.); 2222015024@stmail.ujs.edu.cn (M.S.); 3191603010@stmail.ujs.edu.cn (X.Z.); 3181603070@stmail.ujs.edu.cn (X.D.); 3181603068@stmail.ujs.edu.cn (M.Z.)
[2] Chia Tai Tianqing Pharmaceutical Group Co., Ltd., Nanjing 210046, China
[3] Department of Medical Imaging, Affiliated Hospital of Jiangsu University, Jiangsu University, Zhenjiang 212001, China; locklove@ujs.edu.cn
[4] Jiangsu Sunan Pharmaceutical Group Co., Ltd., Zhenjiang 212400, China
* Correspondence: xying@ujs.edu.cn (Y.X.); 1000003850@ujs.edu.cn (H.L.)

Abstract: Although polymeric platinum(IV) (Pt(IV)) prodrugs can reduce the side effects of cisplatin, the efficacy of the prodrug is still limited by its non-targeted distribution, poor penetration in deep tumor tissue, and low cytotoxicity in tumor cells. To improve the clinical potential of polymeric prodrug micelle, we synthesized amphiphilic polymeric Pt(IV) with high Pt content (22.5%), then developed a theranostic nanocomplex by integrating polymeric Pt(IV) with superparamagnetic $Mn_{0.6}Zn_{0.4}Fe_2O_4$ via simple self-assembly. Due to the high content of $Mn_{0.6}Zn_{0.4}Fe_2O_4$ (41.7% w/w), the theranostic nanocomplex showed high saturation magnetization (103.1 emu g^{-1}) and excellent magnetocaloric effect (404 W g^{-1}), both of them indicating its advantages in efficient magnetic targeting (MT), magnetic hyperthermia (MH), and magnetic resonance imaging (MRI). In vitro, in combination with MH, the theranostic nanocomplex showed as high cytotoxicity as cisplatin because of a significant increase in platinum of cellular uptake. In vivo, the accumulation of theranostic nanocomplex in tumors was increased by MT and confirmed by MRI. Furthermore, MH improved penetration of theranostic nanocomplex in tumors as expanding blackened area in tumors was observed by MRI. Based on these properties, the theranostic nanocomplex, under the assistance of MT and MH, showed the highest tumor growth inhibition rate (88.38%) after different treatments, while the body weight of mice increased slightly, indicating low side effects compared to those of cisplatin. The study provided an advanced theranostic nanocomplex with low toxicity and high efficacy, indicating a great clinical potential of polymeric Pt(IV).

Keywords: polymeric prodrug; theranostic nanocomplex; pH-triggering releasing; magnetic targeting; magnetic hyperthermia; magnetic resonance imaging

1. Introduction

Cisplatin, a classical platinum (Pt) drug with +2 valence (Pt(II)), is one of the most successful antitumor drugs against tumor cells by crosslinking DNA via coordination bond; however, its severe side effects are an inevitable problem in clinics [1]. To overcome the shortcoming of cisplatin, several kinds of polymer-based drug delivery systems have been developed to improve cisplatin pharmacokinetics and enhance its accumulation in tumor sites by enhanced permeability and retention (EPR) effect [2]. As cisplatin is a micromolecule lacking sufficient hydrophobicity and hydrophilicity, physical encapsulation is not suitable for preparing cisplatin-loaded nanocarrier direct. Consequently, a kind of Pt drug with +4 valence (Pt(IV)) has been developed by modifying cisplatin on its axial directions to improve its application potential [3]. The current prevailing view considers the Pt(IV) as a prodrug of cisplatin because its cytotoxicity should be suppressed in blood circulation, then activated by reducing to cisplatin under the effect of intracellular reductants, such as ascorbic acid and glutathione (GSH) [3]. Although Pt(IV) with high hydrophobicity could be encapsulated into micelles by hydrophobic effect easily [4], the physical trapping was unstable, as many studies displayed obvious drug releasing from the nanocarriers under physiological conditions in 24 h, implying the risk of drug leak from corresponding delivery in blood circulation [5,6].

To raise the stability of the Pt(IV)-loaded nanocarrier, an attractive approach is to prepare polymeric prodrug micelle, which immobilizes Pt(IV) on polymers by stimuli-responsive covalent bond and forms prodrug micelle [2]. Because covalent bonding possesses high stability in physical conditions and rapid cleavage in a tumor's extracellular or intracellular environment, polymeric Pt(IV) micelle shows double advantages on long-circulation in blood and targeted accumulation in the tumor. Moreover, high drug content ($\geq$10 wt.%) in prodrug micelle has been achieved by the optimization of the composition and architecture of polymeric prodrug [7,8]. Therefore, the polymeric prodrug micelle should be a competitive option in the clinical application of cisplatin.

However, the high stability of polymeric prodrug micelle is a double-edged sword. In blood circulation, the high binding energy between polymer and Pt(IV) reduced drug leaking, resulting in low side effects. Although the EPR effect has been involved in many studies to improve the accumulation of drug-loaded nanocarriers in tumors, its effect has been limited in small animal models [9]. So far, drug-loaded nanocarriers have almost uniformly failed to improve efficacy in clinics [10]. Much basic research on tumors has found that diffusion of nanoparticles in tumors has been hindered by some barriers, including tortuous tumor blood vessels, high-density extracellular matrix, and consequent elevated interstitial pressure [11]. Meanwhile, differences between tumor and normal tissue on pH [12] and GSH concentration [13] were insufficient for the breakage of covalent bonding efficiently. Therefore, after polymeric Pt(IV) prodrug accumulated in the tumor site by EPR effect, its penetration into deep tumor was more difficult than that of micro-molecular drugs, such as Pt(IV) and cisplatin, which reduced its efficacy in clinics.

In order to overcome the obstacle, hyperthermia should be a promising strategy to promote the permeation of polymeric prodrug micelle. Previous studies have confirmed that regional mild hyperthermia (40–43 °C) can increase tumor blood supply and accelerate the diffusion of macromolecules in solid tumors [14,15]. In addition, hyperthermia can enhance cellular uptake and cytotoxicity of chemotherapeutic drugs significantly, especially for cisplatin and its derivatives. As hyperthermia can interfere reparation of DNA damages caused by platinum-based antitumor drugs [16], the integration of hyperthermia and polymeric Pt(IV) micelles should be an ideal strategy for improving the efficacy of cisplatin in clinics.

According to progress in noninvasive hyperthermia, photothermal treatment and magnetic hyperthermia (MH) have attracted great attention. However, MH possesses a greater clinic potential because an alternating magnetic field (AMF) for MH can penetrate the human body without any loss, in contrast with depth-limited near-infrared ray (NIR) for photothermal treatment [17]. In our previous study, we developed an MH composed of superparamagnetic $Mn_{0.6}Zn_{0.4}Fe_2O_4$ nanoparticles with a high specific adsorption rate (SAR) under AMF and confirmed its efficiency on tumor suppression alone [18] and multi-treatment in combination with chemotherapy [19]. Moreover, magnetic fluid consisting of superparamagnetic nanoparticles (SPIO) has also been used widely in fields of magnetic resonance imaging (MRI) [20] and magnetic targeting (MT) [21]. Therefore, SPIO should be an ideal nanomaterial to combine with polymeric Pt(IV) prodrug, obtaining a versatile nanocomplex for diagnosis and treatment of tumors.

In the study, a theranostic nanocomplex was constructed to promote the clinical potential of polymeric Pt(IV) prodrug by self-assembly of monodispersed $Mn_{0.6}Zn_{0.4}Fe_2O_4$ and amphiphilic polymeric Pt(IV), as shown in Figure 1.

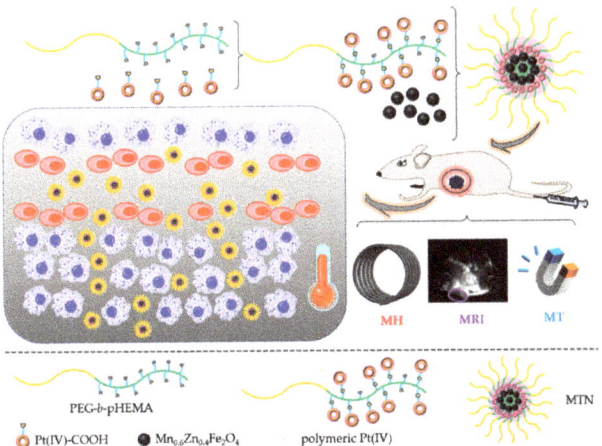

Figure 1. Schematic illustration of the theranostic nanocomplex formation and its cascading effects on diagnosis and therapy of tumors, including efficient magnetic targeting firstly, following magnetic resonance imaging, subsequent magnetic hyperthermia to promote penetration of nanocomplex, and enhanced antitumor efficiency of polymeric Pt(IV) finally.

To prepare the theranostic nanocomplex, we synthesized polymeric prodrugs with high platinum content firstly. A hydrophilic diblock copolymer monomethoxyl poly(ethylene glycol)-block-poly(2-hydroxyethyl methacrylate) (mPEG-*b*-pHEMA) (shown in Figure 1) with suitable hydroxide radical content was synthesized by reversible addition–fragmentation chain-transfer polymerization (RAFT), then a considerable amount of modified Pt(IV) with single carboxyl (Pt(IV)-COOH) combined with hydroxyls of PEG-*b*-pHEMA by esterification reaction, resulting in amphiphilic polymeric Pt(IV). By self-assembly, amphiphilic polymeric Pt(IV) could encapsulate hydrophobic monodispersed $Mn_{0.6}Zn_{0.4}Fe_2O_4$ easily and form the stable micellar theranostic nanocomplex (MTN). MTNs showed advantages in suitable diameter for the EPR effect, high stability under physiological conditions, and obvious acid-triggering drug release. Because of the existence of clustering monodispersed $Mn_{0.6}Zn_{0.4}Fe_2O_4$, the MTN displayed multipotentials on MRI, MT, and MH, also shown in Figure 1. In accordance with relevant properties, cytotoxicity and cellular uptake of MTN in vitro have been enhanced significantly by efficient MH. Furthermore, in vivo studies showed that accumulation of MTN in tumors was enhanced by MT and observed by MRI. What is more, MH of 20 min promoted permeation of MTN in tumors, which was also confirmed by MRI. As the combination of MT and MH benefited accumulation and penetration of the nanocomplex in tumors, as shown in Figure 1, the nanocomplex exhibited high antitumor efficacy and low side effects because of the slight gaining weight of mice, which increased cisplatin potential in clinics.

2. Results and Discussion

2.1. Synthesis and Characterization of Polymeric Pt(IV)

The synthetic route of polymeric Pt(IV) is shown in Figure S1, containing two parts, preparation of Pt(IV)-COOH and synthesis of mPEG-*b*-pHEMA. According to previous studies on Pt(IV) [8,22], we prepared Pt(IV) with two hydroxyl groups (Pt(IV)-(OH)$_2$) at Pt axial positions by oxidization of excessive hydrogen peroxide on cisplatin, then modified the Pt(IV) with a single carboxyl group (Pt(IV)-COOH) by reacting with equimolar succinic anhydride (SA) under mild conditions, also shown in Figure S1. Furthermore, we characterized the structure and molecular weight of Pt(IV)-COOH by Fourier transform infrared (FT-IR) spectrum, H proton nuclear magnetic resonance (¹H NMR), and mass spectrum, as shown in Figures S2–S4. Compared to relative results in previous studies [22–25], Pt(IV)-COOH has been prepared successfully.

At the same time, we synthesized diblock hydrophilic polymer, mPEG-b-pHEMA, by a combination of esterification and RAFT reactions, which was also displayed in Figure S1. In the reaction, S-1-Dodecyl-S′-(α,α′-dimethyl-α″-acetic acid)trithiocarbonate (DDAT) was selected as chain-transfer agent (CTA) for RAFT polymerization and synthesized according to the literature [26]. Then, we prepared macro-CTA by DCC reaction between monomethoxyl poly(ethylene glycol) (mPEG) and DDAT, resulting in mPEG-DDAT. Its structure was characterized by ¹H NMR and is shown in Figure S5. After the successful synthesis of macro-CTA, the successive reaction was to synthesize mPEG-b-pHEMA with repeating units of 2-hydroxyethyl methacrylate (HEAM) by RAFT reaction because hydroxide radical of HEMA could be used to combine with Pt(IV)-COOH. To figure out whether the RAFT reaction was successful or not, we characterized the structure of mPEG-b-pHEMA by ¹H NMR, as shown in Figure 2 (bottom spectrum).

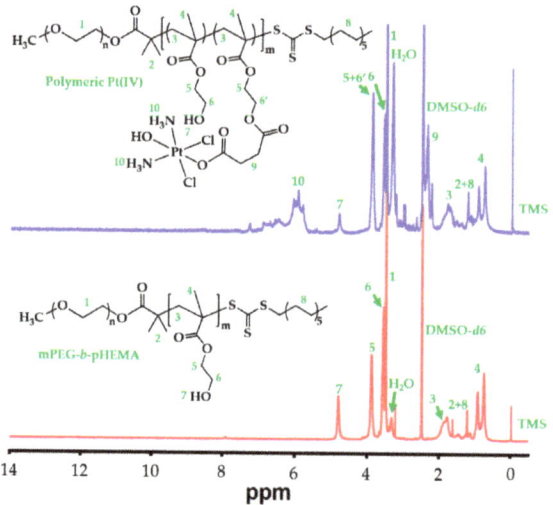

Figure 2. ¹H NMR spectra of mPEG-b-pHEMA and polymeric Pt(IV) in DMSO-d6.

Compared to a previous relative study [27], all characteristic peaks of pHEMA were observed and marked in Figure 2, which confirmed the successful polymerization of pHEMA as a product of mPEG-DDAT chain propagation. Moreover, the average polymerization degree of HEMA was calculated to be 27, resulting from an integral area ratio of peaks between 3.38 ppm (labeled as 1, terminal CH_3 of mPEG) and 4.7–4.9 ppm (labeled as 8, OH of pHEMA).

Based on the structures of Pt(IV)-COOH and mPEG-b-pHEMA, we prepared polymeric Pt(IV) by esterification between carboxyl of Pt(IV) and hydroxy of mPEG-b-pHEMA. Although most previous studies used N,N′-Dicyclohexylcarbodiimide (DCC) reaction to prepare polymer-Pt(IV) conjugation [8,23,25,26,28,29], we modified the reaction process by a combination of 1-(3-Dimethylaminopropyl)-3-ethylcarbodiimide hydrochloride (EDC) and 1-Hydroxybenzotriazole (HOBt) to simplify post-treatment during product purification. The structure of polymeric Pt(IV) was also characterized by ¹H NMR, as shown in Figure 2 (top spectrum). Compared to the counterpart of mPEG-b-pHEMA, polymeric Pt(IV) not only retained all characteristic peaks of mPEG-b-pHEMA but also presented characteristic peaks of Pt(IV) in the ¹H NMR spectrum of polymeric Pt(IV), which was marked in Figure 2. In contrast with that of the bottom spectrum, the intensity of the peak at 4.7–4.9 ppm (labeled as 8) in the top spectrum reduced obviously, which indicated a decrease in the hydroxy amount of polymeric Pt(IV). Meanwhile, the conversion from hydroxy to ester bond was confirmed by increasing peak intensity at 3.83–3.93 (labeled as 5 + 6′) because CH_2 (labeled as 6′) possessed the same chemical environment as CH_2 (labeled as 5) after forming ester bonding. Furthermore, the Pt content was determined precisely by an inductively coupled plasma mass spectrometer (ICP-MS), which was as high as 22.5 wt%. On the basis of the above results, polymeric Pt(IV) with high Pt content was prepared successfully.

2.2. Characterization of Polymeric Pt(IV)-Based Micelles

Using polymeric Pt(IV), we prepared polymeric Pt(IV) micelle (PPM) and MTN; both of them were observed directly by transmission electron microscopy (TEM), as shown in Figure 3A,B, and we further measured their size distributions by dynamic light scattering (DLS), as shown in Figure 3C.

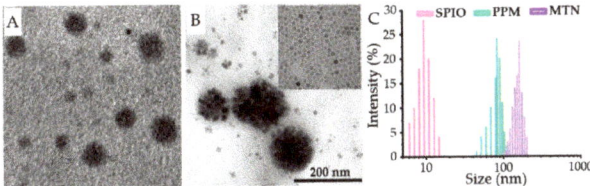

Figure 3. Morphologies (TEM) and particle size distributions (DLS) of PPM, MTN, and SPIO: (**A**) TEM result of PPMs; (**B**) TEM result of MTNs, inset: TEM result of SPIOs; (**C**) DLS results of PPM, MTN, and SPIO.

By self-assembly of polymeric Pt(IV), PPM showed a spherical inner core with high contrast without phosphotungstic acid staining, which implied high content Pt of polymeric Pt(IV). Because of the amphipathy of polymeric Pt(IV), MTN could be prepared to encapsulate $Mn_{0.6}Zn_{0.4}Fe_2O_4$ nanoparticles by the same procedure. Besides PPM and MTN, we also provided a TEM photo of monodispersed $Mn_{0.6}Zn_{0.4}Fe_2O_4$ nanoparticles, which was shown in the inset of Figure 3B and Figure S6. Apparently, MTN exhibited a larger particle size than that of PPM, as MTN possessed a core of $Mn_{0.6}Zn_{0.4}Fe_2O_4$ nanocluster. Therefore, we determined the size distributions of PPMs and MTNs in PBS by DLS. As monodispersed $Mn_{0.6}Zn_{0.4}Fe_2O_4$ nanoparticles displayed high hydrophobicity, their diameter was measured in THF. The size distributions of SPIO, PPM, and MTN increase were 9.8, 86, and 151 nm, respectively (Figure 3C), which were consistent with their TEM results. In order to estimate the stability of MTN, the time-dependent hydrodynamic diameter was studied in PBS further, which was shown in Figure S7, confirming their high stability in physiological buffer. These results not only prove the formation of MTN directly but also suggest the MTN with some potential in clinics, such as suitable size for passive targeting (EPR effect, 10–200 nm) and magnetic properties on magnetic targeting and hyperthermia, because of the existence of highly compacted SPIO cluster in the core of MTN.

After quantifying the content of SPIO in MTN by ICP-MS, the content of SPIO in MTN was calculated as 41.7% w/w, which corresponded to a feed ratio of SPIO in a gross mass of 50%. Because of the existence of SPIO, as expected, MTN displayed excellent magnetism, as shown in Figure 4A.

According to our previous study [18], monodispersed $Mn_{0.6}Zn_{0.4}Fe_2O_4$ nanoparticles exhibited high saturation magnetism (M_s = 74.6 emu g^{-1}) and superparamagnetism, which reappeared in this research, as shown in Figure S8 (M_s = 102.7 emu g^{-1} $_{[Fe+Mn+Zn]}$, corresponding to 74.6 emu g^{-1} $_{[mass\ of\ SPIO]}$). Due to high M_s and superparamagnetism of $Mn_{0.6}Zn_{0.4}Fe_2O_4$ nanoparticles, MTN displayed similar hysteresis loops, as shown in Figure 4A, indicating its high M_s (103.1 emu g^{-1} $_{[Fe+Mn+Zn]}$) and superparamagnetism. Besides high M_s, MTN also exhibits a magnetocaloric effect; the heating profile and corresponding SAR are shown in Figure 4B. It should be noted that we calculated the SAR value of MTN by data of the initial 4 min because a linear correlation was observed between time and temperature in the 4 min. However, the SAR in the research was lower than that of our previous study (SAR = 1102.4 W g^{-1}) [18]. It was caused mostly by low $H_{applied}$ (63.6 kA m^{-1}), which was almost 55.4% of that (114.9 kA m^{-1}) in our previous study. As low $H_{applied}$ can improve biosafety of AMF, meanwhile, SAR of magnetic fluid is proportional to the square of $H_{applied}$ [30], the low SAR value in the study is reasonable.

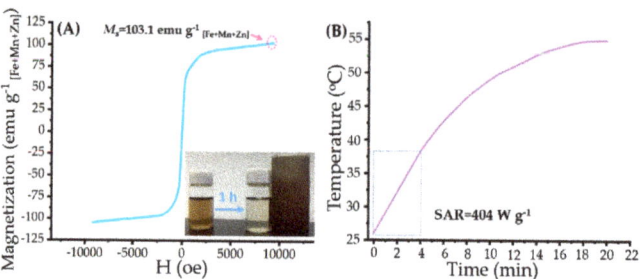

Figure 4. Magnetic property and magnetocaloric effect of MTNs: (**A**) magnetization curve of the MTN at 300 K; inset: photograph of MTN solution and its response to an external magnet at 1 h; (**B**) time-dependent temperature curve of MTN in AMF (corresponding parameters as 114 kHz of frequency and 63.6 kA m^{-1} of strength) and corresponding SAR value.

2.3. Drug Release Studies

To simulate intracellular conditions, an acidic buffer (pH = 5.0) containing acetate and glutathione (GSH, 1 mM) [31] was employed in drug release studies. As a control, other three types of buffers were also employed in drug release studies, including pure acidic buffer (pH = 5.0) without GSH, pure GSH buffer (1 mM), PBS with physiological pH value, and GSH (5 µM) [32]. The drug release profiles of MTN under different conditions were shown in Figure 5, indicating its high stability in the physiological environment and burst release behavior within cells.

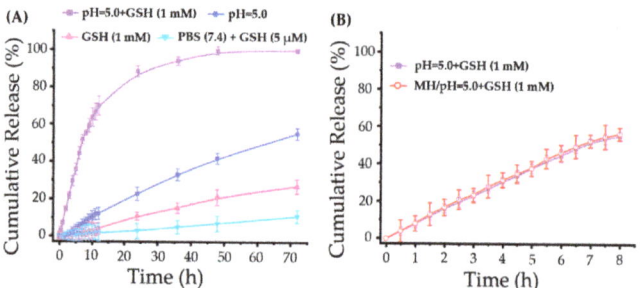

Figure 5. Drug release profiles of MTN under different conditions: (**A**) Pt release profiles of MTN under intracellular environment (pH = 5.0 + 1 mM GSH), physiological condition (pH = 7.4 + 5 µM GSH), pure acid environment (pH = 5.0), and pure reductive environment (1 mM GSH); (**B**) the influence of MH on Pt release under intracellular environment.

As shown in Figure 5A, a small amount of Pt was detected from the outside solution of dialysis tubing in the physiological environment (PBS (pH = 7.4) + GSH (5 µM)) after 72 h incubation, which was consistent with previous studies [33,34]. On the contrary, MTN exhibited rapid release behavior in intracellular environment (pH = 5.0 + GSH (1 mM)). Under the intracellular niche, cumulative Pt release from MTN was rapidly within the initial 10 h, which was 7.27% at 1 h, then up to 63.67% at 10 h. To figure out the weighting of pH value and GSH concentration in platinum release, the Pt release profiles under acid environment (pH = 5.0) were contrasted with that under reductive environment (GSH, 1 mM), also shown in Figure 5A. It was clear that GSH could induce Pt release from MTN because of the high redox sensitivity of Pt(IV) [7]. However, in our study, the intracellular acid environment played a critical effect on triggering Pt release from MTN, as cumulative release in the acid condition is triple that in reductive condition at the same incubation time. The higher pH-sensitive release profile might be attributed to the number of ester bonding, which is triple of number of Pt(IV).

Furthermore, we studied the effect of MH on Pt release from MTN, as shown in Figure 5B. Apparently, MH of 20 min did not influence Pt release, as two release profiles with/without MH almost overlap at all time points. Therefore, the polymeric Pt(IV) is a typical macromolecular prodrug with an intracellular release profile, in which the acid environment is the most important factor involved in drug release. These results will benefit MTN application in vivo by enhancing intracellular release and reducing undesirable side effects.

2.4. Antitumor Efficacy In Vitro

Cytotoxicity experiments were studied by using 4T1. Before evaluation of the tumor inhibition ratio in vitro, biocompatibility of the mPEG-b-pHEMA was investigated and shown in Figure S9. As cell survival rates of mPEG-b-pHEMA at all concentrations (0.2–2 mg mL^{-1}) approximated or even exceeded 100%, mPEG-b-pHEMA was a hydrophilic polymer with excellent biocompatibility.

Antitumor efficacy in vitro is shown in Figure 6, which displays various inhibition rates on 4T1 by different treatments.

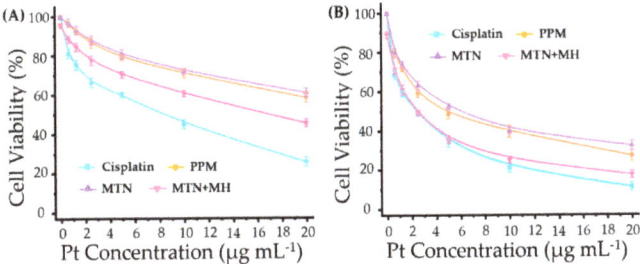

Figure 6. The cytotoxicity of 4T1 treated with cisplatin, PPM, MTN, and MTN + MH (duration time of MH: 20 min per 24 h) for 24 h (**A**) and 48 h (**B**).

Apparently, cisplatin exhibited a higher inhibition rate than that of its macromolecular prodrugs, PPM and MTN, for all tested periods (24 and 48 h). Meanwhile, the cytotoxicities of PPM and MTN on 4T1 were similar because they were prepared by the same macromolecular prodrug. Although periodic MH (20 min per 24 h) suppressed cell viability slightly at 24 h, it could enhance the antitumor efficacy of MTNs obviously. When incubation time reached 48 h, the cell viabilities of cisplatin and MTNs plus MH were almost overlapping at lower Pt concentration ($\leq$5 µg mL^{-1}).

In our previous study, we investigated the synergistic effect between MH and chemotherapy by the mediation of thermo-sensitive drug delivery, in which MH triggered chemotherapy release efficiently. However, in the study, the controlled release of cisplatin from polymeric Pt(IV) is independent beyond the effect of MH, as shown in Figure 4B. Moreover, periodic MH in the study showed limited cytotoxicity on 4T1, as cell viabilities of pure MH were 95.7% at 24 h and 89.1% at 48 h, both of which were lower than those of our previous study [19]. Therefore, the enhancement of polymeric Pt(IV) cytotoxicity by MH should be studied further.

By ICP-MS, we investigated intracellular Pt content after incubating with different formulations for 1 and 4 h, as shown in Figure 7.

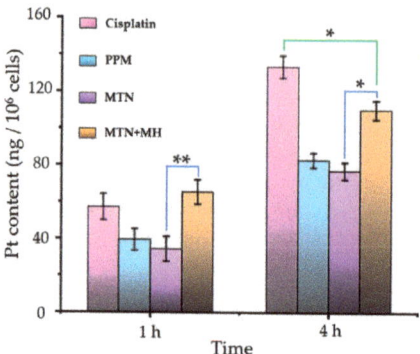

Figure 7. The intracellular Pt contents by treating with cisplatin, PPM, MTN, and MTN + MH for 1 h and 4 h. The MH was operated for the initial 20 min of the study. (* $p < 0.05$; ** $p < 0.01$).

First of all, formulation was a key factor in Pt internalization because cellular uptake of cisplatin showed higher Pt content at 1 and 4 h, in contrast with formulations of PPM and MTN. It is reasonable that cisplatin can enter cells via both passive diffusion and active uptake [35]. On the one hand, cisplatin is small enough to diffuse through cell membranes easily compared to PPM and MTN with larger sizes. On the other hand, copper transporter 1 (CTR-1) can mediate the active uptake of cisplatin efficiently. Because of the high expression of CTR-1 in the kidney proximal tubule [36], nephrotoxicity is the main side-effect of cisplatin in clinics. Unfortunately, 4T1 displayed high CTR-1 expression level (CTR-1/action ≥ 0.5) [37]. Consequently, cisplatin alone displayed efficient internalization (Figure 7) and high cytotoxicity (Figure 6).

Although MTN with the largest size distribution displayed the lowest level of Pt cellular internalization, MH enhanced cellular uptake of MTNs significantly at all time points (1 and 4 h). By stimulation of MH at an initial 20 min, we observed the highest Pt content among all groups at 1 h, which was higher than that of cisplatin. The phenomenon could be explained by thermal-induced increasing lipid fluidity and permeability of cell membranes. However, the influence of MH on MTN internalization is temporary. With prolonging culture time (4 h), Pt internalization in the group of MTN plus MH is still higher than that of MTN but lower than that of cisplatin significantly, as shown in Figure 7, corresponding to its cytotoxicity in Figure 6A. Even so, it is definite that MH is an efficient approach to increasing the cellular uptake of micellar Pt(IV). Therefore, the cytotoxicity of MTN should be improved further by periodic MH (20 min per 24 h) within prolonged culture time (48 h), corresponding to the result shown in Figure 6B.

2.5. Efficient Tumor Diagnosis by a Combination of MT and MRI In Vivo

It is well known that a multifunctional nanocomplex by combining noninvasive imaging and therapy represents the main development trend in tumor treatment because synchronous noninvasive monitoring possesses great advantages in visualizing drug biodistribution, assessing therapeutic responses, and predicting efficacy [38,39]. Among all common noninvasive imaging techniques, MRI is one of the most powerful diagnostic tools because of its high biosafety and remarkable spatial resolution. As nanocluster of SPIO was demonstrated its efficiency in shortening spin–spin relaxation time (T2) of MRI [40], in the study, MTN with a core of $Mn_{0.6}Zn_{0.4}Fe_2O_4$ nanocluster was used as a T2 contrast agent to locate tumors in vivo, as shown in Figure 8.

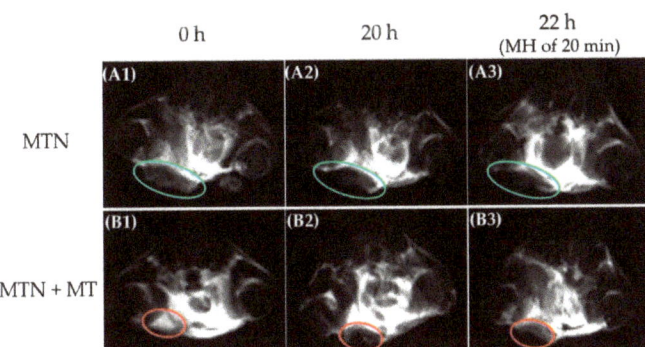

Figure 8. T2-weighted MRI results of orthotopic breast tumor before and after i.v. administration of MTN with corresponding treatments: MTN (**A1–A3**) and MTN + MT (**B1–B3**). Before intravenous injection of MTN, orthotopic breast tumors were scanned by MRI as control (**A1,B1**). After injection, the duration time of MT was 4 h, and the tumors were scanned again at 20 h (**A2,B2**). After MH of 20 min, the third MRI results (**A3,B3**) were obtained at 22 h after intravenous injection of MTN.

Because MTN has a suitable diameter of around 151 nm, MTN could distribute in solid tumors by EPR effect and induce slight darkening in a partial area of the tumor (Figure 8(A2)) compared to the counterpart without MTN injection (Figure 8(A1)). Unfortunately, the EPR effect is inadequate for nanocarrier accumulation in tumor sites, which is confirmed by many previous studies. As MTN exhibited a high M_s value and obvious magnet-induced distribution, as shown in Figure 4A, a button magnet was employed to improve MTN accumulation in tumors specifically. By attracting an external magnet nearby tumors, most areas of the tumor darkened visibly in Figure 8(B2), indicating the effectiveness of MT in increasing MTN biodistribution in tumors.

However, it should be noted that the accumulation of MTN in tumor sites did not equal its uniform distribution in tumor tissue. On the one hand, intrinsic barriers in tumors impeded the diffusion of MTN, as we mentioned previously in the introduction. On the other hand, a permanent magnet is inadequate for attracting MTN completely because the magnetic field of the permanent magnet will attenuate rapidly with increasing distance between tumor tissue and magnet. Meanwhile, the pH value of tumor tissue usually ranged from 6.5 to 6.8 [41], which was much higher than the effective pH value (≤ 5.0) in our drug release studies. It is necessary to promote penetration of MTN in tumor tissue and its endocytosis further. Considering the potential of MH on these aspects, we assessed the influence of MH on MTN distribution in tumors. However, the real-time temperature of tumors could not be monitored during MH in vivo because an overheated copper coil ($\geq 50\ ^\circ C$) interfered with the detection of infrared radiation (IR) thermal camera seriously. The MRI results revealed diffusion of MTN after MH, as darkened areas of tumors in Figure 8(A3,B3) extended, by contrast with the corresponding counterpart before MH (Figure 8(A2,B2)). Especially for the group with MT, the region with T2 enhancement almost covered the whole tumor after MH. Considering high interstitial fluid pressure and dense extracellular matrix within tumors, passive diffusion of nanocarrier around 100 nm is almost impossible [42]. Therefore, we infer that local MH is the only driving force to facilitate the diffusion of MTN with a large diameter within the tumor.

To observe the biodistribution of MTNs directly, all major organs and tumors of mice were stained for iron detection after the MH. As ferric ion (Fe^{3+}) can combine with ferrocyanide, resulting in a bright blue pigment, Prussian blue, we exhibited the distribution of MTN in different organs directly, as shown in Figure 9.

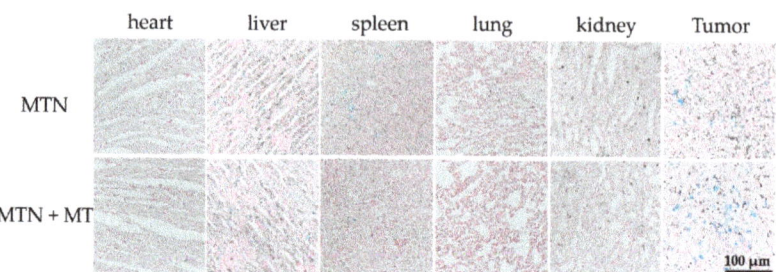

Figure 9. Tissue slices of main organs and tumors after treatments by MTN or MTN + MT. The duration time of MT was 4 h, and those tissues were obtained at 22 h after intravenous injection of MTN. These tissue slices were stained by nuclear fast red and Prussian blue simultaneously.

According to the results, MTN mainly accumulated in tumors and organs such as the liver and spleen after MH, which was consistent with a relative study [43]. In spite of the similar distribution in the liver between the two groups, MT improved the distribution of MTNs in tumors and reduced them in the spleen. As shown in Figure 9, in contrast with passive targeting (MTN alone), visible blue spots in tumors were more obvious in the group combined with MT. Meanwhile, Fe^{3+} content in the spleen showed an opposite trend. Besides the Fe^{3+} content, another marked significance between passive targeting and MT was the dispersion degree of these bright blue spots in tumors after MH. Compared to passive targeting, the group combining with MT exhibited an even distribution of MTN in the tumor section, which corresponded to MRI results after MH.

2.6. Antitumor Efficacy In Vivo

Based on the positive results we mentioned above, MTN not only showed low cytotoxicity alone and enhanced cytotoxicity and cellular internalization by combining with MH in vitro but also displayed MT enhanced tumor accumulation and MH stimulative tumor penetration in vivo. Encouraged by the excellent performance of MTN, we investigated the antitumor efficacy of MTN in vivo, especially under optimized strategy by integrating MT and MH, as displayed in Figure 10.

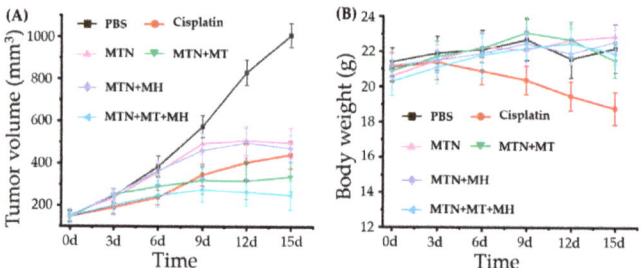

Figure 10. In vivo antitumor activities of different treatments: (**A**) the tumor volume curves after different treatments with the extension of curative time from 0 to 15 d; (**B**) the body weight curves after corresponding treatments with the extension of curative time from 0 to 15 d.

Apparently, the growth of the 4T1 tumor was very rapid, as tumor volume ($n = 6$) of the PBS group developed from 152 to 1008 mm^3 in 15 days. After injection of different formulations with equivalent cisplatin content at 3 mg kg^{-1} body weight via intravenous injection, tumor growth was inhibited obviously, compared to that of the PBS group. Among these groups, MTN alone/MH did not display obvious tumor inhibition in the early stage because tumors in the early phase were too small to exhibit the EPR effect, inducing low accumulation of MTN in tumors and bad antitumor performance. When the tumor reaches a certain volume, low toxic MTN could accumulate in the tumor by the EPR effect and show a certain ability on suppressing tumor growth, as shown in Figure 10A. However, due to the limitation of the EPR effect, the accumulation of MTN was not enough to induce effective MH. The antitumor efficacies between MTN alone and MTN plus MH were similar in the whole study.

Owing to MT, the group of MTN plus MT exhibited more efficiency in suppressing tumor growth by enhancing the accumulation of MTN in tumors. With the repeating MT (4 h per 24 h), the performance of MTN plus MT was even better than that of cisplatin at the later stage. Although cisplatin inhibited tumor growth efficiently at an early stage, its antitumor ability declined rapidly after the third injection. Besides the treatments we discussed above, the group of MTN plus MT plus MH showed the strongest tumor suppression. The phenomenon should be ascribed to the effects of MT and MH on MTN efficacy, in which the former increased MTN accumulation in tumors and the latter improved MTN penetration in dense tumors. Moreover, because of the dual effect of chemotherapy and MH, the group of MTN plus MT plus MH did not only exhibit the smallest tumor size but also displayed a downtrend in shrinking tumor volume at the end of in vivo study, which indicates a possibility of tumor vanishment by prolonged treatment of MTN plus MT plus MH.

Furthermore, we calculated tumor growth inhibition (TGI) at the end of the antitumor study, which reflected the antitumor efficacies of different treatments directly. Corresponding to final tumor volumes, the TGIs of different treatments were 65.73% (cisplatin), 59.67% (MTN), 77.38% (MTN + MT), 62.29% (MTN + MH), and 88.38% (MTN + MT + MH), respectively. Apparently, the group of MTN plus MT plus MH showed the highest TGI up to 88.38%, which could be comparable to those of other cisplatin prodrug systems, such as poly-ermic Pt(IV) with optimal drug/copolymer ratio (75% of TGI) [44], polyermic Pt(IV) plus photothermal therapy (87.89% of TGI) [45], and polyermic Pt(IV) plus another chemotherapy drug (83.4% of TGI) [46]. Therefore, a combination of MTN, MT, and MH should be a promising strategy for polymeric Pt(IV) application in clinics.

Considering high systemic toxicity of cisplatin, a safety evaluation was carried out by weighting the body weight of each mouse after injection, as shown in Figure 10B. Apparently, cisplatin possessed obvious systemic toxicity, as the weight loss of mice could be observed after cisplatin injection. Meanwhile, other mice with MTN injection alone showed a tendency toward gaining body weight, illustrating the high biosafety of MTN. Except for MTN, other MTN-based treatments also exhibited low toxicity, as the mice treated by these strategies, including MTN + MT, MTN + MH, and MTN + MT + MH, showed similar fluctuations of body weights between 20 and 23 g, and all of them fell within the normal weight range of BALB/c mice.

3. Materials and Methods

3.1. Materials

mPEG with an average molecular weight of 5000 Da (mPEG$_{5K}$), HEMA (97%), and SA were purchased from Sigma-Aldrich. DCC (98%), HOBt (97%), 4-Dimethylaminopyridine (DMAP, 99%), and EDC (98%) were purchased from Tokyo Chemical Industry (TCI, Japan). 2,2-Azobis(isobutyronitrile) (AIBN, 99%), anhydrous N,N-Dimethyl sulfoxide (DMSO, 99.9%), anhydrous N,N-Dimethylformamide (99.8%, DMF), cisplatin (c,c,t-[Pt(NH$_3$)$_2$Cl$_2$], 99%), and GSH were purchased from Aladdin (China). 3-(4,5-dimethyl-thiazol-2-yl)-2,5-diphenyl tetrazoliumbromide (MTT) was purchased from Beyotime Biotech. Co., Ltd. (Shanghai, China). Iron(III) acetylacetonate [Fe(acac)$_3$], manganese acetylacetonate [Mn(acac)$_2$], and zinc(II) acetylacetonate [Zn(acac)$_2$] were purchased from Alfa-Aesar. 1,2-Hexadecanediol (97%), oleic acid (technical grade, 90%), oleylamine (technical grade, 70%), and benzyl ether (98%) were purchased from Sigma-Aldrich.

Dialysis tubing, hydrogen peroxide (H$_2$O$_2$, 30%), dichloromethane (DCM), tetrahydrofuran (THF), diethyl ether, acetone, and 1,4-dioxane were purchased from Sinopharm Chemical Reagent Co., Ltd. (Shanghai, China).

AIBN was purified by recrystallization from ethyl alcohol. HEMA was purified by passing through basic alumina to remove monomethyl ether hydroquinone. DCM was desiccated by reflux with calcium hydride (CaH_2) and purified by reduced pressure distillation. Other reagents were used as received. The water used in all experiments was deionized with a Millipore Milli-Qsystem.

The monodisperse magnetic nanoparticles $Mn_{0.6}Zn_{0.4}Fe_2O_4$ were synthesized following our previous study [18]. The typical synthetic procedure was described following. A certain amount of $Fe(acac)_3$, $Mn(acac)_2$, $Zn(acac)_2$, 1,2-hexadecanediol, oleic acid, and oleylamine with molar ratios of 10/3/2/50/30/30 were dispersed successively in benzyl ether. After deoxidizing by argon at 100 °C over 30 min, the mixture was heated to 200 °C for 2 h under an argon atmosphere, then heated further to reflux ($\approx$295 °C) for one and a half hours. The product, monodispersed $Mn_{0.6}Zn_{0.4}Fe_2O_4$ magnetic nanoparticles, was precipitated by excess ethanol, then collected by centrifugation. The purified process was repeated three times. Finally, the magnetic nanoparticles were dispersed in THF with a concentration of 10 mg mL^{-1} for storage under -20 °C.

3.2. Synthesis of Pt(IV) with Single Carboxyl

The preparation of Pt(IV) with a single carboxyl group (-COOH) was performed by oxidization of cisplatin and following reaction with SA, according to previously described [47]. Cisplatin (0.5 g, 1.67 mmol) was suspended in water (10 mL) by magnetic stirring, then excess H_2O_2 (30% w/v, 15 mL) was added to the reaction in dark conditions. The reaction was processed for 5 h at 70 °C with continuous magnetic stirring and dark conditions. The product, hydroxy-modified Pt(IV), named c,c,t-[Pt(NH$_3$)$_2$Cl$_2$(OH)$_2$] or Pt(IV)-(OH)$_2$, was purified by rinsing with water, ethyl alcohol, and diethyl ether, respectively.

After desiccating in vacuum, Pt(IV)-(OH)$_2$ (0.2 g, 0.6 mmol) was dissolved in anhydrous DMSO completely by magnetic stirring, then succinic anhydride (0.06 g, 0.6 mmol) was added to the reaction under nitrogen condition. Under ambient conditions, the mixture was stirred for 12 h. Then, DMSO was removed by vacuum distillation. The final product, Pt(IV) with a single carboxyl group, also named c,c,t-[Pt(NH$_3$)$_2$Cl$_2$OH(OOCCH$_2$CH$_2$COOH)] or Pt(IV)-COOH, was extracted by precipitation in excess acetone. By rinsing with acetone and diethyl ether, respectively, Pt(IV)-COOH was purified and dried under a vacuum oven.

3.3. Preparation of Hydrophilic Block Copolymer mPEG-b-pHEMA

For preparing mPEG-b-pHEMA by RAFT reaction, we prepared mPEG-DDAT as macro-CTA firstly according to our established method [18] and showed the synthetic procedure as follows. A certain amount of mPEG$_{5k}$ (1 g, 0.2 mmol), DDAT (0.22 g, 0.6 mmol), and DMAP (0.024 g, 0.2 mmol) were dissolved in anhydrous DCM (20 mL) completely by magnetic stirring. After that, DCC (0.123 g, 0.6 mmol) was added to the solution at 0 °C and under nitrogen conditions. The reaction was stirred for 30 min at 0 °C and 48 h at room temperature. After the reaction, the solution was concentrated and filtered to remove insoluble by-products. The resulting product was precipitated in an excess amount of diethyl ether to remove excess DDAT. In order to purify the product, the precipitate was reprecipitated other four times by the same process. Finally, the purified mPEG-DDAT was dried by freeze-drying and preserved in argon under low temperatures (-20 °C).

Using mPEG-DDAT as macro-CTA, we synthesized hydrophilic diblock copolymer mPEG-b-pHEMA by RAFT polymerization. Briefly, a certain amount of mPEG-DDAT and HEMA were dissolved in 1,4-dioxane, in which the feed molar ratio of mPEG-DDAT/HEMA was fixed at 1/50. Then, AIBN (10% of macro-CTA molar quantity) was added to the reaction as a catalyst. Under nitrogen conditions, the reaction was processed at 70 °C for 12 h and stopped by cooling down to 0 °C. The final product, mPEG-b-pHEMA, was purified by precipitation in excess diethyl ether three times and dried under vacuum.

3.4. Preparation of Polymeric Pt(IV)

The polymeric Pt(IV) was also prepared by esterification under the assistance of EDC and HOBt. Briefly, Pt(IV)-COOH (200 mg, 0.46 mmol), mPEG-b-pHEMA (76.7 mg, 0.23 mmol hydroxyl group), EDC (83.4 mg, 0.46 mmol), and HOBt (12.4 mg, 0.092 mmol) were dissolved into anhydrous DMF (10 mL) completely under magnetic stirring and nitrogen conditions. Then, the reaction was stirred under ambient conditions for the following 48 h. Thereafter, the solution was dialyzed directly against water to remove DMF, EDC, and HOBt. The lyophilized crude product was dispersed into DCM and centrifuged to remove insoluble by-products and excess Pt(IV)-COOH. Finally, the purified polymeric Pt(IV) was collected by repeated precipitation in an excess amount of diethyl ether and dried in a vacuum oven.

3.5. Characterization of Molecular Structures

The structure of small molecular prodrug Pt(IV)-COOH was characterized by FT-IR (Thermo Scientific, Nicolet iS50, Madison, WI, USA) and ^{1}H NMR spectrum (Bruker, AVANCE II, Zurich, Switzerland). The molecular weight of Pt(IV)-COOH was measured by electrospray ionization mass spectrometer (ESI-MS), which was performed by a high-resolution time-of-flight mass spectrometer (MS, Bruker, MaXis, Karlsruhe, Germany) equipped with electrospray ionization (ESI). The composition and structure of the polymer were characterized by a ^{1}H NMR spectrum with CDCl$_3$ or DMSO-d6 as the solvent and analyzed by their chemical shifts relative to tetramethylsilane (TMS). The Pt content in polymeric Pt(IV) was determined by ICP-MS (Thermo scientific, Xseries II, USA).

3.6. Preparation of Polymeric Pt(IV) Micelles (PPMs) and MTNs

All micelles were prepared by self-assembly technology. For the preparation of PPM, polymeric Pt(IV) was dissolved in THF completely with the concentration of 5 mg mL^{-1}. The mixed solution was then slowly added into excess deionized water under sonication and dialyzed against water for 48 h to remove THF and other impurities, in which a dialysis bag (8–14 KD) was used. The dialysis solution was purified by centrifugation (2000 rmp). After that, PPMs were collected from the supernatant by lyophilization and stored at $-20\ ^\circ$C.

For the preparation of MTNs, a certain amount of magnetic nanoparticles Mn$_{0.6}$Zn$_{0.4}$Fe$_2$O$_4$ and polymeric Pt(IV) were dispersed in THF adequately with the same concentration as 3 mg mL^{-1}. Then, the MTN was prepared by the same procedure.

3.7. General Properties of PPM and MTN

The morphologies of PPM and MTN were characterized by high-resolution transmission electron microscopy (HRTEM, JEOL, JEM-2100, Tokyo, Japan). Particle diameters of PPM and MTN were measured by DLS (Malvern, Nano ZS90, Worcestershire, UK). The content of Mn$_{0.6}$Zn$_{0.4}$Fe$_2$O$_4$ nanoparticles in MTNs was characterized by ICP-MS. The magnetic property of MTN was measured by a vibrating sample magnetometer (VSM, Lake Shore Cryotronics, Inc., LakeShore 7404, Westerville, OH, USA) at 300 K.

We also estimated particle size and colloidal stability of PPMs and MNTs by DLS after they dispersed in phosphate buffer solution (PBS) for 7 d. The concentration of these samples was fixed as 0.5 mg mL^{-1}.

The magnetocaloric effect of MTNs was evaluated by calculating its SAR, according to our previous study [18]. MTNs were dispersed into water with a concentration of Mn$_{0.6}$Zn$_{0.4}$Fe$_2$O$_4$ as 0.1 mg mL^{-1}, which was determined by ICP-MS. The colloidal solution (4 mL) was placed in AMF, which was generated by an alternating magnetic field generator (SPG-20AB, ShuangPing Tech. Ltd., Shenzhen, China). Then, the temperature change of the sample was recorded by a computer-attached fiber optic temperature sensor (FOT-M, FISO, Québec, Canada). Finally, the SAR was calculated by the formula described in our previous study [18].

In this part of the study, the frequency (f) and strength ($H_{applied}$) of the AMF was fixed at 114 kHz and 63.6 kA m^{-1}. The inner diameter of the heating coil was 20 mm.

3.8. Drug Release Studies

In a typical experiment, a certain amount of MTNs (20 mg) was dispersed into 2 mL of the acidic buffer. Then, the solution was placed into dialysis tubing (3 kDa) against 98 mL of the corresponding buffer. The process of drug release was performed at 37 °C in a sharking incubator. At every predetermined time interval, 1 mL sample was withdrawn from outside of the dialysis tubing and measured by ICP-MS to determine the content of Pt. At the same time, an equal volume corresponding buffer was added as a release medium. According to Pt content, the percentage of cumulative Pt release from the MTNs was calculated and determined finally by averaging three measurements.

Furthermore, we also investigated the influence of MH on drug release. In this part, the inner diameter of the heating coil was 40 mm, resulting in constant f (114 kHz) and reduced strength (15.9 kA m^{-1}). Because of the limitation of the heating coil, the study was performed in a 50 mL centrifuge tube. Briefly, MTNs of 10 mg were dispersed into 1 mL of the acidic buffer with 1 mM GSH, followed by 49 mL of the corresponding buffer. To simulate conditions of actual MH in the research, 20 min MH per 1 h was applied and repeated 8 times in a typical study. During the study, the 50 mL centrifuge tube was placed in a sharking incubator at 37 °C after MH until the next MH. At every time interval of 0.5 h, a 0.5 mL sample was withdrawn from the centrifuge tube, and an equal volume of the corresponding buffer was added as a release medium. Finally, the percentage of cumulative Pt release from the MTNs was measured and calculated as we described above.

3.9. Cell Viability Assay In Vitro

The 4T1 was gifted by my colleague, Rui Mengjie, who purchased the cell line from the Chinese Academy of Sciences (Shanghai). 4T1 was cultured in RPMI-1640 medium (Gibco) containing 10% fetal bovine serum (FBS, Biological Industries, Israel), then placed in an incubator at 37 °C, 5% CO_2, and humidified circumstance.

The cell viability in vitro was performed by standard MTT assay in the study. Biocompatibility of magnetic nanoparticle $Mn_{0.6}Zn_{0.4}Fe_2O_4$ has been confirmed by our previous study. In the research, cytotoxicity of hydrophilic copolymer mPEG-b-pHEMA was studied and shown in supporting information (SI).

To evaluate the chemotherapy efficiency of PPMs and MTNs, 4T1 was seeded in 96-well plates at a density of 2×10^4 cells per well in 100 µL of corresponding medium and incubated under standard culture conditions for 24 h. After that, the medium was replaced by a medium containing various drug formations of cisplatin, Pt(IV), PPMs, and MTNs, respectively, in which the final equivalent Pt concentration was varied from 0.625 to 20 µg mL^{-1}. After incubating for 24 and 48 h, cell viabilities were investigated by MTT.

Furthermore, to assess the assistance of MH, 4T1 was seeded in a culture dish (35 mm) at a density of 2×10^5 cells per dish in 2 mL of the corresponding medium. After incubating for 24 h, the culture medium was replaced by a medium containing MTNs (20, 10, 5, 2.5, 1.25, 0.625 µg mL^{-1}). To make sure constant concentration of $Mn_{0.6}Zn_{0.4}Fe_2O_4$ (60 µg mL^{-1}) in the study, we prepared additional magnetic nanocluster fluid according to our previous study [17], then complement shortage of SPIO in groups of Pt concentration as 10, 5, 2.5, 1.25, 0.625 µg mL^{-1}. Afterward, cells were exposed to AMF (20 min per 24 h, 114 kHz, and 15.9 kA m^{-1}) at the beginning of the 24, following culture in an incubator under standard culture conditions. When total culture time reached 24 and 48 h, cell viabilities were also quantified by MTT.

As the culture medium was selected as a negative control, cell survival rates of different treatments were calculated as the percentage of negative control values.

3.10. Cellular Uptake Studies

4T1 were also seeded in culture dish (35 mm) with density of 2×10^6 cells per dish. After incubating for 24 h, cells were treated with cisplatin, PPM, MTN, and MTN plus MH (20 min), respectively. For each formulation, the equivalent Pt content was fixed at 2.5 µg mL^{-1} (2 mL); meanwhile, the SPIO concentration of MTN plus MH was fixed at 60 µg mL^{-1} (2 mL). The drug uptake of Pt was performed by incubating cells with the above-mentioned drug formulations for 1 and 4 h. The cellular uptake of MTN plus MH was treated by exposure to AMF (20 min, 114 kHz, and 15.9 kA m^{-1}) firstly, then incubated under standard culture conditions for prolonged 40 and 220 min, respectively. After removing the supernatant and washing three times, the cells in each culture dish were digested and counted to collect 1×10^6 cells. After repeated freezing and thawing, the intracellular Pt content was determined by ICP-MS.

3.11. Animal Protocol

BALB/c mice (female, 5–7 weeks old, 18–20 g weight) were purchased from the laboratory animal center of Jiangsu University and maintained in the laboratory animal center of Jiangsu University under specific pathogen-free conditions. The orthotopic breast tumor was established by injection of 4T1 cells (1×10^7 cells per mL, 100 µL per mice) into the fourth mammary fat pads of mice. After eight days, the tumor can grow to 100 mm^3. Animals were treated according to the ethical guidelines of Jiangsu University. The animal experiments (approval code: UJS-IACUC-2021092703) were carried out according to the regulations for animal experimentation issued by the State Committee of Science and Technology of the People's Republic of China.

3.12. Biodistribution of MTNs and MRI of Tumor In Vivo

When tumors grew to 200–300 mm^3, these mice were divided into two groups ($n = 5$): MTN alone and MTN plus MT. MRI studies were performed with a 3.0-T clinic MRI imaging system (Siemens Trio 3T MRI Scanner) by using a micro coil for transmission and reception of the signal. The T2-weighted images were acquired by these conditions, which was listed as following: TR = 5000 ms, TE = 10–90 ms, slice thickness = 3 mm, flip angle = 150°, matrix size = 256 × 256, FOV = 100 mm, echo length = 8. Before injection of MTN, tumor-bearing mice were scanned by MRI. Then, the MTN solution prepared by dissolving into PBS at a dose of 4.2 mg kg^{-1} (mFe + mMn + mZn) was injected with 0.1 mL MTN solution from tail-vein for each tumor-bearing mouse. For the group of MT, the button magnet with a surface magnetic intensity of 0.18 T (diameter of 10 mm and thickness of 4 mm) was placed on the tumor area after injection immediately and maintained for 4 h. At 20 h later, after injecting MTNs, an MRI scan was performed to observe the T2 signal of the tumor site.

After that, the influence of MH on the penetration of MTNs within the tumor was also observed by MRI. After the second scanning, mice were treated with MH (20 min of each mouse, 114 kHz, and 15.9 kA m^{-1}), then scanned by MRI following. In reality, the last scanning was performed at 22 h after MTNs injection.

To ensure the distribution of MTNs in vivo, a histological examination was performed after the last MRI scanning. The main organs (heart, liver, spleen, lung, and kidney) and tumors were extracted and fixed in 10% formalin, following treatment with nuclear fast red and Prussian blue stain.

3.13. In Vivo Tumor Inhibition Studies

When tumors grew to 150 mm^3, these mice were divided into 6 groups ($n = 6$), injected with PBS, cisplatin, MTN, MTN plus MT (MTN + MT), MTN plus MH (MTN + MH), and MTN plus MT plus MH (MTN + MT + MH), respectively, in which, the dosage of Pt was calculated as 3 mg kg^{-1} cisplatin. In these groups, the injection was performed every three days, and MH was operated under AMF (114 kHz and 15.9 kA m^{-1}) for 20 min at 20 h after each injection. The MT was carried out as we described in the MRI study. During the treatment, we injected 5 times in each group. Tumor volume and body weight of tumor-bearing mice were measured and recorded every three days, in which tumor volume was calculated by a formula described in a relative study [43]. The TGI rates of different treatments were calculated to assess corresponding antitumor efficacies by a formula described in a relative study [48].

3.14. Statistical Analysis

First of all, all data were presented with mean ± standard deviation (SD). Secondly, a one-way analysis of variance (ANOVA) was used in the research to determine significant differences between pairs of two groups. $p < 0.05$ was considered statistically significant, and $p < 0.01$ was considered as significant extremely.

4. Conclusions

In the study, we developed a versatile MTN successfully with high stability, MH-facilitated accumulation, high-sensitivity MRI, MH-enhanced penetration, and efficacy of Pt(IV) by self-assembly of monodispersed $Mn_{0.6}Zn_{0.4}Fe_2O_4$ and amphiphilic polymeric Pt(IV). First of all, we synthesized macromolecular cisplatin prodrug with Pt content as high as 22.5% polymeric Pt(IV), then used it to prepare MTN by encapsulating superparamagnetic $Mn_{0.6}Zn_{0.4}Fe_2O_4$ nanoparticles. The MTN did not only exhibit the potential for passive targeting by combining a suitable diameter around 151 nm and high stability under physiological conditions but also displayed more abilities on MT, MH, and MRI because it possessed high M_s (103.1 emu g^{-1}) and SAR (404 W g^{-1}). More importantly, the drug release of MTN was sensitive to the intracellular environment, especially for low pH, indicating its low side effects in circulation. According to these properties, polymeric Pt(IV)-based formulations, PPM and MTN alone displayed low cytotoxicity, but the combination of MTN and MH showed as high cytotoxicity as cisplatin. After intravenous injection, targeted accumulation of MTN in tumors could be improved under MT, which facilitated observation of tumor by MRI. The further MH enhanced MTN penetration in tumors, which also could be reflected by MRI directly. By integrating MT and MH, MTN displayed the highest TGI at 88.38% and reduced the side effects of cisplatin simultaneously. Although we did not observe tumor extinction by cascade effects of MT, MH, and chemotherapy of polymeric Pt(IV), the MTN was still a competitive candidate for diagnosis and therapy of tumors in clinics because of its advantages in efficient targeting, high-sensitivity MRI, low toxicity, and high efficacy simultaneously.

Supplementary Materials: The following supporting information can be downloaded at: https://www.mdpi.com/article/10.3390/ph15040480/s1, Figure S1: Synthetic scheme of polymeric Pt(IV); Figure S2: FT-IR spectrum of Pt(IV)-COOH; Figure S3: ^{1}H NMR spectrum of Pt(IV)-COOH; Figure S4: Mass spectrum of Pt(IV)-COOH; Figure S5: ^{1}H NMR spectra of DDAT and mPEG-DDAT; Figure S6: TEM result of monodispersed $Mn_{0.6}Zn_{0.4}Fe_2O_4$ nanoparticles; Figure S7: The time-dependent hydrodynamic diameter of PPM and MTN in PBS; Figure S8: Magnetization curve of the $Mn_{0.6}Zn_{0.4}Fe_2O_4$ at 300 K; Figure S9: The biocompatibility of mPEG-b-pHEMA.

Author Contributions: Conceptualization, Y.Q.; methodology, Y.Q. and Y.X.; software, X.Z.; validation, M.S.; formal analysis, X.D. and M.Z.; investigation, Z.W. and T.Z.; resources, Y.X. and H.L.; data curation, Z.W. and M.S.; writing—original draft preparation, Y.Q.; writing—review and editing, Y.Q.; supervision, Y.Q., Y.X. and H.L. All authors have read and agreed to the published version of the manuscript.

Funding: This research was funded by the National Natural Science Foundation of China, grant number 81602656; Nature Science Foundation of Jiangsu Province, grant number BK 20160546; Postdoctoral Science Foundation of Jiangsu Province, grant number 2018K272C; Jurong Science & Technology program, grant number YF202004 and ZA42109; 2021 Zhenjiang sixth "169 project" scientific research project; and Graduate Research and Innovation Projects of Jiangsu Province, grant number KYCX20-3094.

Institutional Review Board Statement: The animal study protocol was approved by the Institutional Review Board (or Ethics Committee) of Jiangsu University (protocol code UJS-IACUC-2021092703 and 3 September 2021).

Informed Consent Statement: Not applicable.

Data Availability Statement: Not applicable.

Acknowledgments: The authors would like to thank Mengji Rui, who donated the 4T1 cell line.

Conflicts of Interest: The authors declare no conflict of interest.

References

1. Kelland, L. The resurgence of platinum-based cancer chemotherapy. *Nat. Rev. Cancer* **2007**, *7*, 573–584. [CrossRef] [PubMed]
2. Xiao, H.; Yan, B.; Dempsey, E.M.; Song, W.; Qi, R.; Li, W.; Huang, Y.; Jing, X.; Zhou, D.; Ding, J.; et al. Recent progress in polymer-based platinum drug delivery systems. *Prog. Polym. Sci.* **2018**, *87*, 70–106. [CrossRef]
3. Shi, Y.; Liu, S.A.; Kerwood, D.J.; Goodisman, J.; Dabrowiak, J.C. Pt(IV) complexes as prodrugs for cisplatin. *J. Inorg. Biochem.* **2012**, *107*, 6–14. [CrossRef] [PubMed]
4. Guo, D.; Xu, S.; Huang, Y.; Jiang, H.; Yasen, W.; Wang, N.; Su, Y.; Qian, J.; Li, J.; Zhang, C.; et al. Platinum(IV) complex-based two-in-one polyprodrug for a combinatorial chemo-photodynamic therapy. *Biomaterials* **2018**, *177*, 67–77. [CrossRef]
5. Han, Y.; Yin, W.; Li, J.; Zhao, H.; Zha, Z.; Ke, W.; Wang, Y.; He, C.; Ge, Z. Intracellular glutathione-depleting polymeric micelles for cisplatin prodrug delivery to overcome cisplatin resistance of cancers. *J. Control. Release* **2018**, *273*, 30–39. [CrossRef] [PubMed]
6. Ren, Y.; Miao, C.; Tang, L.; Liu, Y.; Ni, P.; Gong, Y.; Li, H.; Chen, F.; Feng, S. Homotypic Cancer Cell Membranes Camouflaged Nanoparticles for Targeting Drug Delivery and Enhanced Chemo-Photothermal Therapy of Glioma. *Pharmaceuticals* **2022**, *15*, 157. [CrossRef]
7. Xiao, H.; Song, H.; Yang, Q.; Cai, H.; Qi, R.; Yan, L.; Liu, S.; Zheng, Y.; Huang, Y.; Liu, T.; et al. A prodrug strategy to deliver cisplatin(IV) and paclitaxel in nanomicelles to improve efficacy and tolerance. *Biomaterials* **2012**, *33*, 6507–6519. [CrossRef]
8. Hou, J.; Shang, J.; Jiao, C.; Jiang, P.; Xiao, H.; Luo, L.; Liu, T. A core cross-linked polymeric micellar platium(IV) prodrug with enhanced anticancer efficiency. *Macromol. Biosci.* **2013**, *13*, 954–965. [CrossRef]
9. Golombek, S.K.; May, J.N.; Theek, B.; Appold, L.; Drude, N.; Kiessling, F.; Lammers, T. Tumor targeting via EPR: Strategies to enhance patient responses. *Adv. Drug Deliv. Rev.* **2018**, *130*, 17–38. [CrossRef]
10. Nichols, J.W.; Bae, Y.H. Odyssey of a cancer nanoparticle: From injection site to site of action. *Nano Today* **2012**, *7*, 606–618. [CrossRef]
11. Dewhirst, M.W.; Secomb, T.W. Transport of drugs from blood vessels to tumor tissue. *Nat. Rev. Cancer* **2017**, *17*, 738–750. [CrossRef] [PubMed]
12. Webb, B.A.; Chimenti, M.; Jacobson, M.P.; Barber, D.L. Dysregulated pH: A perfect storm for cancer progression. *Nat. Rev. Cancer* **2011**, *11*, 671–677. [CrossRef] [PubMed]
13. Kuppusamy, P.; Li, H.; Ilangovan, G.; Cardounel, A.J.; Zweier, J.L.; Yamada, K.; Krishna, M.C.; Mitchell, J.B. Noninvasive imaging of tumor redox status and its modification by tissue gluta-thione levels. *Cancer Res.* **2002**, *62*, 307–312. [PubMed]
14. Li, L.; Hagen, T.L.M.; Bolkestein, M.; Gasselhuber, A.; Yatvin, J.; Rhoon, G.C.; Eggermont, A.M.M.; Haemmerich, D.; Koning, G.A. Improved intratumoral nanoparticle extravasation and penetration by mild hyperthermia. *J. Control. Release* **2013**, *167*, 130–137. [CrossRef] [PubMed]
15. Manzoor, A.A.; Lindner, L.H.; Landon, C.D.; Park, J.Y.; Simnick, A.J.; Dreher, M.R.; Das, S.; Hanna, G.; Park, W.; Chilkoti, A.; et al. Overcoming Limitations in Nanoparticle Drug Delivery: Triggered, Intravascular Release to Improve Drug Penetration into Tumors. *Cancer Res.* **2012**, *72*, 5566–5575. [CrossRef] [PubMed]
16. Mantso, T.; Goussetis, G.; Franco, R.; Botaitis, S.; Pappa, A.; Panayiotidis, M. Effects of hyperthermia as a mitigation strategy in DNA damage-based cancer therapies. *Semin. Cancer Biol.* **2016**, *37–38*, 96–105. [CrossRef]
17. Stolik, S.; Delgado, J.A.; Pérez, A.; Anasagasti, L. Measurement of the Penetration Depths of Red and Near Infrared Light in Human "ex Vivo" Tissues. *J. Photochem. Photobiol. B* **2000**, *57*, 90–93. [CrossRef]
18. Qu, Y.; Li, J.; Ren, J.; Leng, J.; Lin, C.; Shi, D. Enhanced magnetic fluid hyperthermia by micellar magnetic nanoclusters composed of $Mn_xZn_{1-x}Fe_2O_4$ nanoparticles for induced tumor cell apoptosis. *ACS Appl. Mater. Interfaces* **2014**, *6*, 16867–16879. [CrossRef]
19. Qu, Y.; Li, J.; Ren, J.; Leng, J.; Lin, C.; Shi, D. Enhanced synergism of thermo-chemotherapy by combining highly efficient magnetic hyperthermia with magnetothermally-facilitated drug release. *Nanoscale* **2014**, *6*, 12408. [CrossRef]
20. Mazarío, E.; Cañete, M.; Herranz, F.; Sánchez-Marcos, J.; de la Fuente, J.M.; Herrasti, P.; Menéndez, N. Highly Efficient T2 Cobalt Ferrite Nanoparticles Vectorized for Internalization in Cancer Cells. *Pharmaceuticals* **2021**, *14*, 124. [CrossRef] [PubMed]
21. Makharza, S.A.; Cirillo, G.; Vittorio, O.; Valli, E.; Voli, F.; Farfalla, A.; Curcio, M.; Iemma, F.; Nicoletta, F.P.; El-Gendy, A.A.; et al. Magnetic Graphene Oxide Nanocarrier for Targeted Delivery of Cisplatin: A Perspective for Glioblastoma Treatment. *Pharmaceuticals* **2019**, *12*, 76. [CrossRef] [PubMed]
22. Rieter, W.J.; Pott, K.M.; Taylor, K.M.L.; Lin, W. Nanoscale Coordination Polymers for Platinum-Based Anticancer Drug Delivery. *J. Am. Chem. Soc.* **2008**, *130*, 11584–11585. [CrossRef] [PubMed]
23. Xiao, H.; Qi, R.; Liu, S.; Hu, X.; Duan, T.; Zheng, Y.; Huang, Y.; Jing, X. Biodegradable polymer-cisplatin(IV) conjugate as a pro-drug of cisplatin(II). *Biomaterials* **2011**, *32*, 7732–7739. [CrossRef] [PubMed]
24. Song, H.; Wang, R.; Xiao, H.; Cai, H.; Zhang, W.; Xie, Z.; Huang, Y.; Jing, X.; Liu, T. A cross-linked polymeric micellar delivery system for cisplatin(IV) complex. *Eur. J. Pharm. Biopharm.* **2013**, *83*, 63–75. [CrossRef] [PubMed]
25. Pathak, R.K.; Dhar, S. A nanoparticle cocktail: Temporal release of predefined drug combinations. *J. Am. Chem. Soc.* **2015**, *137*, 8324–8327. [CrossRef] [PubMed]
26. Lai, J.T.; Filla, D.; Shea, R. Functional Polymers from Novel Carboxyl-Terminated Trithiocarbonates as Highly Efficient RAFT Agents. *Macromolecules* **2002**, *35*, 6754–6756. [CrossRef]

27. Huynh, V.T.; Chen, G.; Souza, P.; Stenzel, M.H. Thiol-yne and Thiol-ene "Click" Chemistry as a Tool for a Variety of Platinum Drug Delivery Carriers, from Statistical Copolymers to Crosslinked Micelles. *Biomacromolecules* **2011**, *12*, 1738–1751. [CrossRef]
28. Wang, E.; Xiong, H.; Zhou, D.; Xie, Z.; Huang, Y.; Jing, X.; Sun, X. Co-Delivery of Oxaliplatin and Demethylcantharidin via a Polymer–Drug Conjugate. *Macromol. Biosci.* **2014**, *14*, 588–596. [CrossRef]
29. Pathak, R.K.; Basu, U.; Ahmad, A.; Sarkar, S.; Kumar, A.; Surnar, B.; Ansari, S.; Wilczek, K.; Ivan, M.E.; Marples, B.; et al. A designer bowtie combination therapeutic platform: An approach to resistant cancer treatment by simultaneous delivery of cytotoxic and anti-inflammatory agents and radiation. *Biomaterials* **2018**, *187*, 117–129. [CrossRef]
30. Rosensweig, R.E. Heating magnetic fluid with alternating magnetic field. *J. Magn. Magn. Mater.* **2002**, *252*, 370–374. [CrossRef]
31. Forman, H.J.; Zhang, H.; Rinna, A. Glutathione: Overview of its protective roles, measurement, and biosynthesis. *Mol. Asp. Med.* **2009**, *30*, 1–12. [CrossRef] [PubMed]
32. Wang, X.; Chi, D.; Song, D.; Su, G.; Li, L.; Shao, L. Quantification of Glutathione in Plasma Samples by HPLC Using 4-Fluoro-7-nitrobenzofurazan as a Fluorescent Labeling Reagent. *J. Chromatogr. Sci.* **2012**, *50*, 119–122. [CrossRef] [PubMed]
33. Li, J.; Lyv, Z.; Li, Y.; Liu, H.; Wang, J.; Zhan, W.; Chen, H.; Chen, H.; Li, X. A theranostic prodrug delivery system based on Pt(IV) conjugated nano-graphene oxide with synergistic effect to enhance the therapeutic efficacy of Pt drug. *Biomaterials* **2015**, *51*, 12–21. [CrossRef] [PubMed]
34. Wang, Q.; Xiao, M.; Wang, D.; Hou, X.; Gao, J.; Liu, J.; Liu, J. In Situ Supramolecular Self-Assembly of Pt(IV) Prodrug to Conquer Cisplatin Resistance. *Adv. Funct. Mater.* **2021**, *31*, 2101826. [CrossRef]
35. Rottenberg, S.; Disler, C.; Perego, P. The rediscovery of platinum-based cancer therapy. *Nat. Rev. Cancer* **2021**, *21*, 37–50. [CrossRef]
36. Karasawa, T.; Steyger, P.S. An integrated view of cisplatin-induced nephrotoxicity and ototoxicity. *Toxicol. Lett.* **2015**, *237*, 219–227. [CrossRef]
37. Qin, C.; Liu, H.; Chen, K.; Hu, X.; Ma, X.; Lan, X.; Zhang, Y.; Cheng, Z. Theranostics of Malignant Melanoma with 64CuCl2. *J. Nucl. Med.* **2014**, *55*, 812–817. [CrossRef]
38. Imlimthan, S.; Moon, E.S.; Rathke, H.; Afshar-Oromieh, A.; Rösch, F.; Rominger, A.; Gourni, E. New Frontiers in Cancer Imaging and Therapy Based on Radiolabeled Fibroblast Activation Protein Inhibitors: A Rational Review and Current Progress. *Pharmaceuticals* **2021**, *14*, 1023. [CrossRef]
39. Barca, C.; Griessinger, C.M.; Faust, A.; Depke, D.; Essler, M.; Windhorst, A.D.; Devoogdt, N.; Brindle, K.M.; Schäfers, M.; Zinhardt, B. Expanding Theranostic Radiopharmaceuticals for Tumor Diagnosis and Therapy. *Pharmaceuticals* **2022**, *15*, 13. [CrossRef]
40. Zhou, Z.; Yang, L.; Gao, J.; Chen, X. Structure-Relaxivity Relationships of Magnetic Nanoparticles for Magnetic Resonance Imaging. *Adv. Mater.* **2019**, *31*, 1804567. [CrossRef]
41. Wang, Y.; Zhou, K.; Huang, G.; Hensley, C.; Huang, X.; Ma, X.; Zhao, T.; Sumer, B.D.; DeBerardinis, R.J.; Gao, J. A nanoparticle-based strategy for the imaging of a broad range of tumours by non-linear amplification of microenvironment signals. *Nat. Mater.* **2014**, *13*, 204–212. [CrossRef] [PubMed]
42. Sykes, E.A.; Chen, J.; Zheng, G.; Chan, W.C.W. Investigating the Impact of Nanoparticle Size on Active and Passive Tumor Targeting Efficiency. *ACS Nano* **2014**, *8*, 5696–5706. [CrossRef] [PubMed]
43. Chen, L.; Wu, Y.; Wu, H.; Li, J.; Xie, J.; Zang, F.; Ma, M.; Gu, N.; Zhang, Y. Magnetic targeting combined with active targeting of dual-ligand iron oxide nanoprobes to promote the penetration depth in tumors for effective magnetic resonance imaging and hyperthermia. *Acta Biomater.* **2019**, *96*, 491–504. [CrossRef]
44. Chen, Q.; Luo, L.; Xue, Y.; Han, J.; Liu, Y.; Zhang, Y.; Yin, T.; Wang, L.H.; Cun, D.; Gou, J.; et al. Cisplatin-loaded poly-meric complex micelles with a modulated drug/copolymer ratio for improved in vivo performance. *Acta Biomater.* **2019**, *92*, 205–218. [CrossRef]
45. Feng, L.; Gao, M.; Tao, D.; Chen, Q.; Wang, H.; Dong, Z.; Chen, M.; Liu, Z. Cisplatin-Prodrug-Constructed Liposomes as a Versatile Theranostic Nanoplatform for Bimodal Imaging Guided Combination Cancer Therapy. *Adv. Funct. Mater.* **2016**, *26*, 2207–2217. [CrossRef]
46. Lin, C.; Tao, Y.; Saw, P.E.; Cao, M.; Huang, H.; Xu, X. A polyprodrug-based nanoplatform for cisplatin prodrug delivery and combination cancer therapy. *Chem. Commun.* **2019**, *55*, 13987–13990. [CrossRef]
47. Wilson, J.J.; Lippard, S.J. Synthetic Methods for the Preparation of Platinum Anticancer Complexes. *Chem. Rev.* **2014**, *114*, 4470–4495. [CrossRef]
48. Chandra, F.; Zaks, L.; Zhu, A. Survival Prolongation Index as a Novel Metric to Assess Anti-Tumor Activity in Xenograft Models. *AAPS J.* **2019**, *21*, 16. [CrossRef]

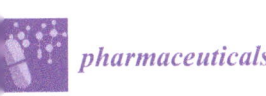

Article

Homotypic Cancer Cell Membranes Camouflaged Nanoparticles for Targeting Drug Delivery and Enhanced Chemo-Photothermal Therapy of Glioma

Yajing Ren [1,†], Chenlin Miao [1,†], Liang Tang [2], Yuxiang Liu [1], Pinyue Ni [1], Yan Gong [1], Hui Li [1], Fuxue Chen [1,*] and Shini Feng [1,*]

[1] School of Life Sciences, Shanghai University, No.381, Nanchen Road, Shanghai 200444, China; yajingren0415@163.com (Y.R.); miaochenlin1002@163.com (C.M.); liuyuxiang1998@126.com (Y.L.); qq310304204@126.com (P.N.); yangong0122@163.com (Y.G.); huili1870805069@126.com (H.L.)
[2] School of Environmental and Chemical Engineering, Shanghai University, No.381, Nanchen Road, Shanghai 200444, China; tang1liang@shu.edu.cn
* Correspondence: chenfuxue@staff.shu.edu.cn (F.C.); fengshini@shu.edu.cn (S.F.)
† These authors contributed equally to this work.

Abstract: Glioma is among the deadliest types of brain cancer, for which there currently is no effective treatment. Chemotherapy is mainstay in the treatment of glioma. However, drug tolerance, non-targeting, and poor blood–brain barrier penetrance severely inhibits the efficacy of chemotherapeutics. An improved treatment method is thus urgently needed. Herein, a multifunctional biomimetic nanoplatform was developed by encapsulating graphene quantum dots (GQDs) and doxorubicin (DOX) inside a homotypic cancer cell membrane (CCM) for targeted chemo-photothermal therapy of glioma. The GQDs with stable fluorescence and a superior light-to-heat conversion property were synthesized as photothermal therapeutic agents and co-encapsulated with DOX in CCM. The as-prepared nanoplatform exhibited a high DOX loading efficiency. The cell membrane coating protected drugs from leakage. Upon an external laser stimuli, the membrane could be destroyed, resulting in rapid DOX release. By taking advantage of the homologous targeting of the cancer cell membrane, the GQDs/DOX@CCM were found to actively target tumor cells, resulting in significantly enhanced cellular uptake. Moreover, a superior suppression efficiency of GQDs/DOX@CCM to cancer cells through chemo-photothermal treatment was also observed. The results suggest that this biomimetic nanoplatform holds potential for efficient targeting of drug delivery and synergistic chemo-photothermal therapy of glioma.

Keywords: graphene quantum dot; targeted drug delivery; photothermal therapy; chemo-therapy

1. Introduction

Glioma is a common primary tumor of the central nervous system [1], accounting for about 45% of intracranial tumors. Glioma has a fast growth rate and a strong invasive ability, and it could infiltrate to the healthy brain tissues by proliferation and invasion, which makes it the most challenging intracranial tumor. Conventional therapy for glioma usually includes surgery, radiotherapy, and chemotherapy [2]. However, the median survival time of glioma patients has so far been only 12 months [3,4]. The current treatment of glioma faces several main obstacles, such as relapse, radiation tolerance, drug tolerance, and the blood–brain barrier [5]. Glioma poses a serious threat to human health and safety. Therefore, it is pivotal to further explore new treatment methods for glioma.

With the development of precision medicine, the nano-sized drug delivery system (NDDS) has become a research hotspot in the treatment of tumors. NDDS can accumulate in tumors via the enhanced permeability and retention (EPR) effects to achieve precise drug release [6–8]. However, the passive aggregation effect of nanoparticles is still limited, depending on the varying degrees of tumor vascularization and the permeability associated with tumor types and development stages [9–11]. To exert pharmacological activities, nano-therapeutics must overcome a cascade of physiological challenges, including blood circulation, cell toxicity, immune evasion, cell internalization, tumor targeting, etc. [12–15]. In recent years, graphene quantum dots (GQDs) nanomaterials have aroused great interest in the scientific community due to their unique physicochemical properties. As a zero micro-nano material, GQDs share some desirable properties of graphene oxide, including water solubility, stable fluorescence, and a variety of attributes, such as size, biocompatibility, excellent photothermal capacity, and the ability to cross the blood–brain barrier [16,17]. These properties make GQDs an excellent drug carrier and could be used in emerging tumor treatments, such as photothermal therapy (PTT) and biological imaging.

Inspired by biological systems in nature, cell membranes are increasingly being used to camouflage nanoparticles, which endow them with properties of natural cells, such as high biocompatibility, low immunogenicity, long circulation, and active targeting [18–20]. The camouflage of the red blood cell membrane for nanoparticles can prolong their circulation time in physical environments and help to escape the phagocytosis of the reticulo-endothelial system so that drugs could reach tumor site at higher concentrations [21–24]. Benefiting from the homing properties of stem cells [25,26], the mesenchymal stem cell membrane was wrapped on nanoparticles to bestow them with a targeting ability, enabling NDDS to escape from phagocytosis by the immune system to play a role upon reaching the tumor site [27–29]. It was reported that the tumor cell could aggregate to form metastatic cells, which was highly dependent on multimolecular-mediated cell–surface interactions, including tumor-specific binding proteins, such as the Thomsen–Friedenreich antigen and E-cadherin presenting on the membrane of the cancer cells [30,31]. Given the ability of homologous adhesion between tumor cells, it was speculated that the cancer cell membrane (CCM) coating could be applied to target the source cancer cells for anti-cancer drug delivery [32–34].

In this study, a novel cancer cell membrane camouflaged NDDS for targeted tumor treatment was developed (Scheme 1). The glioma cell membrane was utilized to camouflage GQDs with anti-cancer drug doxorubicin (DOX). The fabricated GQDs/DOX@CCM were fully characterized. Afterwards, cellular uptake and tumor targeting ability to homotypic glioma cells were investigated. Finally, the chemo-photothermal combination anti-cancer effect of GQDs/DOX@CCM was studied.

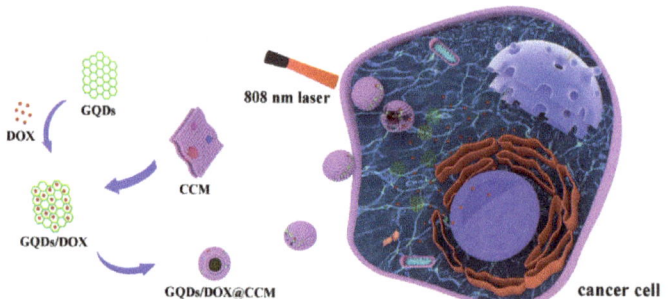

Scheme 1. Schematic illustrating the preparation of GQDs/DOX@CCM for tumor-targeted chemo-photothermal combination therapy of glioma.

2. Results and Discussion

2.1. Characterization of GQDs

GQDs were synthesized according to the previous report [35]. As illustrated in Figure 1a, 1,3,6-trinitropyrene (TNP) and BPEI were dispersed in deionized water for ultrasonic treatment, and then they were reacted at 230 °C for 5 min. Finally, GQDs were obtained after a series of purification and dialysis. After GQDs were prepared, the morphology and structure were characterized. As shown in Figure 1b, GQDs have a broad peak at 23.9°, which corresponds to a wider layer (002) spacing of the graphite structure (3.71 Å), indicating the crystallinity of GQDs. The Raman spectrum shown in Figure 1c suggested that the ordered G band at 1617 cm^{-1} was stronger than the disordered D band at 1376 cm^{-1}, with a large G to D intensity ratio of 1.2, which was consistent with a previous report [35]. The FTIR spectrum in Figure 1d showed a strong vibration at 1646 cm^{-1}, ascribed to the C=C bonds, and a strong, rather broad vibration at 3471 cm^{-1} ascribed to the O-H bonds. The O-H signal was mainly ascribed to the hydroxyl functionalization of the GQDs, which was further confirmed by the XPS. As shown in Figure 1e, GQDs contained three obvious characteristics: C1s at 284.85 eV, N1s at 398.84 eV, and O1s at 531.06 eV, respectively. The C1s spectrum (Figure 1f) exhibited three characteristic peaks corresponding to C=C (284.43 eV), C-N (287.08 eV), and C-OH (287.83 eV). The N 1s spectrum (Figure 1g) showed the binding energy at 398.28 eV and 400.05 eV, corresponding to pyrrolic N and graphitic N, respectively. This result revealed that the fabricated GQDs were nitrogen-doped quantum dots. Besides this, the oxygen-containing species referred to hydroxyl (-OH) (Figure 1h), as confirmed by the C1s and O1s spectra, which further accounted for the good water solubility of GQDs.

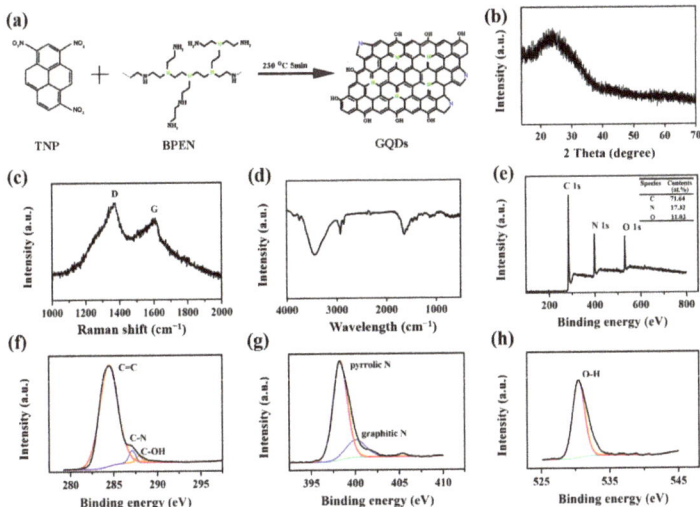

Figure 1. Characterization of GQDs. (a) Schematic diagram of the GQDs synthesis pathway. (b) XRD pattern of GQDs. (c) Raman spectrum of GQDs. (d) FTIR spectra of GQDs. (e) Survey XPS spectrum. (f) High-resolution C1s spectrum. (g) High-resolution N1s spectrum. (h) High-resolution O1s spectrum.

As a novel fluorescent probe, the photoluminescence properties of GQDs were investigated. As shown in Figure 2a, the maximum excitation and emission wavelength of GQDs were 490 nm and 520 nm, respectively. The emission peak of GQDs hardly moved, while the excitation wavelength changed from 390 to 490 nm (Figure 2b). The distinguished luminous performance endowed GQDs with a potential application in tumor tracing and diagnosis. Thereafter, the photothermal performance of GQDs was verified. The GQDs solution with a concentration of 500 µg/mL was exposed to the near-infrared (NIR) laser (808 nm, 1.44 W/cm^2), and the photothermal curves were recorded. As shown in Figure 2c, the temperature of the GQDs solution rose to 84 °C after 8 min of laser irradiation, while the aqueous solution did not change significantly. This result was further verified and visualized in Figure 2d. Results in Figure 2e,f suggested that the photothermal performance of

GQDs exhibited concentration and laser power-dependent manner. After six cycles of laser irradiation, the photothermal conversion capability of GQDs remained stable (Figure 2g). After the photothermal sensitivity of GQDs was characterized, we further explored the photothermal conversion efficiency of GQDs. It was seen from Figure S1a that GQDs have a clear absorption peak in the near-infrared region, which was due to the doping of nitrogen and the presence of oxygen-containing functional groups. The absorbance of GQDs at 808 nm was 0.160. Then, the GQDs solution was exposed to a NIR laser (808 nm, 1.44 W/cm^2) for 300 s and cooled naturally. The temperature change in Figure S1b showed that under the irradiation of the 808 nm laser, the temperature of the GQDs solution rose from 25 to 66 °C, and after 600 s of natural cooling, it dropped to 30 °C. The time constant (τs) of GQDs was calculated to 204.66 s (Figure S1c), and the photothermal conversion efficiency of GQDs was further calculated to be 49.97%. After cell membrane encapsulation, the photothermal ability of GQDs@CCM and GQDs/DOX@CCM showed only slight changes compared with GQDs (Figure 2h). These results demonstrated the excellent photothermal sensitivity of GQDs and their promising potential for application in the photothermal therapy of tumors.

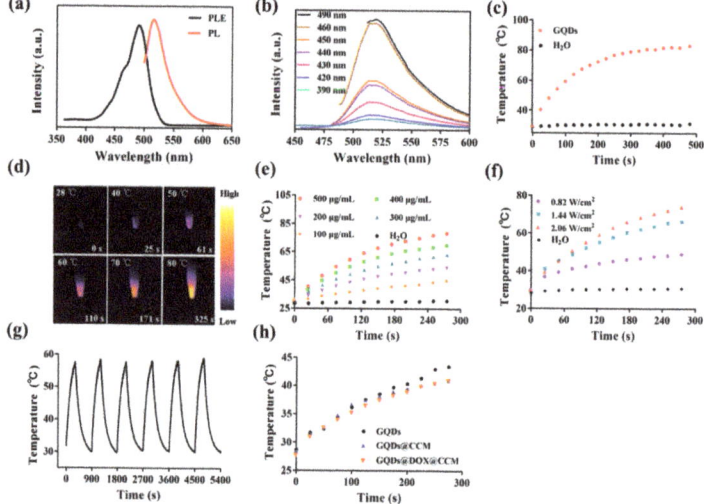

Figure 2. Characterization of GQDs. (**a**) PL and excitation (PLE) spectra of GQDs. (**b**) PL spectra of GQDs excited at different wavelengths varied from 390 to 490 nm. (**c,d**) The temperature change of the GQDs solution (500 µg/mL) under NIR laser irradiation (808 nm, 1.44 W/cm^2) for 8 min. (**e**) The temperature change of the GQDs solution under NIR laser irradiation (808 nm, 1.44 W/cm^2) with different concentrations for 5 min. (**f**) The temperature change of the GQDs solution of 300 µg/mL under 808 nm laser irradiation with different power for 5 min. (**g**) The photostability of GQDs of 200 µg/mL under NIR laser irradiation (808 nm, 1.44 W/cm^2). (**h**) The temperature change of GQDs, GQDs@CCM, and GQDs/DOX@CCM solutions under NIR laser irradiation (808 nm, 1.44 W/cm^2), and the GQDs concentration in all groups was 100 µg/mL.

2.2. Preparation and Characterization of GQDs/DOX@CCM

The biomimetic drug delivery nanoplatform GQDs/DOX@CCM was synthesized as follows: GQDs were mixed with the anticancer drug hydrochloride doxorubicin (DOX) for π-π stacking and electrostatic interaction at room temperature for 24 h. Then, the mixture was co-extruded with CCM, which was gained from freshly harvested BV2 cells. After ultracentrifugation, the GQDs/DOX@CCM was obtained and characterized.

The morphology and structure of GQDs and GQDs/DOX@CCM were visualized by transmission electron microscopy (TEM). As a zero-dimensional nanomaterial, GQDs exhibited a clear lattice structure with an ultra-small particle size of 5.8 ± 2 nm (Figure 3a). After being encapsulated in CCM with DOX, GQDs/DOX@CCM showed an increased particle size of approximately 130 ± 10 nm, which was further confirmed by the hydrodynamic particle size measured by DLS (Figure 3b,c). As shown in Figure 3d, the surface charge of the CCM was determined to be −18.76 ± 1.41 mV, which was consistent with previous reports [36,37]. The GQDs/DOX@CCM exhibited a surface potential (−19.8 ± 1.34 mV) similar to that of CCM, suggesting a successful membrane coating. Subsequently, the protein contents of GQDs/DOX@CCM were assessed by SDS-PAGE. Figure 3e indicated that the compositions of membrane proteins were mostly retained on GQDs/DOX@CCM.

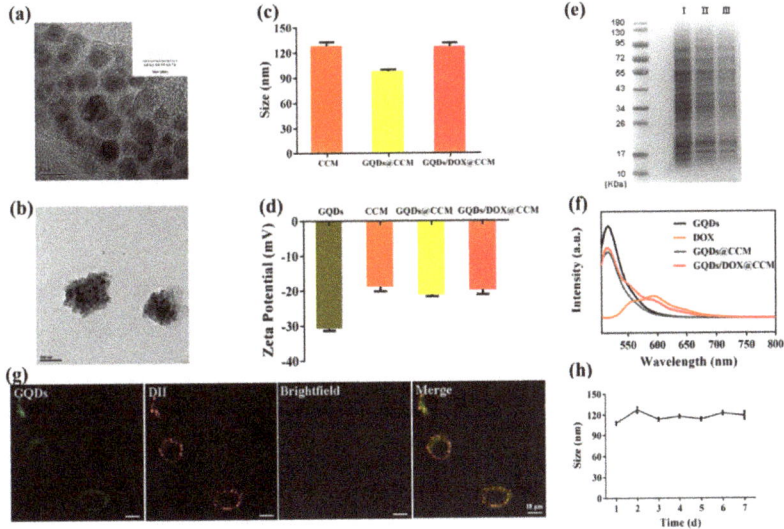

Figure 3. Characterization of GQDs/DOX@CCM. (**a**) TEM image of GQDs. Scale bar = 5 nm. (**b**) TEM image of GQDs/DOX@CCM. Scale bar = 100 nm. (**c**) DLS analysis of CCM, GQDs@CCM, and GQDs/DOX@CCM. (**d**) Zeta potentials of GQDs, CCM, GQDs@CCM, and GQDs/DOX@CCM. (**e**) SDS-PAGE protein analysis of I CCM, II GQDs@CCM, and III GQDs/DOX@CCM. (**f**) PL spectra of GQDs, DOX, GQDs@CCM, and GQDs/DOX@CCM. (**g**) CLSM images of the GQDs@CCM illustrating the colocalization of the GQDs and CCM (DII channel). Scale bar = 10 µm. (**h**) Stability of GQDs/DOX@CCM in PBS (pH = 7.4) by measuring the particle size.

To further verify the integrity of the core-shell particle structure, fluorescent dye DII was used to stain the CCM of GQDs@CCM. Figure 3f showed that the emission peak of GQDs was around 480 nm when excited at 405 nm, and the emission peak of DOX was around 600 nm. The characteristic peaks of GQDs and DOX were both shown in GQDs/DOX@CCM, which indicated the successful loading of GQDs and DOX. After being co-cultured with BV2 cells for 1 h, GQDs@CCM was visualized by CLSM. As shown in Figure 3g, the green fluorescent signals from the GQDs and red fluorescence from the membrane exhibited a high degree of colocalization, indicating the structural integrity of GQDs@CCM. Moreover, the long-term stability of GQDs/DOX@CCM was measured by DLS, which revealed that the GQDs/DOX@CCM was stable at around 33–36 °C within 7 d (Figure 3h). These results demonstrated the successful synthesis of GQDs/DOX@CCM with an intact natural surface membrane protein and long-term stability.

2.3. Biocompatibility In Vitro

Considering the importance of the biocompatibility of nanomaterials for clinical applications, we investigated the biosafety of GQDs and GQDs-based membrane camouflaged nanoparticles through blood compatibility and cell cytotoxicity. It was reported that incompatible materials can break the red blood cells, activate and aggregate platelets, and then induce the formation of thrombosis when entering the blood [38]. Therefore, a hemolysis assay is an important index to explore the biocompatibility of materials. The results of blood compatibility (Figure 4a,b) showed that the hemolysis rate was less than 5% after incubating with GQDs@CCM or GQDs/DOX@CCM of different concentrations for 4 h. To further verify the cytotoxicity of GQDs@CCM, cells from different sources were co-cultured with GQDs or GQDs@CCM for 24 h. The CCK-8 result (Figure 4c,d) showed that cell viability in all groups remained above 95%, even at a high concentration of 200 µg/mL. These results suggested the high biosafety and bio-compatibility of GQDs and GQDs@CCM.

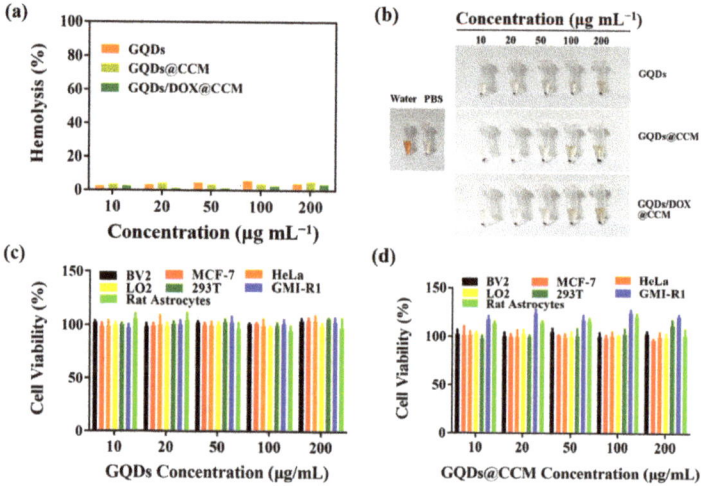

Figure 4. Biocompatibility in vitro. (**a,b**) Hemolysis quantification of red blood cells incubated with deionized water, PBS, GQDs, GQDs@CCM, and GQDs/DOX@CCM. (**c,d**) Cytotoxicity of GQDs and GQDs@CCM to various cell lines with different concentrations for 24 h.

2.4. DOX Encapsulation and Releasing

Drug loading efficiency was investigated under the presence of DOX with different concentrations. It was shown that the DOX encapsulation efficiency was calculated to be 89% ± 6.37, 88% ± 6.19, and 74% ± 6.54 when the initial added DOX concentration was 300 µg/mL, 400 µg/mL, and 500 µg/mL, respectively (Figure 5a). Next, the drug release behavior of GQDs/DOX@CCM was detected at about 33–36 °C. As shown in Figure 5b, the drug release rate in a pH 5.0 solution was about 46% ± 0.4 at 72 h, which was significantly higher than that in pH 7.4 (22% ± 2.1), suggesting pH-dependent drug release behavior of GQDs/DOX@CCM. Moreover, the release rate of DOX from GQDs/DOX@CCM with NIR laser irradiation (808 nm, 1.44 W/cm^2) was significantly improved compared with the non-irradiated group (48% ± 1.2 vs. 78% ± 2.0) (Figure 5c). The laser irradiation induced amhigh temperature, which helped boosting DOX release. These results suggest the favorable controlled release behavior of GQDs/DOX@CCM for reducing the side effects of DOX to normal tissues.

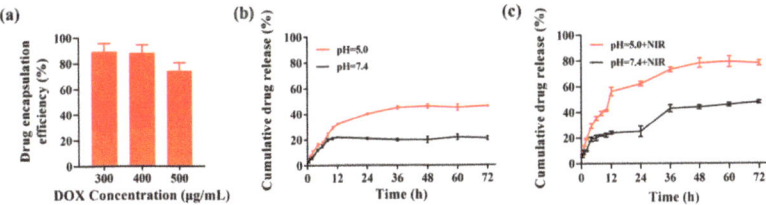

Figure 5. Drug loading capacity and release behavior of GQDs/DOX@CCM. (**a**) Encapsulation efficiency of DOX with initial concentrations of 300, 400, and 500 µg/mL. (**b**) DOX release from GQDs/DOX@CCM at pH 5.0 and pH 7.4. (**c**) DOX release from GQDs/DOX@CCM after 5 min of NIR laser irradiation (808 nm, 1.44 W/cm^2).

2.5. In Vitro Homologous Targeting

When cultured with BV2 cells, GQDs tended to locate at the cytoplasm and exhibit stable green fluorescence (Figure 6a). The cellular internalization of GQDs and GQDs@CCM in BV2 cells were investigated by CLSM and FCM. As displayed in Figure 6a, GQDs could be internalized and located in the cytoplasm of cancer cells. However, after being wrapped by the BV2 cell membrane, a stronger green fluorescence was observed in BV2 cells at the same incubation time. This result was further verified by the quantitative analysis of FCM (Figure S2a–c). After 60 min of co-culturing, the fluorescence intensity of intracellular GQDs@CCM was 1.6 times that of GQDs at the same GQDs concentration of 200 µg/mL (Figure 6b). The enhanced cellular uptake of GQDs@CCM could be attributed to the surface adhesion molecules in the cell membrane, which endowed the nanocomposites with the homotypic tumor self-recognition ability.

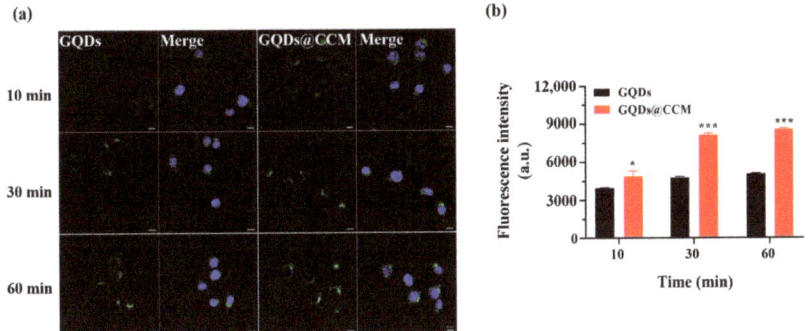

Figure 6. Cellular uptake of GQDs and GQDs@CCM. (**a**) CLSM images of BV2 cells incubated with GQDs or GQDs@CCM at a GQD concentration of 200 µg/mL for different time periods. Scale bar = 10 µm. (**b**) Quantitative analysis of BV2 cell uptake by FCM in different time periods. The differences among groups were determined by a one-way ANOVA analysis followed by the Tukey's post-test: * $p < 0.05$, *** $p < 0.001$.

To further demonstrate the self-recognition ability of cancer cell membrane camouflaged GQDs with homotypic cancer cells, cellular internalization of BV2 cell membrane coated GQDs@CCM by BV2 cells and MCF-7 cells was studied. It was found that the fluorescence intensity originating from BV2 cell membrane coated NPs was far superior in the source BV2 cells than in heterotypic cells MCF-7 after co-culturing for 1 h, which approximated to 2.0–2.3-fold in terms of the mean fluorescence intensity inside cells (Figure 7a,b). These results were also validated by FCM (Figure S2d–f). Besides this, a more rapid cell internalization by the source cell membrane coated GQDs@CCM was found when the incubation period was further prolonged. These results proved the high specific self-recognition affinity of GQDs@CCM to the source tumor cells.

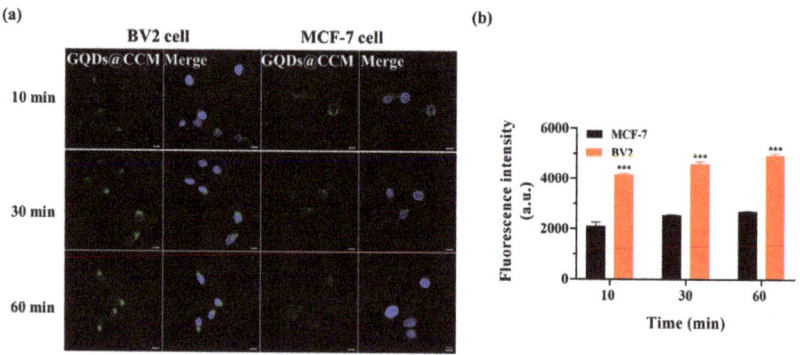

Figure 7. Homologous targeting of GQDs@CCM. (**a**) CLSM images of BV2 and MCF-7 cells incubated with GQDs@CCM at a GQDs concentration of 200 μg/mL for different time periods. Scale bar = 10 μm. (**b**) Quantitative analysis of cell uptake by FCM in different time periods. The differences among groups were determined by a one-way ANOVA analysis followed by the Tukey's post-test: *** $p < 0.001$.

2.6. Antitumor Efficacy In Vitro

Encouraged by the aforementioned results, we further investigated the anticancer effect of GQDs/DOX@CCM in vitro. Then GQDs were co-cultured with BV2 cells and subjected to different laser treatments. The cell survival situation was studied by using Calcein-AM and PI as probes to indicate the live (green) and dead (red) cells, respectively (Figure 8a). The result showed that GQDs treatment did not cause obvious cell death. However, after laser treatment, the red fluorescence of dead cells increased with the increase of the GQDs concentration and irradiation time, indicating their excellent photothermal performance in cancer treatment. Subsequently, the antitumor activity of GQDs/DOX@CCM by the combination of chemo-phototherapy in vitro was investigated. BV2 cells were treated with free DOX and GQDs/DOX@CCM for 24 h, and cell viability was evaluated through a CCK-8 assay (Figure 8b). The reduction in BV2 cell viability was dose-dependent in all groups. Both GQDs (under NIR) and free DOX could effectively inhibit cell proliferation. After being co-encapsulated in CCM, there was a slight reduction in the cytotoxicity of GQDs/DOX@CCM, which was mainly caused by the relatively long drug release time in cancer cells. However, after being irradiated by an external laser, less than 10% of cells survived. The significantly enhanced toxicity to cancer cells could be attributed to the cooperation of the homologous targeted delivery, superior photothermal effect, and controlled drug release responding to the temperature increment. These results were further confirmed by Calcein-AM/PI staining, which was consist with the viability assay (Figure 8c). The above results demonstrated that GQDs/DOX@CCM possess superior therapeutic performance in homogeneous cancer cells. However, further in vivo experiments are still needed before making a final statement on their antitumor effect.

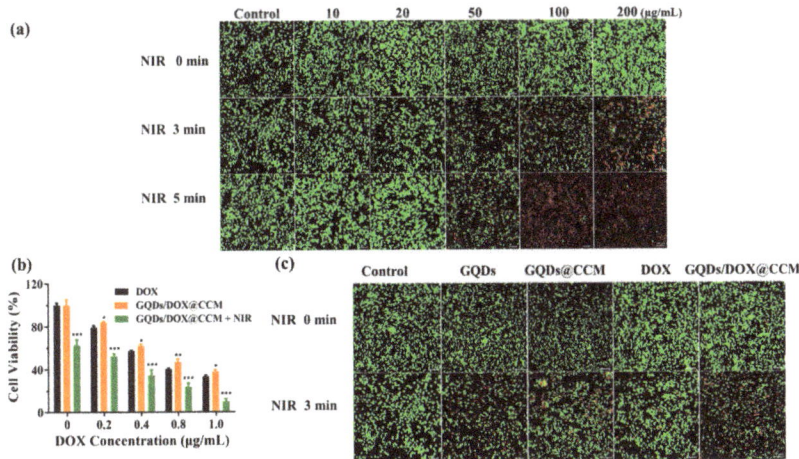

Figure 8. Antitumor efficacy in vitro. (**a**) The cytotoxicity of BV2 cells treated with different concentrations of GQDs for 4 h with NIR laser irradiation (808 nm, 1.44 W/cm^2). Scale bar = 10 µm. (**b**) Relative BV2 cells viability after treatment with different concentrations of DOX, GQDs/DOX@CCM, and GQDs/DOX@CCM (NIR) for 24 h. (**c**) Calcein-AM/PI cell staining of BV2 cells subjected to different treatments. Scale bar = 10 µm. The differences among groups were determined by a one-way ANOVA analysis followed by the Tukey's post-test: * $p < 0.05$, ** $p < 0.01$, *** $p < 0.001$.

3. Materials and Methods

3.1. Materials

Pyrene (purity > 98%) was obtained from TCI (Tokyo Chemical Industry, Tokyo, Japan). Polymers of branched polyethylenimine (BPEI) were obtained from Aladdin (Shanghai, China). A Cell Counting Kit-8 (CCK-8) and Calcein-AM/PI Double Staining Kit were purchased from dojindo (Dojindo Laboratories, Kumamoto, Japan). Dulbecco's modified Eagle's medium (DMEM), heat-inactivated fetal bovine serum (FBS), Doxorubicin (DOX), and trypsin were purchased from BI (Shanghai, China). Furthermore, 4,6-diamidino-2-phenylindole (DAPI) and DII were purchased from beyotime (Shanghai, China).

3.2. Cell Culture

Mouse glioma cells (BV2), human cervical carcinoma cells (HeLa), human breast cancer cells (MCF-7), human normal liver cells (LO2), human embryonic kidney cells (293T), rat microglia (GMI-R1), and rat astrocytes cells were obtained from the Chinese academy of sciences. All cells were cultured in a DMEM medium supplemented with 1% penicillin–streptomycin and 10% fetal bovine serum at 37 °C in a humidified atmosphere of 90% humidity and containing 5% CO_2.

3.3. Isolation of Cancer Cell Membrane

When BV2 cells grew to 90% confluence in culture flasks, cells were collected and suspended in a hypotonic cell lysis buffer, placed in 4 °C for 12 h, then disrupted by a D-130 homogenizer (Beijing, China) for 20 passes. The cell suspensions were centrifuged at 3000 rpm for 20 min at 4 °C; the resulting supernatant was collected and centrifuged again at 100,000× g for 30 min. The plasma membrane pellet was resuspended in PBS with PMSF and stored in −80 °C for further experiments.

3.4. Preparation of GQDs and GQDs/DOX@CCM

According to the previous report [39], the 1,3,6-trinitropyrene (TNP) was firstly prepared by the nitrification reaction of pyrene. Then, TNP and BPEI were dispersed in deionized water for ultrasonic treatment and placed in a dedicated reactor at 230 °C for 5 min. Finally, the pure GQDs were obtained after filtration and dialysis.

A total of 1 mL of DOX (800 µg/mL) was added to 1 mL of GQDs (400 µg/mL) at room temperature in the dark for 24 h. The mixture was co-extruded with 2 mL of BV2 cancer cell membrane vesicles through a 200 nm polycarbonate membrane for 20 passes. The unloaded DOX and GQDs were removed by centrifugation at 13,000× g for 10 min.

3.5. Characterization

Transmission electron microscopy (TEM) images were carried out by a G2F20 microscope (Thermo Fisher Scientific, Wyman Street, Waltham, MA, USA). Raman spectra were recorded on a horiba evolution laser Raman spectrometer (Horiba Scientific, Piscataway, NJ, USA). X-ray photoelectron spectroscopy (XPS) measurements were performed using a K-Alpha+ X-ray photoelectron spectrometer (Thermo Fisher Scientific, Wyman Street, Waltham, MA, USA). X-ray diffraction (XRD) patterns were obtained with a D8 Advance X-ray diffractometer (Showa, Tokyo, Japan). The fluorescence spectrum was recorded with an LS55 fluorophotometer (PerkinElmer Inc., Waltham, MA, USA). UV-Vis-NIR spectroscopy was recorded on a U-4150 Ultraviolet visible near infrared spectrophotometer (Hitachi, Tokyo, Japan). The FTIR spectrum was recorded on the VERTEX70 Fourier infrared spectrometer (Bruker, Karlsruhe, Germany). Particle size and surface zeta potential were measured by dynamic light scattering (DLS) using Zetasizer equipment (Zetasizer Nano ZN, Malvern Analytical Ltd., Malvern, UK). The protein components were analyzed by sodium dodecyl sulfate-polyacrylamide gel electrophoresis (SDS-PAGE).

3.6. Photothermal Performance Measurements

GQDs with different concentrations were exposed to a near-infrared laser (808 nm) for 5 min with different power densities; the temperature of the solution was measured and recorded with an E53 infrared thermal imager (FLIR Systems Inc, Portland, OR, USA). In the photothermal stability experiment, the solution of GQDs was radiated with the near-infrared laser (808 nm, 1.44 W/cm^2) for 5 min, and then the solution was cooled to room temperature naturally. After being repeated 6 times, the temperature was recorded, and the temperature curve was drawn. Different concentrations of GQDs were co-cultured with BV2 cells for 4 h and then irradiated by a near-infrared laser (808 nm, 1.44 W/cm^2) for 3 or 5 min. Cell mortality was measured through the Calcein-AM/PI Double Staining Kit.

3.7. Photothermal Conversion Efficiency Measurement

The photothermal conversion efficiency of GQDs was investigated by irradiating the centrifuge tube containing a dispersion of GQDs at 300 µg/mL (808 nm, 1.44 W/cm^2). The temperature of the GQDs solution was measured every 25 s by an infrared thermal imager (FLIR Systems Inc, Portland, OR, USA).

Q_{Dis} can be determined by the following Equation [40,41]:

$$Q_{DIS} = \frac{m_D c_D \Delta_T}{t} \quad (1)$$

where Q_{Dis} represents the baseline energy input of water, m_D is the mass of aqueous solution, c_D is the specific heat capacity of aqueous solution, Δ_T is the temperature change of aqueous solution during the 5 min laser irradiation (808 nm, 1.44 W/cm^2), and t is the irradiation time (5 min).

h represents heat-transfer coefficient, A represents the surface area of the container, and hA can be determined by the following equation:

$$\theta = \frac{T - T_{surr}}{T_{max} - T_{surr}} \quad (2)$$

$$t = -\tau_s (\ln \theta) \quad (3)$$

$$\tau_s = \frac{m_D c_D}{hA} \tag{4}$$

Here, θ is a dimensionless parameter, and τ_s is the time constant of the sample system. c_D and m_D represent the mass of GQDs (0.5 g) and heat capacity (4.2 J/g), T_{max} represents the maximum temperature of GQDs solution, and T_{surr} represents the ambient temperature.

Photothermal conversion efficiency (η) can be determined by the following equation:

$$\eta = \frac{hA(T_{max} - T_{surr}) - Q_{DIS}}{I(1 - 10^{-A\lambda})} \times 100\% \tag{5}$$

I is the laser power, and Aλ is the absorption value at 808 nm.

3.8. Biocompatibility In Vitro

The blood of healthy Kunming mice was collected from the eyeball and then centrifuged several times to obtain red blood cells and suspended in PBS. A total of 0.2 mL of erythrocytes were mixed with I 0.2 mL PBS (negative control), II 0.2 mL of deionized water (positive control), and III 0.2 mL of GQDs, GQDs@CCM, or GQDs/DOX@CCM solutions of different concentrations. The mixtures were placed at room temperature (33–36 °C) for 4 h. Then, the supernatants were collected and measured at 540 nm to calculate the hemolysis rate after centrifugation at 10,000× g for 5 min.

$$\text{Hemolysis rate} = \frac{A_{sample} - A_{Negative\ control}}{A_{Positive\ control} - A_{Negative\ control}} \times 100\% \tag{6}$$

The cell viability was investigated by Cell Counting Kit (CCK)-8 assays. BV2, MCF-7, HeLa, LO2, 293T, GMI-R1, and rat astrocyte cells were seeded into 96-well plates (n = 5) at a density of 4000 cells per well. After adhering, the medium was taken out, and 100 μL of fresh medium containing GQDs or GQDs@CCM with various GQDs concentrations (10, 20, 50, 100, and 200 μg/mL) were added and co-cultured for another 24 h. Then, 10 μL of the CCK-8 solution was added to each well and incubated for 2 h. Finally, the absorbance at 450 nm was detected by a VICTOR X3 Multifunctional microplate reader (PerkinElmer Inc., Waltham, MA, USA).

3.9. Drug Encapsulation Efficiency and Drug Release In Vitro

To assess the drug loading capacity, GQDs/DOX@CCM was centrifuged to remove the unloaded DOX. The unloaded DOX was determined by measuring absorption at 480 nm using a Multifunctional microplate reader (Perkin Elmer, Waltham, MA, USA). The drug encapsulation efficiency was calculated using the following formula:

$$\text{Drug encapsulation efficiency (\%)} = \frac{\text{Initial mass of drug} - \text{Mass of unload drug}}{\text{Initial mass of drug}} \times 100\% \tag{7}$$

To measure the profile of drug release, 1.5 mL of GQDs/DOX@CCM (DOX concentration of 300 μg/mL) were dialyzed in 8 mL PBS with a different pH (7.4 or 5.0) at about 33–36 °C in the dark (MWCO = 3.5KD). At different time intervals, 500 μL of dialysis buffer was withdrawn to detect the amount of DOX released. After the measurement, the solution was poured back to maintain the constant total amount.

3.10. Cellular Uptake

BV2 cells were seeded into a 35 mm confocal dish (n = 3) at a density of 4000 cells per well and cultured for 24 h. Then, cells were cultured with GQDs or GQDs@CCM for 10 min to 60 min. Cells were washed three times and treated with paraformaldehyde for 20 min. After that, DAPI was added to label the nuclei for 5 min. Then, cells were washed with PBS and visualized by confocal laser scanning microscopy (CLSM) (Occult International Ltd., DE). For quantitative analysis, BV2 cells were seeded into 12-well plates (n = 3) at a density of 40,000 cells per well and cultured for 24 h; then, GQDs or GQDs@CCM were added with a final GQDs concentration of 200 µg/mL for 10 to 60 min; after the cells were washed and digested, the fluorescence of GQDs and GQDs@CCM were observed with a Flow cytometer (Beckman Coulter, Inc., S. Kraemer Boulevard Brea, CA, USA) at the PB450A channel.

3.11. Homologous Recognition In Vitro

BV2 cells and MCF-7 cells were seeded into a 35 mm confocal dish (n = 3) at a density of 4000 cells per well and cultured for 24 h. Then, cells were incubated with GQDs@CCM at a final GQDs concentration of 200 µg/mL from 10 to 60 min. After the cells were washed and fixed with paraformaldehyde for 20 min, the cells were stained with DAPI for 5 min. The internalization of GQDs or GQDs@CCM by cells was observed via CLSM. Simultaneously, flow cytometry (FCM) was also used to evaluate the specific targeting of cells. BV2 cells and MCF-7 cells were seeded into 12-well plates (n = 3) at a density of 40,000 cells per well and cultured for 24 h. Then, cells were incubated with GQDs@CCM from 10 to 60 min. After the cells were washed and digested, the fluorescence of BV2 and MCF-7 cells were observed with a Flow cytometer (Beckman Coulter, Inc., S.Kraemer Boulevard Brea, CA, USA) at the PB450A channel.

3.12. Anti-Tumor Effect In Vitro

BV2 cells were seeded into 96-well plates (n = 5) at a density of 4000 cells per well and cultured for 24 h. The cell culture medium was replaced with 100 µL of fresh medium containing an increased concentration of DOX and GQDs/DOX@CCM complexes, respectively. The treatment concentration of GQDs was 100 µg/mL in the GQDs/DOX@CCM group. After co-cultivation for 24 h, the cells were washed twice with PBS, and then they were incubated with 10 µL of CCK-8 solution for another 2 h. The absorbance at 450 nm was detected using a Multifunctional plate reader ((PerkinElmer Inc., Waltham, MA, USA). The PTT groups were exposed to an 808 nm laser with a power density of 1.44 W/cm^2 for 3 min after co-cultivation for 4 h, with other conditions kept the same. The formula for calculating the cell viability (%) was listed as follows:

$$\text{Cell viability} = \frac{A}{A_0} \times 100\% \qquad (8)$$

Note: A is the OD$_{450}$ of the treated BV2 cells; A$_0$ is the OD$_{450}$ of the untreated BV2 cells.

For the Calcein-AM/PI double-staining assay, BV2 cells were seeded in 35 mm confocal dishes (n = 3) at a density of 40,000 cells per well and co-cultivated with free DOX, GQDs, GQDs@CCM, and GQDs/DOX@CCM for 4 h. The concentration of GQDs was kept consistent at 100 µg/mL. Then, cells were washed three times with PBS and subjected to the light irradiation (808 nm, 1.44 W/cm^2) for 3 min. After being washed by PBS, cells were stained with Calcein-AM and PI for 15 min at 37 °C. Finally, cells were visualized by CLSM.

3.13. Statistical Analysis

Data was reported as mean ± SD. The differences among groups were determined by a one-way ANOVA analysis followed by the Tukey's post-test: (*) $p < 0.05$, (**) $p < 0.01$, (***) $p < 0.001$.

4. Conclusions

In summary, a cancer cell membrane biomimetic drug delivery system for chemo-photothermal combination therapy of homogeneous cancer cells was developed. The synthesized GQDs with favorable properties of excellent dispersibility, controllable size, stable fluorescence, and superior photothermal performance was utilized as a therapeutic agent and co-encapsulated with DOX in a BV2 cell membrane. The GQDs were not only capable of converting near-infrared light to heat for photothermal therapy, but they also improved the release of DOX for chemotherapy. Besides this, benefiting from the homologous targeting of the cancer cell membrane, the GQDs/DOX@CCM can actively target BV2 cells in vitro, resulting in a higher cellular uptake. The antitumor results demonstrated the superior killing efficiency of GQDs/DOX@CCM to cancer cells through chemo-photothermal treatment. Based on this study, the fabricated GQDs/DOX@CCM are capable of providing an effective combination strategy for precision oncology therapy.

Supplementary Materials: The following supporting information can be downloaded at https://www.mdpi.com/article/10.3390/ph15020157/s1: Figure S1: characterization of GQDs. (a) UV-Vis-NIR spectrum of GQDs. (b) Photothermal effect of the GQDs solution (300 µg/mL) exposed to the NIR laser (808 nm, 1.44 W/cm^2). The lasers were shut off after 300 s irradiation. (c) Plot of cooling time versus negative natural logarithm of the temperature driving force obtained from the cooling period after the NIR irradiation (808 nm, 1.44 W/cm^2). Figure S2: Flow cytometry analysis. (a–c) Mean fluorescence intensity of BV2 cells after 10, 30, and 60 min incubation with GQDs or GQDs@CCM; the final concentration of GQDs was 200 µg/mL. (d–f) Mean fluorescence intensity of MCF-7 and BV2 cells after 10, 30, and 60 min incubation with GQDs@CCM; the final concentration of GQDs was 200 µg/mL. Figure S3. Homologous targeting of GQDs@CCM. (a) CLSM images of GMI-R1 and Rat astrocytes cells incubated with GQDs@CCM at GQDs concentration of 200 µg/mL for different time period. Scale bar = 10 µm. (b,c) Quantitative analysis of cell uptake by FCM in different cell lines.

Author Contributions: Conceptualization, F.C., S.F., Y.R. and C.M.; writing—review and editing, Y.R. and C.M.; methodology, Y.R., C.M. and L.T.; project administration and funding acquisition, F.C. and S.F.; formal analysis, Y.L. and P.N.; software, H.L. and Y.G. All authors have read and agreed to the published version of the manuscript.

Funding: This research was funded by the National Natural Science Foundation of China (52002239).

Institutional Review Board Statement: The animal study protocol was approved by the Ethics Committee of Shanghai University (protocol code ECSHU-2020-030).

Informed Consent Statement: Not applicable.

Data Availability Statement: The data are contained within the article and Supplementary Materials.

Conflicts of Interest: The authors report no conflict of interest.

References

1. Wang, X.; Hua, Y.Q.; Xu, G.Y.; Deng, S.Y.; Yang, D.K.; Gao, X. Targeting EZH2 for glioma therapy with a novel nanoparticle-siRNA complex. *Int. J. Nanomed.* **2019**, *14*, 2637–2653. [CrossRef] [PubMed]
2. Mizuno, Y.; Naoi, T.; Nishikawa, M.; Rattanakiat, S.; Hamaguchi, N.; Hashida, M.; Takakura, Y. Simultaneous delivery of doxorubicin and immunostimulatory CpG motif to tumors using a plasmid DNA/doxorubicin complex in mice. *J. Control Release* **2010**, *141*, 252–259. [CrossRef] [PubMed]
3. Zheng, J.; Liu, X.B.; Xue, Y.X.; Gong, W.; Ma, J.; Xi, Z.; Que, Z.Y.; Liu, Y.H. TTBK2 circular RNA promotes glioma malignancy by regulating miR-217/HNF1β/Derlin-1 pathway. *J. Hematol. Oncol.* **2017**, *10*, 52. [CrossRef] [PubMed]
4. Wang, K.Y.; Huang, R.Y.; Li, G.Z.; Zeng, F.; Zhao, Z.; Liu, Y.W.; Hu, H.M.; Jiang, T. CKAP2 expression is associated with glioma tumor growth and acts as a prognostic factor in high-grade glioma. *Oncol. Rep.* **2018**, *40*, 2036–2046. [CrossRef] [PubMed]
5. Xiong, Y.; Kuang, W.; Lu, S.G.; Guo, H.; Wu, M.J.; Ye, M.H.; Wu, L. Long noncoding RNA HOXB13-AS1 regulates HOXB13 gene methylation by interacting with EZH2 in glioma. *Cancer Med.* **2018**, *7*, 4718–4728. [CrossRef] [PubMed]
6. Yin, Q.; Yu, H.J.; Zhang, Z.W.; Cao, M.; Zhang, Y.Y.; Li, Y.P. Shrapnel nanoparticles loading docetaxel inhibits metastasis and growth of breast cancer. *Biomaterials* **2015**, *64*, 10–20. [CrossRef] [PubMed]
7. Feng, S.N.; Zhang, H.J.; Zhi, C.Y.; Gao, X.D.; Nakanishi, H. pH-responsive charge-reversal polymer-functionalized boron nitride nanospheres for intracellular doxorubicin delivery. *Int. J. Nanomed.* **2018**, *13*, 641–652. [CrossRef]
8. Feng, S.N.; Zhang, H.J.; Xu, S.; Zhi, C.Y.; Nakanishi, H.; Gao, X.D. Folate-conjugated, mesoporous silica functionalized boron nitride nanospheres for targeted delivery of doxorubicin. *Mater. Sci. Eng. C* **2019**, *96*, 552–560. [CrossRef]
9. Bertranda, N.; Wu, J.; Xu, X.Y.; Kamaly, N.; Farokhzad, O.C. Cancer nanotechnology: The impact of passive and active targeting in the era of modern cancer biology. *Adv. Drug Deliv. Rev.* **2014**, *66*, 2–25. [CrossRef]
10. Yu, M.K.; Park, J.; Jon, S. Targeting strategies for multifunctional nanoparticles in cancer imaging and therapy. *Theranostics* **2012**, *2*, 3–44. [CrossRef]
11. Furman, N.E.T.; Lupu-Haber, Y.; Bronshtein, T.; Kaneti, L.; Letko, N.; Weinstein, E.; Baruch, L.; Machluf, M. Reconstructed stem cell nanoghosts: A natural tumor targeting platform. *Nano Lett.* **2013**, *13*, 3248–3255. [CrossRef]

12. Adiseshaiah, P.P.; Crist, R.M.; Hook, S.S.; McNeil, S.E. Nanomedicine strategies to overcome the pathophysiological barriers of pancreatic cancer. *Nat. Rev. Clin. Oncol.* **2016**, *13*, 750–765. [CrossRef] [PubMed]
13. Khawar, I.A.; Kim, J.H.; Kuh, H.J. Improving drug delivery to solid tumors: Priming the tumor microenvironment. *J. Control Release* **2015**, *201*, 78–89. [CrossRef] [PubMed]
14. Rosenblum, D.; Joshi, N.; Tao, W.; Karp, J.M.; Peer, D. Progress and challenges towards targeted delivery of cancer therapeutics. *Nat. Commun.* **2018**, *9*, 1410. [CrossRef] [PubMed]
15. Ji, T.J.; Zhao, Y.; Ding, Y.P.; Karp, J.M.; Peer, D. Using functional nanomaterials to target and regulate the tumor microenvironment: Diagnostic and therapeutic applications. *Adv. Mater.* **2013**, *25*, 3508–3525. [CrossRef]
16. Campbell, E.; Hasan, M.T.; Rodriguez, R.G.; Akkaraju, G.R.; Naumov, A.V. Doped graphene quantum dots for intracellular multicolor imaging and cancer detection. *ACS Biomater. Sci. Eng.* **2019**, *5*, 4671–4682. [CrossRef]
17. Geng, B.J.; Shen, W.W.; Fang, F.L.; Qin, H.; Li, P.; Wang, X.L.; Li, X.K.; Pan, D.Y.; Shen, L.X. Enriched graphitic N dopants of carbon dots as F cores mediate photothermal conversion in the NIR-II window with high efficiency. *Carbon* **2020**, *162*, 220–233. [CrossRef]
18. Wu, M.L.; Le, W.L.; Mei, T.X.; Wang, Y.C.; Chen, B.D.; Liu, Z.M.; Xue, C.Y. Cell membrane camouflaged nanoparticles: A new biomimetic platform for cancer photothermal therapy. *Int. J. Nanomed.* **2019**, *14*, 4431–4448. [CrossRef] [PubMed]
19. Zhen, X.; Cheng, P.H.; Pu, K.Y. Recent advances in cell membrane-camouflaged nanoparticles for cancer phototherapy. *Small* **2019**, *15*, e1804105. [CrossRef]
20. Fang, R.H.; Jiang, Y.; Fang, J.C.; Zhang, L.F. Cell membrane-derived nanomaterials for biomedical applications. *Biomaterials* **2017**, *128*, 69–83. [CrossRef]
21. Gao, W.W.; Hu, C.M.; Fang, R.H.; Luk, B.T.; Su, J.; Zhang, L.F. Surface functionalization of gold nanoparticles with red blood cell membranes. *Adv. Mater.* **2013**, *25*, 3549–3553. [CrossRef] [PubMed]
22. Rao, L.; Cai, B.; Bu, L.L.; Liao, Q.Q.; Guo, S.S.; Zhao, X.Z.; Dong, W.F.; Liu, W. Microfluidic electroporation-facilitated synthesis of erythrocyte membrane-coated magnetic nanoparticles for enhanced imaging-guided cancer therapy. *ACS Nano* **2017**, *11*, 3496–3505. [CrossRef]
23. Sun, L.H.; Li, Q.; Hou, M.M.; Gao, Y.; Yang, R.H.; Zhang, L.; Xu, Z.G.; Kang, Y.J.; Xue, P. Light-activatable Chlorin e6 (Ce6)-imbedded erythrocyte membrane vesicles camouflaged prussian blue nanoparticles for synergistic photothermal and photodynamic therapies of cancer. *Biomater. Sci.* **2018**, *6*, 2881–2895. [CrossRef] [PubMed]
24. Chai, Z.L.; Ran, D.; Lu, L.W.; Zhan, C.Y.; Ruan, H.T.; Hu, X.F.; Xie, C.; Jiang, K.; Li, J.Y.; Zhou, J.F.; et al. Ligand-modified cell membrane enables the targeted delivery of drug nanocrystals to glioma. *ACS Nano* **2019**, *13*, 5591–5601. [CrossRef]
25. Huang, X.X.; Guo, B.; Liu, S.; Wan, J.; Broxmeyer, H.E. Neutralizing negative epigenetic regulation by HDAC5 enhances human haematopoietic stem cell homing and engraftment. *Nat. Commun.* **2018**, *9*, 2741. [CrossRef]
26. Karp, J.M.; Teo, G.S. Mesenchymal sctem chell homing: The devil is in the details. *Cell Stem Cell* **2009**, *4*, 206–216. [CrossRef]
27. Yang, N.; Ding, Y.P.; Zhang, Y.L.; Wang, B.; Zhao, X.; Cheng, K.M.; Huang, Y.X.; Taleb, M.; Zhao, J.; Dong, W.F.; et al. Surface functionalization of polymeric nanoparticles with umbilical cord derived mesenchymal stem cell membrane for tumor-targeted therapy. *ACS Appl. Mater. Interfaces* **2018**, *10*, 22963–72293. [CrossRef] [PubMed]
28. Gao, C.Y.; Lin, Z.H.; Jurado-Sánchez, B.; Lin, X.K.; Wu, Z.G.; He, Q. Stem cell membrane-coated nanogels for highly efficient in vivo tumor targeted drug delivery. *Small* **2016**, *12*, 4056–4062. [CrossRef] [PubMed]
29. Gao, C.Y.; Lin, Z.H.; Wu, Z.G.; Lin, X.K.; He, Q. Stem cell membrane camouflaging on near-IR photoactivated upconversion nanoarchitectures for in vivo remote-controlled photodynamic therapy. *ACS Appl. Mater. Interfaces* **2016**, *8*, 34252–34260. [CrossRef] [PubMed]
30. Fidler, I.J. The pathogenesis of cancer metastasis: The 'seed and soil' hypothesis revisited. *Nat. Rev. Cancer* **2003**, *3*, 453–458. [CrossRef]
31. Sultan, A.S.; Xie, J.W.; LeBaron, M.J.; Ealley, E.L.; Nevalainen, M.T.; Rui, H. Stat5 promotes homotypic adhesion and inhibits invasive characteristics of human breast cancer cells. *Oncogene* **2005**, *24*, 746–760. [CrossRef] [PubMed]
32. Zhu, J.Y.; Zheng, D.W.; Zhang, M.K.; Yu, W.Y.; Qiu, W.X.; Hu, J.J.; Feng, J.; Zhang, X.Z. Preferential cancer cell self-recognition and tumor self-targeting by coating nanoparticles with homotypic cancer cell membranes. *Nano Lett.* **2016**, *16*, 5895–5901. [CrossRef] [PubMed]
33. Li, S.Y.; Cheng, H.; Qiu, W.X.; Zhang, L.; Wan, S.S.; Zeng, J.Y.; Zhang, X.Z. Cancer cell membrane-coated biomimetic platform for tumor targeted photodynamic therapy and hypoxia-amplified bio reductive therapy. *Biomaterials* **2017**, *142*, 149–161. [CrossRef] [PubMed]
34. Rao, L.; Yu, G.T.; Meng, Q.F.; Bu, L.L.; Tian, R.; Lin, L.S.; Deng, H.Z.; Yang, W.J.; Zan, M.H.; Ding, J.X.; et al. Cancer cell membrane-coated nanoparticles for personalized therapy in patient-derived xenograft models. *Adv. Funct. Mater.* **2019**, *29*, 1905671. [CrossRef]
35. Geng, B.J.; Qin, H.; Shen, W.W.; Li, P.; Fang, F.L.; Li, X.K.; Pan, D.Y.; Shen, L.X. Carbon dot/WS2 heterojunctions for NIR-II enhanced photothermal therapy of osteosarcoma and bone regeneration. *Chem. Eng. J.* **2020**, *383*, 123102. [CrossRef]
36. Feng, S.N.; Li, H.; Ren, Y.J.; Zhi, C.Y.; Huang, Y.X.; Chen, F.X.; Zhang, H.J. RBC membrane camouflaged boron nitride nanospheres for enhanced biocompatible performance. *Colloids Surf. B Biointerfaces* **2020**, *190*, 110964. [CrossRef]
37. Sun, H.P.; Su, J.H.; Me, Q.S.; Yin, G.Q.; Chen, L.L.; Gu, W.W.; Zhang, P.C.; Zhang, Z.W.; Yu, H.J.; Wang, S.L.; et al. Cancer-cell-biomimetic nanoparticles for targeted therapy of homotypic tumors. *Adv. Mater.* **2016**, *28*, 9281–9288. [CrossRef]

38. Tran, D.L.; Thi, P.L.; Lee, S.M.; Thi, T.T.H.; Parka, K.D. Multifunctional surfaces through synergistic effects of heparin and nitric oxide release for a highly efficient treatment of blood-contacting devices. *J. Control Release* **2021**, *329*, 401–412. [CrossRef] [PubMed]
39. Geng, B.J.; Shen, W.W.; Li, P.; Fang, F.L.; Qin, H.; Li, X.K.; Pan, D.Y.; Shen, L.X. Carbon dot-passivated black phosphorus nanosheet hybrids for synergistic cancer therapy in the NIR-II window. *ACS Appl. Mater. Interfaces* **2019**, *11*, 44949–44960. [CrossRef]
40. Lin, H.; Gao, S.S.; Dai, C.; Chen, Y.; Shi, J.L. A two-dimensional biodegradable niobium carbide (MXene) for photothermal tumor eradication in NIR I and NIR-II biowindows. *J. Am. Chem. Soc.* **2017**, *139*, 16235–16247. [CrossRef]
41. Lin, H.; Wang, X.G.; Yu, L.D.; Chen, Y.; Shi, J.L. Two-dimensional ultrathin MXene ceramic nanosheets for photothermal conversion. *Nano Lett.* **2017**, *17*, 384–391. [CrossRef] [PubMed]

MDPI
St. Alban-Anlage 66
4052 Basel
Switzerland
Tel. +41 61 683 77 34
Fax +41 61 302 89 18
www.mdpi.com

Pharmaceuticals Editorial Office
E-mail: pharmaceuticals@mdpi.com
www.mdpi.com/journal/pharmaceuticals

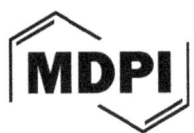

www.ingramcontent.com/pod-product-compliance
Lightning Source LLC
LaVergne TN
LVHW070743100526
838202LV00013B/1293